Introduction
to
Clinical Nursing

Introduction to Clinical Nursing

MYRA ESTRIN LEVINE, R.N., M.S.N.

Assistant Professor of Nursing, Loyola University School of Nursing, Chicago. Formerly Chairman of Department of Clinical Nursing, Cook County School of Nursing, Chicago

F. A. DAVIS COMPANY
PHILADELPHIA, PA.

 Printed in the United States of America. Library of Congress Catalog Card Number 68-16817

To the memory of
Doris Phillips Wheeler, M.D.

And since, to look at things in bloom,
Fifty springs are little room . . .

A. E. HOUSMAN, *A Shropshire Lad*

Preface

Nursing is learned at the bedside. But modern nurse educators, painfully aware of the apprentice tradition in early nursing education and its continuing threat in a technological age, have rightfully insisted that the knowledge of nursing be transmitted in an educational environment. Very early in nursing education, the emphasis on "how to do it" was fortified by "why it is done." But tradition fades slowly, and the continuing emphasis on procedures for the beginning student of nursing has persisted even in a time when the scientific and technological structure of nursing knowledge defies easy analysis and organization. Furthermore, the teaching of basic skills (i.e., procedures) has traditionally taken place quite out of the context of the sick. A nurse learned to bathe a *patient* by following the "rules" as established in a bath procedure, and the unique needs of the individual himself were not, and unfortunately still are not, matters of emphasis.

Beginning courses in nursing—nursing arts, fundamentals of nursing, or foundations of nursing—remain characterized by a rigid dependence on procedures. The "why" is not entirely neglected, but it is often applied after the fact, as if such justification invested the procedure with a special scientific holiness. Nurses cherish "applied science principles" in an era when nursing is deeply involved in scientific research, but even the lessons learned from nurse researchers are too often ignored.

Individual nurses, as mobile as the rest of the population in these days of rapid transport, have learned that the rigidity of their procedure orientation has hampered their ability to practice satisfactorily. Every hospital has a personality of its own, and every hospital procedure manual clings to variations and idiosyncrasies, even in fundamental nursing activities, which are peculiarly its own. It is sometimes difficult to discover the logic in such variants, although many of them reflect the intensely localized administrative realities of the hospital itself. It is, for example, displayed in as common an area of practice as in the use of linens at the bedside. If a hospital has its own laundry facilities, the handling of linens, both clean and used, will vary considerably from that of an organization that must send its linens to a commercial laundry in the community. Invariably, nursing procedures are statements of administrative policy arising from fiat and reality, and the tradition of padding them with so-called applied principles has made them not less but more confining.

In order to learn nursing at a beginning level, it is essential that the aspects of nursing care which are administratively determined be separated from those aspects which are basic nursing practice and thereby valid everywhere that nurses practice. The fitting of nursing practice into the policy structure of any institution is the clearcut obligation of in-service orientation and teaching and must take place in any event. But the nurse who comes armed with nursing knowledge focused on the patient and his individual needs is a practitioner who can readily adapt to the administrative demands in any institution.

This text is a beginning course in nursing. It is based on an analysis of the content that has traditionally been offered in the introductory course in nursing but organized within a structure of science principles *from which* nursing processes are derived. In this way, sciences fundamental to nursing from many disciplines—biological, physical, and behavioral-social—are offered as the organizing foundation for many kinds of nursing activity. Such an analysis has resulted in the formulation of nine models. Each model is a structural framework which establishes a conceptual pattern so that a wide variety of nursing processes, all related to each other through a generic cluster of science principles and ideas, can be understood. The model is constructed of three major parts: a Statement of Objectives, Essential Science Concepts, and Nursing Processes. The objectives are intended to focus the student's attention on the broad goals of nursing practice which fall into the general category of the subject of the model itself. They are intended to provide an intellectual framework for analysis and understanding of the scientific nature of nursing activity. The essential science concepts develop the rationale, using ideas from all areas of knowledge that contribute to the development of the nursing process in the specific area of the model. By this means, a generalization of nursing approach becomes possible, but always related to the scientific foundation which determines the nature of the nursing activity. For example, Model IV: Pressure Gradient Systems in Nursing Intervention (Fluids) establishes the scientific base for the performance of many nursing processes. This model, describing the knowledge that illuminates and directs nursing care, is essential to the understanding of every nursing activity that deals in pressure gradient systems with fluids: blood pressures, parenteral injections (including intravenous), enemas, catheterization and irrigation of organs via body orifices, gastrointestinal decompression, and spinal taps. The specific, and often highly localized, *technique* for the performance of each of these procedures can only be learned in the clinical setting, but the fundamental rationale in the performance of each skilled activity rests on this scientific base. The models offer a new approach to nursing skills, because they substitute broad concepts for the procedural rules and allow for variation in practice which is sound and scientific and, therefore, safe for individualizing the care of every patient.

It must be emphasized that the author does not underestimate the importance of technical skill. On the contrary, such skills are, in fact, the *"silent language"* of the nurse, and without them all of the book knowledge is useless. The practitioner must develop technical skill as *one* essential means of communication with the patient. In the beginning student such communication is often the most meaningful and relevant. It is only with increasing knowledge and experience that the student learns, finally, to communicate with patients in all the complex and subtle realities of human interaction. The technical skills afford the most immediate satisfactions to the beginning student of nursing, but they must not be allowed to become the entire *raison d'être* of the nurse.

The models thus represent but a single dimension of nursing knowledge. Nursing skills in themselves have no reality unless they are clearly related to the care of the sick. Each chapter of this text is designed to present the beginning level of pathophysiologic and psychosocial understanding which, in effect, also makes this a first course in medical-surgical nursing. Once more, specific emphasis is made on the larger concepts which allow for understanding of a broad spectrum of disease conditions. The organization along pathophysiologic lines permits intensive study of a prototype disease entity so that nursing concepts may be drawn from it which may be utilized in the care of patients suffering from many different diagnostic categories of disease. Individual chapters have a definitive relationship to the model that follows it so that the student may develop a conceptual base upon which beginning technical and intellectual skills can take shape. The model concerned with administration of personal hygiene needs is related to the chapter dealing with the diabetic patient. The very essential nursing care which maintains the personal hygiene of the diabetic patient emphasizes the importance of such nursing intervention for all individuals, diabetic or not.

The serious study of any discipline requires a theoretical baseline which gives it substance and meaning. The theoretical framework used in this text visualizes nursing intervention as a conservation activity. This "keeping-together" function of the nurse emphasizes the wholeness and integrity of every individual patient. The Conservation Principles of Nursing are used as a structural design in the development of the prototype diagnostic entity in each chapter. The development of this conceptual structure is described in Chapter 1.

The evolution of this approach to nursing has necessarily resulted from a constant exchange of ideas with colleagues, students, and consultants. The author is deeply indebted to the students of the Cook County School of Nursing, Chicago, Illinois, who took this knowledge to the bedsides of their patients and nursed them with confidence, knowledge, and insight. I acknowledge, with gratitude, the faith and freedom invested in the development of this text by Miss F. Pauline Gesner, R.N., of the Cook County School of Nursing. The assistance and dedication of the instructors in Clinical Nursing of the Cook County School of Nursing brought depth and dimension to the development of the text, and I must especially thank Beulah Gingrich, R.N., Ruby A. Roberts, R.N., and Lita Vigilia, R.N. I am grateful to Professor Rachel Bliss and Doctor Jerome Handler for reading the manuscript and offering sensible counsel and advice. I especially thank Esther Kopaczewski, R.N., for incisive and perceptive criticism that sharpened the focus and the encouragement and dedication which has left its mark on the text and its author. I am indebted to Mr. Wyatt Peterson and the staff of the F. A. Davis Company for their willing support in this creative effort. I acknowledge gratefully the permission of the *American Journal of Nursing* and *Nursing Forum* to include concepts in Chapter 1 which originally appeared in those publications. Finally, a maternal thanks to Patsy and Bill because they did the dishes, and abiding gratitude to Professor Edwin B. Levine, who tempered scholarly demand with unending devotion.

MYRA ESTRIN LEVINE

Evanston, Illinois

Contents

1 Introduction to Patient-Centered Nursing Care

Theories of Disease as a Basis for Nursing Practice

Introduction

Nursing is a human interaction. It is a discipline rooted in the organic dependency of the individual human being on his relationships with other human beings. An "interaction" by its very nature presupposes a system of exchange between individuals: it can occur only if *communication* can occur. Language represents only one mode of communication, and, indeed, the ability to respond to the behavior of other individuals often requires no exchange of words at all. Hall says, "Culture is communication," and, within this view, the artifacts of every culture become useful and relevant only when they are placed within the perspectives of the individual's response to them. In every generation, meaningful interaction has taken place with utilization of the knowledge, tools, skills, and ideas unique to that time and place. The scientific knowledge of the modern world provides exciting avenues for the essential dialogue between human beings. It is not a substitute for the fundamental relationships which they must establish with each other. It is the means by which such relationships can be constituted. Nursing knowledge, thoroughly grounded in modern scientific concepts, allows for a sensitive and productive relationship between the nurse and the individual entrusted to her care. In the care of the sick, this has always been true, but never before has there been available to the nurse so rich and demanding a body of knowledge to use in the patient's behalf.

Nursing practice has always mirrored the prevailing theories of health and disease because such theories pervade every culture. Every society has made provision for the care of the sick based upon the ideas shared by the group about disease and its meaning to the individual and to the society. The earliest concepts of health and disease developed from man's seeming

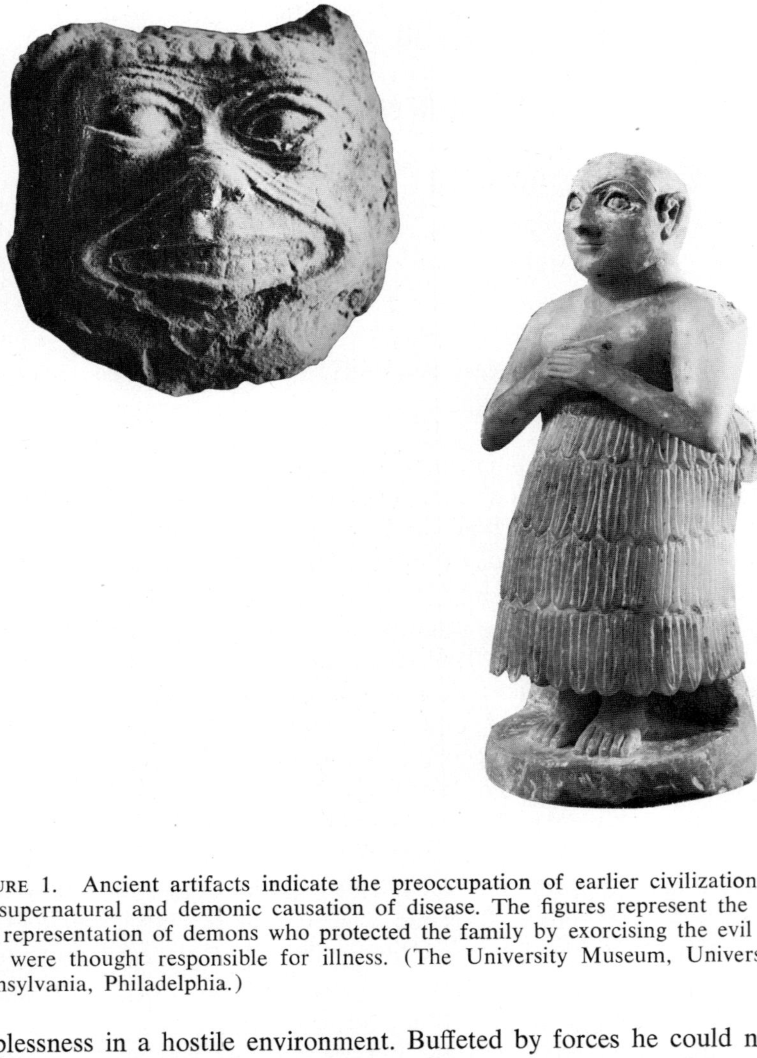

FIGURE 1. Ancient artifacts indicate the preoccupation of earlier civilizations with the supernatural and demonic causation of disease. The figures represent the priests and representation of demons who protected the family by exorcising the evil forces that were thought responsible for illness. (The University Museum, University of Pennsylvania, Philadelphia.)

helplessness in a hostile environment. Buffeted by forces he could neither explain nor understand, he turned to supplication and endowed nature with supernatural qualities.

The care of the sick is closely associated with societal attitudes towards the value that the group places on individual human life, and the economic and political structure of the group strongly influence these values. In many social groups, individual members are valued according to their role in the group. In some societies, throughout history, when the aging member is no longer productive, his loss through illness or injury is not as disastrous as the loss of a younger person who fulfills a useful and essential economic role. Some of the value placed on the lives of the very young may reflect the society's need for productive workers.

The factors that influence the attitudes of any group towards its sick members are very complex. In any individual member, such attitudes are further complicated by the fact that they arise from the several sources that influence his life. His ethnic affiliation is one such fundamental tie, but subcultural attitudes, religious beliefs, and his unique life experiences also leave their mark on his concern for health and his response to disease.

In a real sense, nursing itself is a subculture, possessing ideas and values which are unique to nurses, even though they mirror the social template which created them. And like all other social institutions, the practice of nursing has faithfully reflected the changing currents of knowledge and belief within the human communication systems of which it is a part.

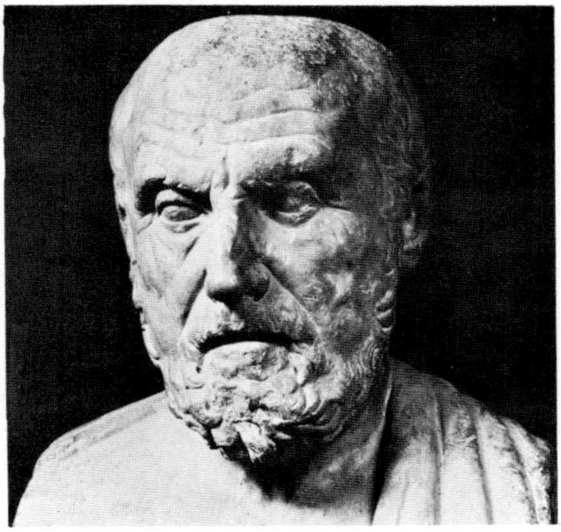

FIGURE 2. Hippocrates (460-357 B.C.) recognized the influence of environmental interactions on the well-being of the individual and established guidelines for the observation, diagnosis, and care of the sick that have influenced all medical practice since his time. (The Bettmann Archive.)

NATURE AS THE GREAT HEALER

The healing power of natural forces, still a part of all superstitious belief, strongly influenced the development of scientific medical thought. The concept of Nature as the Great Healer (*vis medicatrix naturae*) was enunciated clearly by Hippocrates, and persisted through centuries of evolving scientific knowledge. Man fortified himself in his hostile environment, and knowledge changed fear to awesome wonder.

A benevolent healing power in Nature was fundamental doctrine in the rise of the humanitarians and sanitarians of the nineteenth century. Florence Nightingale was their greatest spokesman. Perhaps no historical figure has been so poorly understood as has Florence Nightingale. She was called a "legend" in her own time, and the fantasies perpetuated about her have reinforced a legendary aura which belies the incisive, perceptive, and honest excellence of her thinking and her contribution to modern health theory. Her writings were primarily aimed at the establishment of a system of hospital care based on effective sanitation practices, and such practice, in turn, arose from an unceasing concern for the integrity and decency of the individual. *Notes on Nursing* was written for the "layman," and, in fact, Miss Nightingale never wrote a "textbook" of nursing. But this delightful volume is a treasury of wisdom and insight, and much of it is as relevant today as it was in 1859. Miss Nightingale wrote, "Shall we begin by taking it as a general principle—that all disease, at some period or other of its course, is more or less a reparative process. . ."

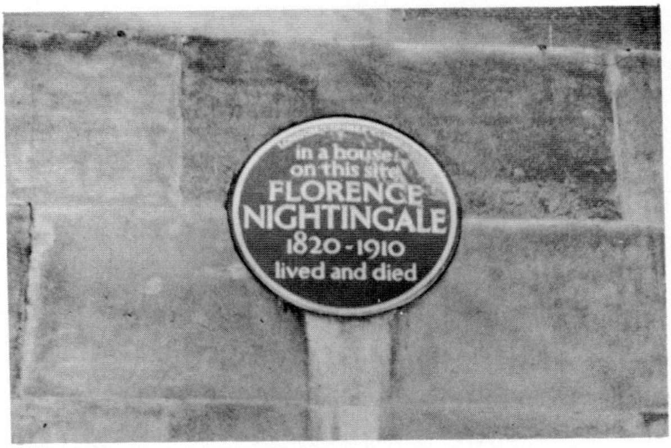
in a house
on this site
FLORENCE
NIGHTINGALE
1820-1910
lived and died

FIGURE 3. The plaque on the site of the South Street home of Florence Nightingale where for fifty years the vital nucleus of modern nursing thought was centered. (Photo by Assoc. Prof. Rachel Bliss, University of Illinois College of Nursing, Chicago.)

With this mandate, the direction of nursing care became remarkably clear: the nurse created an environment in which healing could occur. Nursing responsibility focused on procedures to establish an environment of cleanliness, safety, and comfort, both physical and mental. Thus protected and nurtured, the "reparative process" within the patient was enhanced. It was in this way that the "procedure-orientation" in nursing began. Its persistence to this day has accompanied the growth of technology in nursing, as indeed nursing has shared in technological expansion in every area of modern life. But the tradition of the procedure—of "how-to-do-it"—has become so deeply imbedded in the nursing psyche that it is almost "holy."

The Theory of Specific Causation

The great microbiological discoveries of Koch and Pasteur took place during Miss Nightingale's lifetime. She never accepted the "Germ Theory," but even her unwillingness to do so could not stop the radical change in nursing practice demanded by it. Now a single organism could be demonstrated as the cause of a single disease, and therapy became specific and definitive. Once more, nursing responsibility was clear and unequivocal. Curing a disease required indentification of its specific cause, and the use of the specific agent which would eliminate it. Nurses learned about the disease, its manifestations, and its progress. The patient was merely the repository, however temporary, for the disease organism. Nursing education became "disease-oriented" because the disease, not the patient, was treated.

The microbiological discoveries permitted the development of aseptic techniques which, coupled with the discovery of anesthetic agents, vastly expanded the practice of surgery. The communicable diseases of childhood became controllable, and the control of infection affected the entire hospital structure. Lower morbidity and mortality rates produced widespread sociological change: more infants grew to maturity and more adults lived to old age. All kinds of improved techniques and therapies—many arising in the pressure of war—enabled individuals with previously fatal disorders to live. They now survived their acute illnesses, but required continuing treatment and care for chronic ailments. In fact, some diseases, such as diabetes, were understood for the first time, because the "natural" progress of the disease had never unfolded, since the individual stricken with it died quickly when treatment was so inadequate.

The Theory of Multiple Factors

The avalanche of increasing knowledge and discovery soon showed that specific causation had very limited scope. Notably, the behavioral sciences drew attention to the multiple factors that always play upon any single disease process in any single individual. Although some remnants of faith in specific causation exist today in the hope for a "cure" for many ills, such wistful simplicity is obviously naive.

In response to the multiple factors theory, nursing became concerned with the complexities of providing "total patient care." Recognition of the psychosocial determinants to health and of the alarming social pressures at the bedside has given emphatic new directions to nursing learning and practice. The myriad factors relevant to every patient's care have vastly complicated the nurse's task. With no rationale for truly unifying its application to patients, nursing care tends, indeed, to become an unsynthesized "total," a sum of many disparate parts. The urgency for knowledge that allows the use of sophisticated technology in an arena where sensitivity to psychological and emotional factors must also be acknowledged, creates the danger of serious sins of omission in the care of individual patients. An approach to patient care which recognizes multiple factors has no validity unless there are some unifying directions that clarify the ultimate goals.

The Unified Theory of Health and Disease

A great theologian, Paul Tillich, summarized the problem confronting the modern nurse when he said that the "multidimensional unity of life in man calls for a multidimensional concept of health, of disease and of healing, but in such a way that it becomes obvious that in each dimension all the others are present."

The human being responds to the forces in his environment in a singular yet integrated fashion. The specific symptoms of a disease may emphasize some bodily functions more than others, but even to such a localized cluster of events, the afflicted person responds in a way peculiar to him and to him alone.

There are no magic scales which allow nurses to weigh the multiplicity of factors operating in a single individual. Ultimately, decisions for nursing intervention must be based on the unique behavior of the individual patient. It is the nurse's task to bring a body of scientific principles on which decisions depend into the precise situation that she shares with the patient. Sensitive observation and the selection of relevant data form the basis for her assessment of his nursing requirement. A theory of nursing must recognize the importance of unique detail of care for a single patient within an empiric framework which successfully describes the requirements of *all* patients.

The integrated function of the human organism has been described in the scientific literature since the nineteenth century. Claude Bernard recognized the interdependence of bodily function in his description of the *milieu interne*—the internal environment. Bernard identified the primordial seas, captured within the integument of the human body and providing the organism with a tightly regulated solution of substances essential to its continuing well-being. In the pursuit of understanding that accompanied Darwinian thought in the late nineteenth century, this significant contribution underscored the remarkable ability of the human organism to survive successfully in widely variant external environments. Man carried the essentials with him, safely packaged inside his skin. But it was apparent to Bernard, and to the army of investigators who followed him, that the internal environment was susceptible to constant change. In 1915, Walter Cannon, an outstanding American physiologist, coined the word "homeostasis" (*homeo,* equal and *stasis,* condition) to describe the remarkable equilibrium that was maintained in the internal environment in the face of constant change.

The concept of homeostasis recognized that the balance maintained within the internal environment took place on a continuum of relationships, with an upper and a lower limit between which the balance was normally struck. In fact, the concept of "normal" presupposes that the values for the many different substances dissolved in the body fluids will fall somewhere between those upper and lower limits, and a value either above or below the limits indicates an abnormal condition. The well-being of the organism is thus dependent upon the balance, and in general, when the value exceeds the limits, it must be promptly restored or the life of the organism is threatened.

The physiologists have identified many of the interactions that the body is called upon to make when the internal environment is threatened by alterations in the value of vital substances. By and large, such revisions depend on "negative feedback" mechanisms resulting in "autoregulation" of the internal environment. A negative feedback exercises control by reinserting into the system the results of its past performances. Wiener has described this effect as "patterns that perpetuate themselves." They are control systems, designed to maintain the balance—and thereby the well-being—of the organisms. Thus it is that the factors influencing a person's response to illness do not exist as discrete entities which may be selected and used at will. All of the forces within him exist in a dynamic relationship to each other, seeking a state of equilibrium or balance that will best maintain a uniformity of function.

The exquisite internal balance responds constantly to external forces, however. There is an intimate relationship between the internal and the external environments, much of it vividly understood in recent years by research in physiological periodicity and the circadian cycles. Some of the earliest attention to the periodic nature of physiological function was devoted to studies of sleep and wakefulness, and the familiar experience of every individual emphasizes, even in this single area, how individual well-being is dependent upon external environmental experience. The fundamental integrative ability of the human organism illuminates all understanding of human structure, function, and response to disease.

The total life process of the entire organism is dependent upon the inter-relatedness of its component systems. In fact, the organism is a sys-

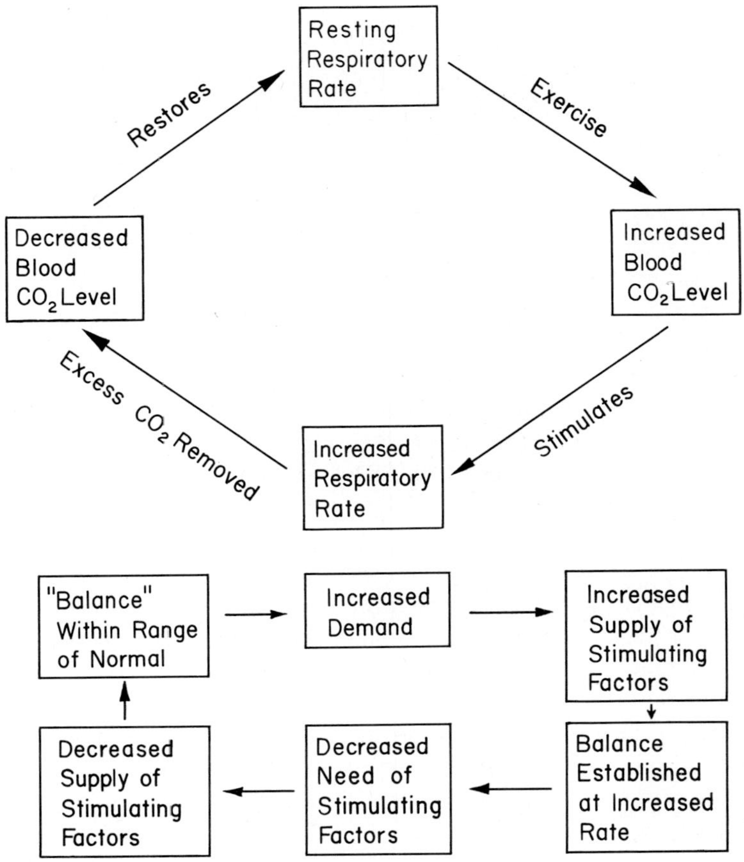

FIGURE 4. The controls exercised by "negative feedbacks" result in a regulatory system in which a balance is maintained because alterations in the variables increase or decrease the rate of function of the entire system. Most physiological systems are "autoregulated" by this kind of mechanism.

tem of systems, and in its wholeness expresses the organization of all the contributing parts. Organization means an orderly sequence, and so the organism represents a pattern of orderly, sequential *change.* Because it is both ordered and sequential, the pattern is a *message.* So long as the pattern is consistent, it is also understandable. If change in the organism were to occur in an undisciplined and unregulated way, then anarchy would result, and the pattern would be so disrupted that it could no longer successfully support life. Such anarchy, in fact, occurs in disease processes, and unless the pattern can be restored, the organism will die.

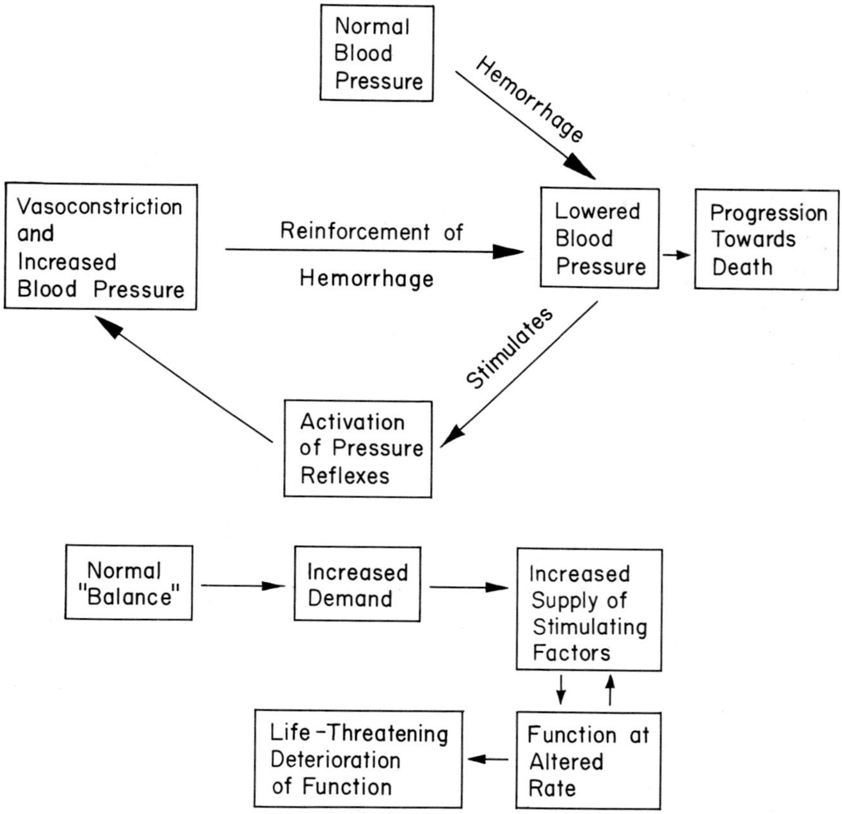

FIGURE 5. A positive feedback results in an increasing rate of function without the regulatory control that restores balance. Thus a "vicious cycle" is instituted which produces more and more disruption of function. The process must be stopped before the changes become irreversible. Many pathological processes result in a positive feedback.

Change is the essence of life, and it is unceasing as long as life goes on. Such change is not a random activity. It is directed, purposeful, and meaningful, and it is also eminently understandable. The change which supports the well-being of the organism can be predicted, measured, and observed, and therefore is a cogent message. It must be emphasized that the message is not a single sentence. It is far too complex for that. It is always at least a paragraph and may indeed as often be equivalent to a book or a library filled with books.

Change is characteristic of life, and adaptation is the method of change. The organism retains its integrity in both the internal and external environment through its adaptive capability. Adaptation is the process of change whereby the individual retains his integrity within the realities of his environments. Adaptation is basic to survival, and it is an expression of the integration of the entire organism. The measure of effective adaptation is compatibility with life. A poor adaptation may threaten life itself, but at the same time the degree of adaptive potential available to the individual may be sufficient to maintain life at a *different level of effectiveness.* Adaptation is not "all-or-none." It is susceptible to an infinite range within the continuum of life compatibility. Within that range, there are numerous possible degrees of adaptation.

Thus, the dynamic processes establishing balance along the continuum are adaptations. All the processes of living are processes of adaptation. Survival itself depends upon the *quality* of the adaptation possible for the individual. Health and disease are patterns of adaptive change. Engel argues that the study of disease must be grounded in knowledge of it as a "natural phenomenon." Wolf says that "physicians now consider most diseases to be distinct from one another insofar as they represent patterned responses or adaptations to noxious forces in the environment."

The nurse participates actively in every patient's environment, and much of what she does supports his adaptations as he struggles in the predicament of illness. Nursing intervention means that the nurse interposes her skill and knowledge into the course of events that affects the patient. Thus, nursing intervention must be founded not only on scientific knowledge, but specifically on recognition of the individual's organismic response which indicates the *nature of the adaptation taking place.* The nurse must learn to read the message. Such assessments provide the only rational basis for judicious decision-making by the nurse in the patient's behalf. Furthermore, nursing intervention must be designed so that it fosters successful adaptation whenever possible.

When nursing intervention influences adaptation favorably, or toward renewed social well-being, then the nurse is acting in a *therapeutic* sense. When nursing intervention cannot alter the course of the adaptation — when her best efforts can only maintain the status quo or fail to halt a downward course—then the nurse is acting in a *supportive* sense.

The organismic nature of the human response to the environment provides the rationale for substantive principles of nursing. A principle is a fundamental concept that forms the basis for a chain of reasoning. Formulated on a broad base, it establishes the relationships between apparently otherwise unrelated facts. Nursing principles are fundamental assumptions which provide a unifying structure for understanding a wide variety of nursing activities.

Nursing principles are all "conservation" principles. Conservation means "keeping together" (L. *conservatio*), but this does not imply *minimal* activity. "To keep together" means to maintain a proper balance between active nursing intervention coupled with patient participation on the one hand and the safe limits of the patient's ability to participate on the other. The four conservation principles have as a postulate the unity and integrity of the individual, recognizing that every response to every environmental stimulus results from the integrated and unified nature of the human organism. In effect, this entire text is designed to explain and illuminate the four conservation principles of nursing. They are, therefore, listed here, and frequent reference to them will be made.

I. The principle of the conservation of patient energy
Nursing intervention is based on the conservation of the individual patient's energy.

II. The principle of the conservation of structural integrity
Nursing intervention is based on the conservation of the individual patient's structural integrity.

III. The principle of the conservation of personal integrity
Nursing intervention is based on the conservation of the individual patient's personal integrity.

IV. The principle of conservation of social integrity
Nursing intervention is based on the conservation of the individual patient's social integrity.

The Hospital as an Environment

The Sociology of the Hospital

All social institutions have an organizational structure that identifies and distinguishes them. No social institution springs up fully formed. All have their roots in their historical past, and all possess patterns of function that reflect the established traditions of their past as well as the practices arising from the interactions with the community of which they are a part.

The modern hospital is a recent social institution. Its growth has paralleled the changing nature of medical practice in the past hundred years and reflects the evolving social attitudes towards illness in modern communities. Many large public institutions began as "poorhouses" or "poor farms" which were established to absorb the indigent sick of rapidly expanding urban areas. The standards of care in such institutions were closely correlated with their purpose: they provided minimal, custodial care for those who could not care for themselves. It is no wonder that hospitals were originally places to which people went to die.

The development of aseptic knowledge and social institutions that took over the role of the care of the indigent in a community contributed to progressive change in hospital function. The hospital gradually became the center for technological and scientific learning, and only as health resources expanded did they become places of healing. Even though people today come to hospitals in order to be healed, an undercurrent of tradition persists. For many persons, admission to a hospital is viewed as a dire and catastrophic event, fraught with danger.

The widespread availability of hospitalization insurance, both private and government-financed, has added another function to the complex social role fulfilled by the hospital. The hospital has become a central agent in the planning for community health, and its obligations to the world beyond its walls have increased as new insights into the need for continuity of care of the individual have been developed. The dissemination of knowledge of exciting advances in the treatment of disease has created an informed lay public and an increasing demand that expensive equipment, requiring the services of highly skilled professionals, be available for all patients. The economic tensions that confront the modern hospital are responsible for continuing public concern and have stimulated a necessary social debate. The astronomical cost of electronic equipment, modern drug therapy, and sophisticated technological components for diagnosis and treatment requires the devoted attention of the community as well as of the individuals within it who are directly responsible for the direction of the hospital program. It is almost a paradox that the growing excellence of hospital care has in itself caused the crisis in financing and supporting the modern hospital.

The Patient's Perception of the Roles of Hospital Personnel

The individual entering the hospital leaves behind him the familiarity and comfort of his daily life and must substitute for it a complicated routine which bears little resemblance to his activities outside the hospital. The impersonal reality of the hospital itself — the strange surroundings and the mysterious routines — are ameliorated only through the personal relationships which are so vital to the welfare of all human beings. The individual can quickly become adjusted to the physical surroundings in which he finds himself. The crucial adjustments must involve the other human beings, most of them utter strangers, whom he recognizes at once as participants in the most intimate aspects of his life. Some of his expectations of the behavior of these important strangers are predetermined. In fact, his expectations may be as unique as any of the individualizing aspects that define him and set him apart from all other persons. But, in some ways, the hospitalized patient carries expectations which reflect the social and professional roles of the hospital personnel with whom he comes in contact.

The physician, and particularly if he is a private physician, represents to the hospitalized patient his tie with the life he has temporarily abandoned in the world outside the hospital. The physician is part of the hospital staff, and in fact, exercises a strong controlling force in the policies of the hospital. But, at the same time, he functions out in the community, and the patient has a relationship with him that often begins before hospitalization and will continue after it is terminated. The patient is well aware that it is the knowledge and judgement of this individual upon which his future well-being depends. He looks to the physician as his representative in the hospital hierarchy, confident that his rights and privileges will be protected by his personal relationship with the physician.

The nurse, on the other hand, embodies the very image of the hospital and all it means to the patient. The nurse *belongs* to the hospital; she is the spokesman through whom the hospital, its policies, its demands, its provocation of fear and anxiety — and its hope for his future — are interpreted by the patient. The nurse may remain at his bedside for much longer than the physician actually does, but three times a day all the nurses are changed, and there is never any assurance that the same nurse will return to care for him the next day. In the physician's absence, he recognizes the nurse as the physician's agent and quickly learns that he must depend upon the nurse to fulfill the therapeutic plan the doctor has outlined for him. He may, in fact, be frustrated by the limitations the nurse expresses in making certain decisions concerning his care, even while he recognizes the importance of her responsibilities for him. As the hospital's representative, the nurse often bears the brunt of his disaffection. Complaints about food, for example, are socially acceptable ways in which to express anger and hostility that arise from the threat of the illness and the discomfort of its treatment, and, even when the food service is quite separate, the patient may still vent his wrath to the nurse.

Other hospital personnel, and especially those who perform nursing tasks in the patient's presence, are also closely identified with the hospital itself. The responsibility for their actions is invested in the nursing staff that supervises them, and they are therefore extensions of the patient's perception of the nursing role.

The Administrative Realities of the Hospital Structure

The Bedridden Individual The independence of action that characterizes the individual's social life is rigorously restricted when he is admitted to the hospital. His immediate personal environment is restricted to the hospital bed and whatever articles of furnishings surround his "unit." Those essential activities which are most personal and private must now depend upon the willing assistance of other persons. He must be provided with food and with the means to maintain personal hygiene and cleanliness and to satisfy his elimination needs; also, because he is ill, he must be provided with the necessary medications and treatments the physician has ordered for him.

Every aspect of his personal comfort and safety rests in the hands of other persons. For each individual patient, the hospital must provide the necessary equipment, linens, food, medications, and services which are specifically and uniquely his own, and such provision must be made within a defined time limit and with scrupulous accuracy. In addition, his particular psychological and emotional needs become the concern of those who are caring for him; these persons are further charged with fortifying his integrity as a human being and his responsibility as a member of a family and a social group.

Caring for a Patient Census When one patient is multiplied by ten or a hundred, the problems of providing individualized service for many individuals in the safest and most economical way create the need for a well-planned administrative structure. The problems of caring for a single patient become multiplied into very large problems, and the solutions are dependent upon the entire organization. The administration of the hospital must, by its very nature, devote its efforts to the care of all patients within its walls. The complex organizational framework required to fulfill this essential responsibility must be "impersonal." The hospital administration functions within the demands of the goals of the community of which it is a part, and no small determinant of its success depends upon its financial resources and its budgetary limitations.

The administrative policy of every institution inevitably influences the basic activities of its nursing personnel. The daily activities of the nursing staff in a hospital where bathing utensils are kept in the individual's unit throughout his hospitalization will vary considerably from those in one where a central supply of utensils is utilized for many patients. The use of disposable equipment will differentiate bedside nursing care in one hospital from that in another where equipment must be cleaned, sterilized, and stored after each usage.

A clear-cut distinction must be made between those aspects of care that are dictated by administrative necessity and those that are dependent upon nursing principles which would be the same in any institution. The care of a large patient census does not eliminate the individual requirement for the safety of each patient from cross-contamination. Establishing routines which will minimize the danger of cross-contamination is clearly an administrative responsibility, but the specific instances of prevention of infection remain dependent upon fundamental aseptic techniques effectively performed by the nurse. The individual safety of the patient from such hazards as falling, or receiving the wrong medication or the wrong treatment, will continue to be charged to excellence of nursing care, even though the administrative policy must place patient safety as one of its fundamental considerations.

Individualization of care rests with the nurse's appreciation of the patient's unique requirements, but it must take place within the depersonalized framework of the administrative structure. Recognition of the importance of administrative policy in providing for all patients is an essential part of learning to provide individualized nursing care. The nurse may have many opportunities to help the patient to understand that the apparently irrational "rules" and "regulations" of the hospital routine have a purpose as immediate to the patient's well-being as the nurse's studied efforts in his behalf.

The hospital is the community of the sick. Many persons enter the hospital with life-threatening disease, and even those who are not so realistically threatened may interpret their hospitalization as if they were. The hospital environment is one in which fear and anxiety are daily experiences. The discomfort, pain, and dislocation of illness can best be met by a nursing staff able to recognize and face the reality with the patient in a sensible, sympathetic, and helpful way.

Patient-Centered Nursing Intervention

The Vital Importance of Sound Observation

Patient-centered nursing care means *individualized* nursing care. It is predicated on the reality of common experience: every man is a unique individual, and as such he requires a unique constellation of skills, techniques, and ideas designed specifically for him. Such nursing intervention can take place only when the nurse has made an accurate assessment of his unique needs, and this, in turn, is possible only through the formulation of all relevant factors that contribute to the patient's predicament at a given time and place. There are numerous sources of information available in the determination of any single patient's requirements. The ability to utilize all the information about a patient comes with increasing knowledge and maturity in nursing, but even the beginning student can contribute to, and utilize important determinants in, the planning of nursing care.

The fundamental interaction between nurse and patient presupposes that the nurse brings to the relationship the objectivity and discipline of the professional practitioner. The nurse bears a responsibility for evaluation of the patient's condition at the time of actual contact, as well as the ability to anticipate the course of events in the immediate, and often the distant, future. Equipped with all the information available about the patient, the nurse functions in his behalf effectively only in direct proportion to her ability to make relevant observations of him and then to initiate activity that may be required as a result of the observations.

Miss Nightingale wrote, "In dwelling upon the vital importance of *sound* observation, it must never be lost sight of what observation is for. It is not for the sake of piling up miscellaneous information or curious facts, but for the sake of saving life and increasing health and comfort." In the century that has passed since these words were written, the importance of accuracy and relevance of observations has never been stated better. Because we are constantly in contact with our environment, all kinds of signals and stimuli reach us continuously. It is in the selection of those perceptions which bear relevance to the patient's progress that the nurse demonstrates the judgement that permits sound professional decisions.

The word "observation" is defined as "faculty or habit of taking notice." But the Latin noun from which the English word is derived, *observatio,* originally meant "guarding against" or "watching over." Those observations which form the structure of professional assessment are distinguished by the importance that active involvement places upon them. The skills of observation are subservient to the guardian responsibilities of the nurse who makes them. From the outset, the student of nursing should be constantly aware of the signals, both obvious and hidden, which come from her interaction with the patient. Abdellah has called these "overt" and "covert" needs, because the apparent intent of a patient's behavior may often substitute for a real intent of far greater importance and relevance to his well-being.

The professional skill of "observations" requires that the test of "relevance" always be intrinsic to the act. All observations of patient behavior take place within an environment which influences his behavior, and thus the relevance may well reflect the environment as well. A patient may not have displayed any behavior that suggested anxiety until another patient within his milieu became noisy or desperately ill, or, perhaps, died. On the other hand, a patient may become increasingly fearful as the time for an operative procedure draws near. A patient may be rested and relaxed on a morning after a good night's sleep, but irritable and tired on another morning when his sleep has been interrupted because of some distraction during the night. Nurses frequently can see measurable relaxation in patients following their morning care. There are countless situations in the environmental exchange which influence the patient's response, and they must be identified when they occur.

Another important dimension in observation is the passage of time. The expectation of change characterizes all medical and nursing goals, and therapy is decidedly based on deliberate anticipation of change. The entire semantics of medical care is formulated on concepts of change. The patient is described by relating his "progress." He may be "improving" or he may be "going downhill." He "reacts" or "responds" to a therapeutic intervention, such as a medication or a treatment. His disease is a "process" which includes the idea of an onset, a course, and a termination. Thus an observation which is relevant at one time may no longer be accurate at another. Some responses are almost instantaneous, and some are gradual and subtle. Observations of his reactions at the onset of his disease should be quite different from those when he is nearing convalescence. And observations before a treatment or a nursing process is accomplished will not be the same as those evaluating the effects of such activity after it is completed. Observations are continuous, repetitive, and changing, because they must, to retain their validity and usefulness, reflect the constant and changing nature of the individual's response to his illness. Many therapeutic designs, in fact, include a time factor as an aspect of their success. If one treatment does not bring the desired results in a specific time, then another may be tried in its stead. Only cautious observation can provide the data for making decisions of such importance.

Observations become relevant when they fit into a pattern of orderly relationships. If the patient's condition has been altered by the administration of a drug, the importance of the drug to the change is a basic part of the observation. This is true of any active intervention in the patient's progress, but it may be equally essential in assessment of the disease process. Knowledge of the expected course of a disease influences the relevance of observations because an unexpected development may presage great danger if it goes unobserved. Recognition of priorities of importance in the changing pattern of the patient's response depends on thorough knowledge of disease processes and their pathophysiological implications. Of equal importance is knowledge of the expectations of the therapeutic purpose in the medical and nursing plan for the patient. Here, too, an unexpected or untoward response may demand intervention not previously indicated.

If observation is practiced as a "guardian" activity, it is successful only when it is, in fact, used to initiate activity on the part of the nurse. Some observations are important because they contribute information that *the doctor* must have in planning the medical care. Others are important because they contribute information which *both the nurse and the doctor* may use in planning care. Still other observations are important because they contribute information which *the nurse* must have in planning care. Whatever their ultimate contribution to the patient's care, the measure of usefulness is dependent upon the institution of the necessary action they indicate. Observation is not an end in itself, but a tool that is used to guide patient care. As a guide to action, it constitutes an important part of the nurse-patient interaction. There is a mutuality of response which assures the patient that he is in safe hands and a continuing assessment by the nurse of the effects of her ministrations.

In addition, the sharing of knowledge gained by observation assures the necessary continuity of care from one group of nurses to the next, and from the nursing personnel to the medical personnel responsible for the patient's care. As information is accumulated, it serves as a continuing evaluation of the patient's progress. And because, for all its genius, modern health care is constantly learning and appraising, the consistent recording of observations contributes to the furtherance of knowledge. The precision of description of the patient's response to his disease and its treatment illuminates and enlarges the knowledge available concerning that disease. Thus, observations correctly made, sensibly utilized, and diligently recorded extend the "guardian" role of the observer beyond the individual who benefits directly to many who may benefit in the future.

Modes of Communication

Nursing skills of all kinds represent a "language" which speaks more eloquently to the sick than words can possibly do. The certainty and sureness of what the nurse does for the patient tells him he is safe. The knowledge the nurse brings to bear on his problems tells him he is secure. Attentiveness and prompt fulfillment of his needs tell him that he is respected and cherished as a person.

Verbal communication between patient and nurse may range from the most casual social exchange to a complex teacher-learner relationship, and skilled verbal communication is often therapeutic as well. Frequently the beginning student finds verbal communication awkward and difficult. But, as knowledge grows, and the ability to assess patient needs increases, the uses of verbal communication become more comfortable and productive for both the patient and the nurse. The nurse becomes a teacher when her confidence in her own knowledge allows her to recognize the patient's need to learn. This, too, becomes easier with experience and increasing maturity.

Communication between other members of the health team concerned with the patient's welfare is vital to the provision of a consistent plan for care. A basic exchange must always exist between the nurse and the doctor. The nurse acts as the doctor's agent in his absence and is directly responsible for the actual performance of the therapeutic measures he prescribes. Each contributes the special knowledge and skill which defines the respective roles of the physician and the nurse, and, of course, the patient is

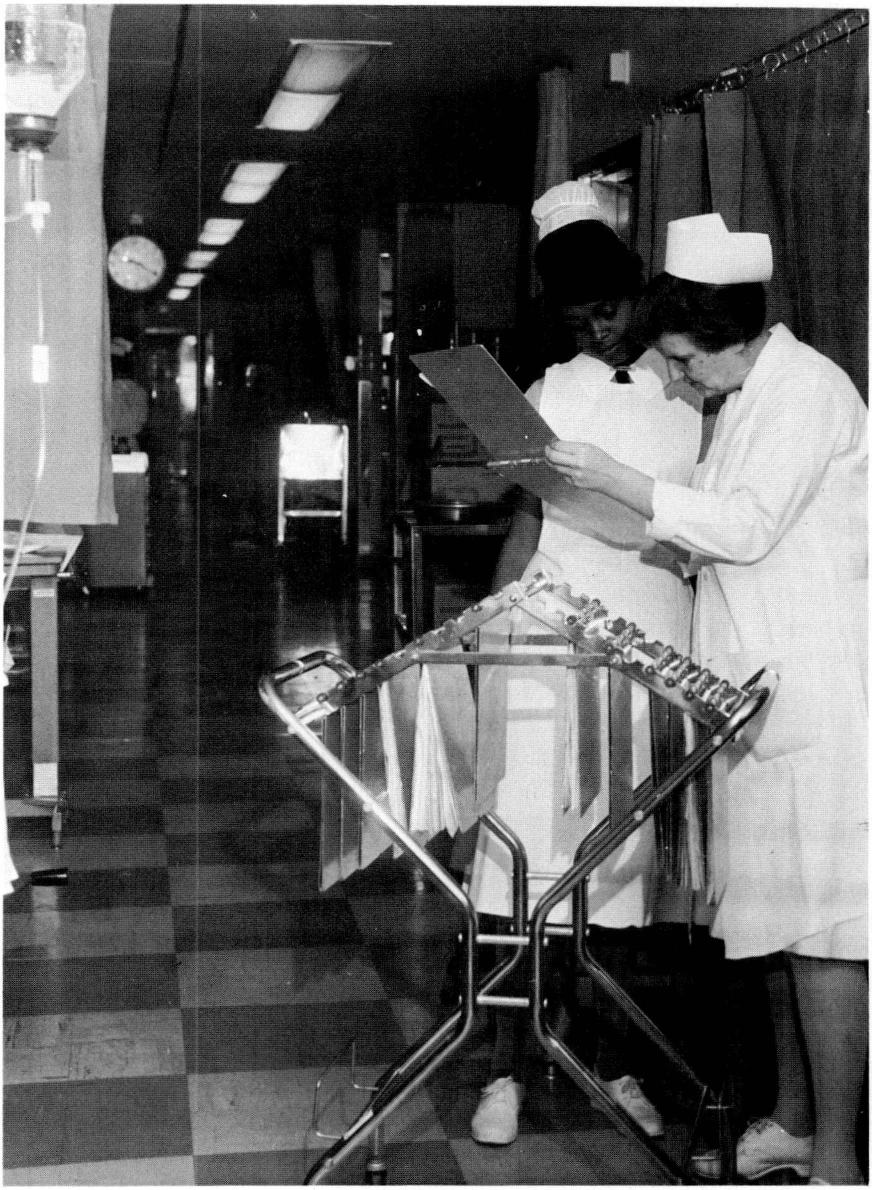

FIGURE 6. Effective nursing care depends upon the transmission of essential information concerning the patient's progress to all individuals charged with responsibility for his welfare. Such communication is not only a characteristic of the learning process but represents a constant professional obligation for every nurse. (Photo courtesy of the Cook County School of Nursing, Chicago.)

central to their mutual concern. The nurse is obligated to fulfill the doctor's orders in an accurate and precise way, including meeting the specifications as to time and place that may contribute to the treatment.

Medicine and nursing share their historical growth in modern hospitals. Both disciplines have become increasingly complex, and both demand an exacting educational preparation. The demands of new knowledge, coupled with the technological progress of the past fifty years, have resulted in shifting to the nurse many responsibilities that once were performed only by doctors. There is good evidence that such shifting roles continue and, in fact, seem accelerated in the age of electronics. But the focus of both doctors and nurses remains on the patient and his predicament of illness. With this central concern in both professions, a fruitful dialogue, grounded in continuing communication, is possible and essential.

Many other professional workers function in the patient's interests too. These include the dietitian, the social worker, the physical and occupational therapists and, in some hospitals, the professional hospital administrator, both in the ward setting and in the hospital as a whole. Here, too, continuing communication is essential in the patient's interest, and frequently the nurse becomes the focus of communication because of her intimate involvement with the patient. The hospital chaplain, or private religious advisor, is another individual who may contribute to the dialogue that assures quality patient care.

Nonprofessional hospital workers who are concerned with many aspects of nursing care can make significant contributions to the information about a patient. Regular seeking of such communication is part of many hospital routines. The licensed practical nurse, ward aide, or attendant, and sometimes the volunteer worker are participants in regular conferences that promote the exchange of information and observation which may aid in the care of the patient.

The patient's family are concerned witnesses to his welfare, and they often can provide the staff with information that cannot be obtained in any other way. Even their expressions of disaffection or dissatisfaction may bring important knowledge to the staff, because they may communicate distressing fears and anxieties which they share with the patient. They are, in any event, so essential to his well-being that the nurse must have free channels of communication with them as part of the routine seeking of information which will benefit the patient.

In addition to the variety of ways in which information is disseminated by verbal means, the use of written records and charts represents another important method of communication. Every hospital ward has a variety of record-keeping duties that are designed to promote the free exchange of essential information about the patient between those who must participate in his care. In the past few years, the recording of nurses' observations has been severely criticized because it lacks substance and relevance. The oft-repeated accusation that nurses spend too much time on "paperwork" frequently fails to recognize that the recording of information is absolutely essential to the patient's continuing welfare. Nurse records should be succinct, but they should also be meaningful; efforts to provide shortcuts by reducing the amount of recording must be planned so that essential knowledge is still transmitted. The written record bears the additional burden of becoming a legal record, and this simply adds to the importance of relevant but accurate selection of observations recorded by the nurse. A well-kept patient history is a gold mine for every student in the care of the patient. Each individual nurse bears a responsibility to add to the record so that the clarity and incisiveness make it the valid communication system it should be.

Model I: Vital Signs (Temperature, Pulse, Respiration)

OBJECTIVES

1. To recognize the inter-relationships of the vital signs as measurements of physiological activity and pathophysiological change.
2. To recognize the periodic nature of physiological activity as a basis for evaluation of the measurement of vital signs.
3. To utilize the information offered by the measurement of vital signs as a determinant of patient progress, response to therapy, and a basis for nursing intervention.
4. To recognize and evaluate the response of the individual patient to environmental factors, internal and external, as indicated by the measurement of vital signs.
5. To assure safety and comfort of the patient during measurement of the vital signs by cautious aseptic technique and appropriate use of equipment.
6. To recognize, through accurate observation of the individual patient, the necessity to measure vital signs above and beyond the prescribed periodic recording of such information.
7. To understand the necessity for proper communication of the single measurement of vital signs as part of a graphic record providing essential information concerning the patient's progress.
8. To recognize changes in the vital signs that require urgent medical and/or nursing intervention.

ESSENTIAL SCIENCE CONCEPTS

1. Vital signs are measurements of the effectiveness of cellular oxygenation.
   - 1.1 Oxygen is absolutely indispensable to life.
     - 1.11 Central nervous system tissue can withstand hypoxia for a maximum of 3 to 5 minutes without irreversible damage.
     - 1.12 Cellular respiration demands a continuing supply of oxygen.
     - 1.13 Chemical activities of metabolism depend on the oxygen supply.
       - 1.131 Biochemical activity produces the energy for all body processes while providing the homeostatic range of body heat.
         - 1.1311 Normal body temperature is regulated by physiological control systems within specific environmental conditions.
           - 1.13111 Optimal effectiveness of body processes takes place within a range of 97.6 to 99.6°F (36.5 to 37.5°C).
           - 1.13112 Body loses 300 to 5000 BTU per hr relative to activity.

1.1312 Increase of 1°F body temperature results in a 7% increase of basal metabolic rate.

1.132 Adaptation permits a wide range of balance between heat production and heat loss.

1.2 Oxygen is absorbed only across the alveolar membrane of the lungs.

1.21 The patency of the airway must be insured at all times.

1.211 Upper respiratory passages warm, filter, and humidify the air.

1.212 Cilia and mucosal sheet protect lower passages from microorganisms and contaminants.

1.213 Cough and sneeze reflexes are defense activities to keep airway clear and clean.

1.22 Breathing is an act involving muscular work.

1.221 On inspiration, muscles of respiration increase the size of the thoracic cage.

1.222 On expiration, muscles of respiration decrease the size of the thoracic cage.

1.23 Respirations are involuntary but are influenced by voluntary components.

1.231 Alveolar ventilation is regulated by respiratory feedback systems.

1.2311 Carbon dioxide blood levels regulate respiratory center in the thalamus.

1.2312 Stretch reflexes in the lungs regulate limit of pulmonary expansion.

1.2313 Normal adult rate is 14 to 16 respirations per minute at rest.

1.232 Voluntary activities alter respiratory rate.

1.2321 Physiological adjustment accompanies swallowing, defecating, laughing, and crying.

1.2322 Somesthetic influences are reflected in change of respiratory rate.

1.23221 Pain tends to increase the rate of pulmonary ventilation.

1.23222 Rapid external temperature change (especially sudden cold) results in immediate alteration of respiratory rhythm.

1.2323 Emotional influences on respiratory rate.

1.23231 Fear, anxiety, apprehension increase rate.

1.23232 "Chronic" alteration of rate may be related to emotional disturbance (hysteria).

1.3 Oxygen can be brought to the individual body cells only via transport by the circulatory system.

1.31 Effective circulatory function depends on an intact system.

1.311 Rhythmic contractility of the heart results in its function as a pulsatile pump.

1.312 Blood is transported under pressure through a closed system of patent, distensible tubes of varying diameter.

1.32 Optimal effectiveness of body processes takes place within a cardiac rate of 60 to 100 beats per minute.

1.321 Adaptations permit variation in circulatory function within a homeostatic range.

1.322 Physiological variables influence circulatory effectiveness.

1.3221 Cardiac output responds to variations in the internal environment.

1.3222 External environmental influences may result in altered cardiac rate.

1.33 Oxygen transport is accomplished by adequate hemoglobin concentration in an adequate number of red blood cells.

2. Vital signs are measurements of the individual's integrated and unique response to internal and external environmental stimuli.

2.1 Alteration in one parameter is accompanied by corresponding alteration in the others.

2.11 Body temperature is a measure of metabolic activity.

2.111 Increase in temperature requires increased oxygen with resultant increase in pulse and respiratory rates.

2.112 Decrease in temperature slows oxygen demand with resultant decrease in pulse and respiratory rates.

2.12 Altered cardiac activity influences tissue oxygenation, resulting in compensatory respiratory efforts.

2.121 Muscular effort is the result of *work* (Work = force × distance).

2.1211 The kinetic energy of the mass of blood is imparted to it by cardiac pumping action.

2.1212 Cardiac action in a closed system takes place against resistance.

2.12121 Friction of vessel walls.

2.12122 Pressure gradients related to diameter of vessels.

2.12123 Viscosity of moving stream of blood.

2.12124 Total blood volume.

2.122 Variation in tissue oxygen demand is immediately reflected in cardiac effort.

2.1221 Increased pulse rate means increased work of the heart.

2.1222 Decreased pulse rate means decreased work of the heart.

2.2 Circadian nature of physiological function results in expected periodic curve of vital sign measurements.

2.21 Hours of slowed metabolic activity produce lowered readings in the absence of pathological or therapeutic alteration.

2.22 Hours of increased metabolic activity produce higher readings in the absence of pathological or therapeutic alteration.

2.23 Establishment of normal variation for the individual patient depends on accurate comparison with his own periodic pattern.

2.3 Individual energy resource in health and disease is influenced by every aspect of activity, both physical and emotional.

2.31 Awareness of the external environment is accompanied by alterations in the economy of the internal environment.

2.311 Fight-flight syndrome is characterized by immediate metabolic response.

2.312 Stress responses (Selye) produce long-term metabolic changes.

2.313 Muscular activity of all kinds is reflected in metabolic demand of the tissues.

2.32 Pathophysiological changes are characterized by altered energy utilization by the body.

2.33 Individual interpretation of environmental factors results in physiological change.

2.331 Realistic evaluation of threat, presence of pain, or adaptation to unfamiliar surroundings and routines.

2.332 Unrealistic evaluation arising from anxiety, fear, loneliness, and vague discomfort.

3. Vital signs are valid only when measured and recorded in a recurrent daily pattern for every patient.

3.1 Accuracy of individual measurements assures validity of graphic summary.

3.11 Physical characteristics of instrument for recording temperature determines its use.

3.111 Maximum-reading thermometer is calibrated in a 16° range compatible with life (94-110°F).

3.1111 Capillarity of extremely fine bore results in retention of final reading unless forcibly shaken down.

3.1112 Surface area (shape) of bulb influences the rate at which expansion of confined fluid can take place.

3.1113 Magnification allows reading within 0.2°F.

3.112 Electric thermometer utilizes a thermocouple so that value is recorded instantaneously.

3.12 Since the rate is the same in all parts of the body, pulse may be counted wherever an artery is close enough to the body surface to be palpated.

3.13 Respiratory rate is influenced by conscious awareness of environmental factors.

3.2 Safety factors are essential in all areas of nursing intervention.

3.21 Physical characteristics of glass thermometers.

3.211 Hollow glass tube is brittle and fragments when broken.

3.212 Size and shape of bulb determine orifice in which it is safely used.

3.213 Engraved surface provides harbor for micro-organisms

3.22 Aseptic handling of instruments prevents cross-contamination with microorganisms.

3.221 Maximum-reading thermometer cannot be sterilized by heat methods.

3.222 Presence of protein contaminants limits choice of chemical disinfection.

3.2221 Mechanical removal of protein contaminants precedes sterilization of glass surface.

3.2222 Chemicals must be effective against flora of mouth and rectum.

3.23 Selection of site for taking temperature includes evaluation of individual's ability to participate.

3.3 Recording of data contributes to assessment of individual patient's response to disease process and therapeutic regime.

NURSING PROCESS

1. Nursing and medical intervention may be directed by the evidence disclosed in the measurement of vital signs.

1.1 Individualized conservation of patient energy is guided by specific values of the vital signs.

1.11 All nursing activities are paced to the individual patient's tolerance.

1.12 Evidence of rapid metabolic activity determines nursing measures to promote rest, minimize activity and fatigue.

1.121 Enhance body's compensatory mechanisms when cellular oxygen needs are not being met.

1.1211 Positioning to support a hard-working heart and/or difficult respirations.

1.1212 Maintenance of a clear airway.

1.1213 Utilization of measures to lower elevated temperature.

1.122 Determination of nursing activities during bedrest that support cardiac and respiratory function.

1.2 Recognition of vital signs as indices of the expected course of the individual's disease process.
  1.21 Identification of precise patterns may aid in diagnosis.
  1.22 Differential diagnosis may depend on changing pattern of vital signs.
1.3 Evaluation of vital signs as indices of the individual patient's response to medical and nursing therapy.
  1.31 Determination of a "resting" value of vital signs for the individual patient.
    1.311 Checking of pulse and respiratory rates during nursing activities provides nurse with information that will guide further care.
    1.312 Checking of pulse and respiratory rates, when prescribed activity is increased, to provide safe convalescence towards ambulation.
    1.313 Recognition of precipitate change in values of vital signs as a basis for urgent or immediate medical intervention.
  1.32 Knowledge of expected results of prescribed medication and treatments as reflected in response of vital signs.
  1.33 Continuing assessment of patient's progress with emphasis on change for better or worse.
1.4 Evaluation of the influence of environmental factors on vital signs.
  1.41 Knowledge of influence of temperature and humidity on cardiac rate and body temperature.
  1.42 Elimination of noise, distraction, and fear-provoking episodes in immediate patient environment.
  1.43 Provision for comfortable, restful posture for patient during taking of vital signs.

2. Meaningful data are provided when assessment of vital signs is accurate.
  2.1 All three measurements are standardized by unit time.
    2.11 Pulse rate is determined by convention for one minute with patient at rest.
      2.111 Count is gauged by second hand of watch.
      2.112 Full count allows certainty that rhythm is recognized.
        2.1121 Regular rhythm contributes to effective cardiac action.
        2.1122 Irregular rhythm has diagnostic and therapeutic importance.
        2.1123 Regular irregularity assists in diagnosis.
      2.113 Quality of pulse provides important information about cardiac function.
    2.12 Respiratory rate is determined by convention for one minute with patient at rest.
      2.121 Large voluntary component in respiratory rate requires counting when individual is not aware it is being done.

2.122 Quality of respiratory excursion should be fully described.

2.1221 Presence of irregularity in rate aids in assessment of intervention required.

2.12211 Distinction between dyspnea (subjective) and hyperpnea (objective).

2.12212 Periodic variation in rate (Cheyne-Stokes) indicates serious respiratory difficulty.

2.1222 Muscular activity involved in respiratory excursion provides clues as to problem.

2.13 Thermometer records maximum reading when left in position for sufficient time.

2.131 Elongated bulb (oral) thermometer registers in minimum of one minute.

2.1311 Bulb must be in close approximation to mucosal surface in order to register properly.

2.1312 Food, drink, and smoking should not precede oral temperature by less than 10 minutes.

2.1313 Oral temperature is not indicated when individual is NPO, receiving oxygen, or has nasogastric tubes in place.

2.1314 Individual patient must be able to understand and participate in holding thermometer in place for prescribed time.

2.132 Pear-shaped bulb (rectal) thermometer registers in minimum of two minutes.

2.1321 Rectal site is prescribed by physician.

2.1322 Patient should be competent to understand his participation.

2.1323 Position of patient allows safety and comfort as well as adequate visualization of anus before insertion.

2.1324 Nurse remains with patient while thermometer is inserted to preclude accident or injury.

2.2 Accuracy is vouchsafed by adherence to specific procedural requirements.

2.21 Aseptic technique is determined by availability of necessary material.

2.211 All sterilization of maximum-reading thermometers is chemical, following careful mechanical removal of protein contaminants.

2.212 Instruments used for many patients are sterilized between use for time period required by selected chemical disinfectant.

2.22 Lubrication of rectal thermometers assures comfort and prevents injury on insertion.

2.23 Site for measurement of temperature is usually specified by physician.

3. Continuity of the vital sign record assures the continuing validity of individual readings in the patient's behalf.

3.1 Recording of individual measurements assures communication of essential information for the subsequent record.

3.11 Variation in "normal" reading of temperature from differing sites requires recording from same site for a valid record.

3.12 Circadian variations establish expectation of vital sign measurements.

3.121 Lowest readings usually occur in early morning.

3.122 Highest readings usually occur in late afternoon.

3.1221 Single daily recording usually performed in late afternoon to insure highest daily reading.

3.1222 Alterations in pattern indicate clinical problem requiring medical attention.

3.123 Complete records for each individual over several days establish his unique circadian pattern.

3.2 Comparison with previous readings provides information which may require prompt nursing and/or medical attention.

3.21 Sudden alteration in pulse or respiratory rate or quality may indicate life-threatening change in condition.

3.22 Gradual change over a period of time in the vital sign measurements indicates patient's changing response to disease process and/or therapeutic plan.

3.23 Temperature reading above 100°F (oral) or 101°F (rectal) is immediately reportable.

3.231 Standing orders for medication or treatment may be instituted.

3.232 Repetition of vital sign measurements every four hours is essential to watch continuing response of the patient.

4. Nurse-patient interaction during measurement of vital signs is a profitable nursing activity.

4.1 Contact allows for observation of the patient's condition.

4.11 Assessment of individual's general appearance.

4.12 Awareness of his emotional tone and state of mind.

4.13 Identification of changes which are relevant to his care.

4.2 Contact with the nurse may be supportive in itself.

4.21 Familiar, nontraumatic experience indicates to patient nurse's continuing concern and interest in his progress.

4.22 Physical contact during checking of pulse can be reassuring to individual patient.

4.23 Expressed anxiety over the results of measurement of vital signs allows immediate response from nurse.

4.231 Teaching may be performed on the spot if it is required.

4.232 Reassurance is immediately available.

4.24 Requests or complaints relating to other facets of care may be dealt with at once.

4.3 Plans for nursing care to follow, or alterations in the nursing care plan, may be made on the basis of this nurse-patient interaction.

Vocabulary

acute
adaptation
administration
aseptic
assessment
autoregulation
chronic
communicable
communication
conservation
contagious
continuum
culture
diagnostic
disease
environment
equilibrium
ethnic
feedback
germ theory
health
homeostasis
individualized
infection
integrative
integrity
interaction
intervention
milieu interne
mortality
morphology
multiple factors
nurse
nursing
observation
organismic
orientation
parameter
perception
principles
reparative
social
specific causation
supportive
technical
technique
therapeutic

General Bibliography

BELAND, IRENE: Clinical Nursing: Pathophysiological and Psychosocial Implications. Macmillan Co., Inc., New York, 1965.

BROWN, ESTHER LUCILLE: Newer Dimensions of Patient Care (Parts I, II, III). Russel Sage Foundation, New York, 1961-1964.

CANNON, WALTER B.: The Wisdom of the Body. W. W. Norton & Co., Inc., New York, 1939.

DUBOS, RENE: Mirage of Health. Doubleday & Co., Inc., Garden City, New York, 1961.

GOODMAN, LOUIS S., AND GILMAN, ALFRED: The Pharmacological Basis of Therapeutics, ed. 3. Macmillan Co., Inc., New York, 1965.

GREENWOOD, MAUD E.: An Illustrated Approach to Medical Physics. F. A. Davis Co., Philadelphia, 1963.

GUYTON, ARTHUR C.: Textbook of Medical Physiology, ed. 3. W. B. Saunders Co., Philadelphia, 1966.

HALL, EDWARD T.: The Silent Language. Fawcett World Library, Greenwich, Conn., 1959.

HOPPS, HOWARD: Principles of Pathology, ed. 2. Appleton-Century-Crofts Inc., New York, 1964.

JACO, E. GARTLY, ED.: Patients, Physicians and Illness. Macmillan Co., Inc., New York, 1958.

MODELL, WALTER: Relief of Symptoms, ed. 2. C. V. Mosby Co., St. Louis, 1961.

NIGHTINGALE, FLORENCE: Notes on Nursing (facsimile edition). J. B. Lippincott, Philadelphia, 1946.

ORLANDO, IDA J.: The Dynamic Nurse-Patient Relationship. G. P. Putnam's Sons, New York, 1961.

SIMMONS, LEO W., AND WOLFF, HAROLD G.: Social Science in Medicine. Russel Sage Foundation, New York, 1954.

SKIPPER, JAMES K., JR., AND LEONARD, ROBERT C.: Social Interaction and Patient Care. J. B. Lippincott Co., Philadelphia, 1965.

SODEMAN, WILLIAM, AND SODEMAN, WILLIAM, JR.: Pathologic Physiology: Mechanisms of Disease, ed. 4. W. B. Saunders Co., Philadelphia, 1967.

SELYE, HANS: Stress. Acta, Inc., Montreal, 1950.

TRAVELBEE, JOYCE: Interpersonal Aspects of Nursing. F. A. Davis Co., Philadelphia, 1966.

WIENER, NORBERT: The Human Use of Human Beings. Doubleday & Company, Inc., Garden City, N.Y., 1954.

Articles

ABDELLAH, FAYE, AND LEVINE, EUGENE: Future directions of research in nursing. Amer. J. Nurs. 66:112-116, Jan. 1966.

AMBURGEY, PAULINE I.: Environmental aids for the aged patient. Amer. J. Nurs. 66:2017-2018, Sept. 1966.

CRATE, MARJORIE A.: Nursing functions in adaptation to chronic illness. Amer. J. Nurs. 65:72-76, Oct. 1965.

DUBOS, RENE: Man and his environment–Biomedical knowledge and social action. Perspect. Biol. Med. IX:523-536, Summer 1966.

DUBOS, RENE: Hippocrates in modern dress. Perspect. Biol. Med. IX:275-288, Winter 1966.

ENGEL, GEORGE L.: A unified concept of health and disease. Perspect. Biol. Med. III:459-485, Summer 1960.

KEEZER, WILLIAM S.: The clinical thermometer. Amer. J. Nurs. 66:326-327, Feb. 1966.

LEVINE, EDWIN B., AND LEVINE, MYRA E.: Hippocrates, father of nursing, too? Amer. J. Nurs. 65:86-88, Dec. 1965.

LEVINE, MYRA E.: Florence Nightingale: The legend that lives. Nurs. Forum II:22-35, 1963.

LEVINE, MYRA E.: Adaptation and assessment: A rationale for nursing intervention. Amer. J. Nurs. 66:2450-2453, Nov. 1966.

LEVINE, MYRA E.: The four conservation principles of nursing. Nurs. Forum VI:45-59, 1967.

LEWIS, OSCAR: The culture of poverty. Sci. Amer. 215:19-25, Oct. 1966.

LINDER, FORREST E.: The health of the American people. Sci. Amer. 214:21-29, June 1966.

MacGregor, Frances D.: Uncooperative patients: Some cultural interpretations. Amer. J. Nurs. 67:88-91, Jan. 1967.

Piore, Nora K.: Metropolitan medical economics. Sci. Amer. 212:19-27, Jan. 1965.

Sjoberg, Gidean: The origin and evolution of cities. Sci. Amer. 213:55-63, Sept. 1965.

Stewart, William A.: Medical education and the community. Perspect. Biol. Med. 10:462-470, Spring 1967.

Storlie, Frances J.: Message for Marcia. Amer. J. Nurs. 67:1682-1683, Aug. 1967.

Taylor, Carl E., and Hall, Marie-Francoise: Health, population and economic development. Science 157:651-657, Aug. 1967.

Taylor, Carol D.: The hospital patient's social dilemma. Amer. J. Nurs. 65:96-99. Oct. 1965.

Tillich, Paul: The meaning of health. Perspect. Biol. Med. IV:92-100, Autumn 1961.

Vaillot, Sister Madeleine Clemence: Existentialism: A philosophy of commitment. Amer. J. Nurs. 66:500-505, March 1966.

Wolf, Stewart: Disease as a way of life: Neural integration in systemic pathology. Perspect. Bial. Med. IV:288-303, Spring 1961.

2 Nursing the Patient Who Has a Failure of Nervous System Integration

Neural Integration Insures the Individual's Integrity in His Environments

All living things are in unceasing contact with their environment. Such contact can never be entirely passive, and as long as the life processes go on, the exchange between the individual and the environment involves incessant activity. In "Adventures of Ideas," Whitehead wrote, " . . . the living organ of experience is the living body as a whole. . . . We cannot determine with what molecules the brain begins and the rest of the body ends. Further, we can not tell with what molecules the body ends and the external world begins. The truth is that the brain is continuous with the body, and the body continuous with the rest of the natural world." Despite the organic relationship that exists between the living being and its environment, identification of the individual is not only possible, but a necessary aspect of environmental awareness. In fact, the concept of continuity *with* the environment is difficult to grasp because discrete knowledge of self-identity and individual awareness is the common vantage point of environmental experience. The evolution of individual identity accompanies the process of maturation in the child, and the recognition of the "self" grows out of the learning processes of life itself. Successful interaction with the environment depends upon the integrity—or wholeness—of the individual, and his ability to conserve and defend his integrity depends upon a responsive and unifying regulatory system. In turn, regulation implies a communication system through which the transmission of messages between the organism and the environment—in both directions—can take place. The transmission of information, which insures individual integrity, must be accurate, swift, and complete.

All living organisms have some kind of message-transmittal system. In the unicellular organism, it is a biochemical reaction which permits prompt response to alterations in the environmental milieu. In more complex individuals, the message transmission systems become more complex, reflecting, as they must, the interactions within the organism as well as its response to environmental factors.

All of the responsiveness to the environment, as well as all of the stimuli arising from it, are exchanges that involve the production, transmission, and utilization of energy in some form. The ultimate source of all the energy of the organism-environment interchange is the sun, but the specific forms of energy may be electrical, physical, mechanical, or chemical, as well as thermal. The individual is equipped with a message-transmittal system capable of responding to all of these forms of energy. The initial energy exchange in the living organism depends upon the presence of tissues that are capable of receiving the stimuli and are, therefore, *receptors.* In the unicellular organism, the receptor may be a participant in the actual alteration of the chemical structure, which produces a change in the behavior of the entire organism. But, in the complex individual, reception of the stimuli is only the first step in a coordinated process that ultimately involves many, many cells. Thus, the receptor is associated with a *transmitter,* a tissue capable of carrying the energy package (that is, the message) to the cells that organize, coordinate, interpret, collate, and direct the interactions of all of the body tissues. The *organizer,* in order to coordinate the effect of the stimulus or message in the interest of the whole individual, sends the instruction along another transmission pathway to the specific tissues that must be stimulated to perform or behave in response to the original stimuli. The tissues which must respond for the organism are the *effectors,* or doers. The cycle is thus completed. The original environmental message, in the form of an energy package, is translated into an alteration in the behavior of the individual organism, a process that is achieved only because the energy can be transmitted within the closed circuit of the system.

The integrating, or "wholeness," system of the human body is, of course, the nervous system. The receptors are the organs which make the living individual a "sentient being" (feeling being). The body depends upon receptors to assess and respond to the variety of stimuli in the environment. The kinds of energy may stimulate a receiving organ that is designed to "recognize" mechanical energy such as pressure or touch. The energy may be thermal, so that the organ responds to temperature. It may be light and thus stimulate visual receptors, or sound and thereby stimulate auditory receptors. The mere stimulation of the receptor cells, however, only initiates the process. The response of the entire body to the stimulus next depends on an intact transmitter; this is an afferent (towards or going to) nerve tract. The afferent fibers carry the message progressively towards the cells of the spinal cord and brain, and it is, of course, in these sites that the interpretative activity takes place. The instructions then must traverse an efferent (away from) nerve fiber that terminates in the effector organ, which may be a muscle or a gland. The analogy between the nervous system and a closed electrical system is often made, but it must be emphasized that the "decision making" of the control tissues in the nervous system (in the brain) reflects the simultaneous occurrence of thousands of stimuli, and no man-made machine has yet achieved the astounding capability of the human brain to integrate and direct body function.

The ability of the nervous system to regulate the body economy as it adapts to the variety of stimuli from the external environment is not a simple cause and effect arrangement. In the eye, for example, adjustment of the size of the pupil, involving the activity of several muscle groups, allows for some control of the amount of light energy permitted to enter the eye. But pupillary changes have also been demonstrated in response to emotional stimuli. The subject which is viewed therefore also affects the size of the pupil. Sounds also create specific response in the individual. Many persons react vigorously to the noise of chalk squeaking on a blackboard, and the use of pleasant music as a means of influencing emotional response in an environment is quite common, even on a therapeutic level. Even in the seemingly simple and discrete response, the organism displays the interpretative effect of its higher centers.

In addition, the effective response of the individual to stimuli from the environment is restricted by the limits of tolerance of living tissue to the strength of the energy that impinges upon its receptor organs. The human eye cannot tolerate the direct energy source of sunlight, and, during every eclipse of the sun, cases of permanent blindness are reported because individuals have looked directly at the energy source. Extremely loud noise can deafen the listener, sometimes permanently. And, of course, tolerance to heat and cold involves not only the local effect on tissues, but the systemic response of the entire body to excesses in the environmental temperature. Within the range of tolerance, the adaptation of the body to the environment depends upon the interpretation by the nervous system, which permits a defensive posture. The small child quickly learns not to touch a hot stove, and crossing a busy intersection requires the alert and inter-related activity of many body systems.

The nervous system protects the individual from noxious forces in the environment by mobilizing the organism to the threat, and instigating the necessary behavior to escape it. But not all danger is real. The anticipation of a threat elicits the same response in the individual and prepares him to defend himself in advance of the reality. The anxious individual responds in precisely the same physiological way as if the danger were present and real, even though it may have been imagined in the first place or never actually materializes. The intensity of the nervous system reaction to imagined threat emphasizes that the individual is also capable of selecting stimuli from the vast number that are always present in the environment and responding only to some of them. This ability to select is essential to integrated function of the body because it would be impossible to respond to all of the stimuli simultaneously present in the environment.

The Central Nervous System

The structural unit of the nervous system is the nerve cell, or *neuron*. The neuron is capable of receiving the package of energy (or stimulus) and of sending the energy on to another cell. In other words, it is excitable. Like the old-time fire fighters who passed the bucket of water from one man to the next, the neuron passes the energy package from one cell to the next. It accomplishes this by transmission of an electrochemical impulse that involves an exchange of ions (electrically-charged particles) across its cell membrane. The electrical charge immediately inside the cell membrane is different from that immediately outside the cell membrane. The difference in the electrical charge is called a *membrane potential* because the difference makes it always possible that a movement of electricity will take place in an effort to equalize the charge on either side of the membrane. The membrane itself is semipermeable, thus allowing some changed particles to pass through the membrane while not permitting

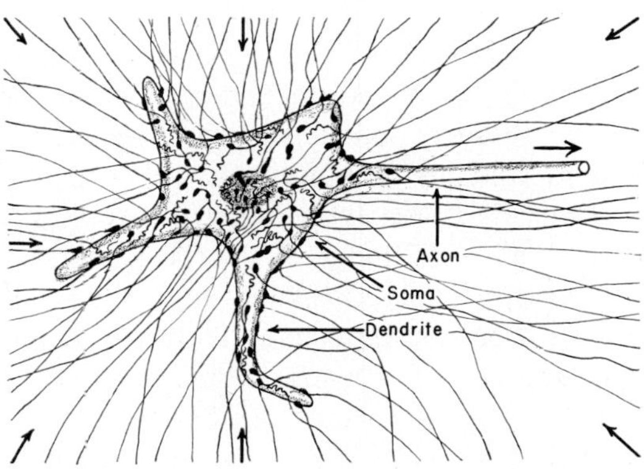

FIGURE 7. The structural unit of the nervous system is the neuron. The *soma* is the cell body, the *dendrites* bring impulses to the cell, while the *axon* carries the stimulus away from the cell. The individual is born with all the neurons he will ever have. (From Guyton, A.C.: *Textbook of Medical Physiology,* 3rd ed. W.B. Saunders Co., Philadelphia, 1966.)

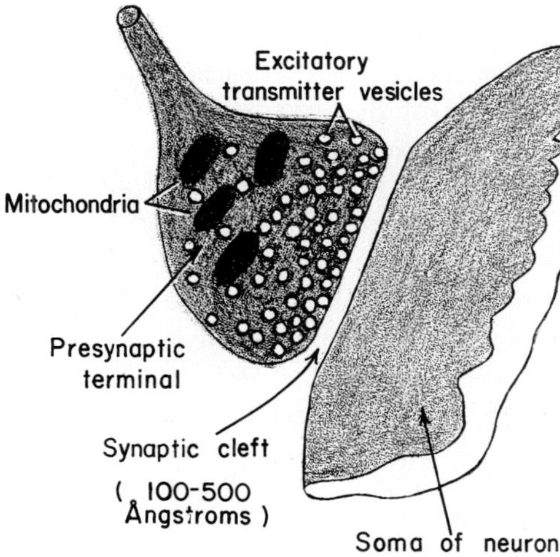

FIGURE 8. The synapse. Acetylcholine is elaborated in the vesicles and this substance transmits the energy exchange across the synaptic cleft. It is promptly inactivated by the enzyme cholinesterase, so that the stimulus is discrete and terminated, thus allowing for a "rest" or refractory period in preparation for the next transmission of impulse. (From Guyton, A.C.: *Textbook of Medical Physiology,* 3rd ed. W.B. Saunders Co., Philadelphia, 1966.)

the passage of other particles. When the cell is excited, there is a movement of positively charged particles out of the cell, leaving a negative electrical charge inside the membrane. The difference in charge is a measurable one, and, although very small (only 70 millivolts), it is sufficient to cause a movement of positive ions back into the cell in order to equalize the charge once again. The movement of ions in and out of the cell through the membrane involves—as does all motion of any kind—an energy exchange. The change in permeability of the cell membrane, which allows the passage of the ions in and out, is essential to the entire process, and the change itself is influenced by many chemical factors. The transmission of the nerve impulse is dependent upon the presence of chemicals at the site where the neuron meets another neuron, or when the neuron meets an effector cell, such as a muscle cell. The meeting place where one cell transmits its electrical impulse to the next is called the *synapse.* In the central nervous system and its peripheral branches, the chemical substance, acetylcholine, alters the permeability of the cell membrane to permit passage of ions across the synapse. The effect lasts for a fraction of a millisecond, and then it is stopped by another substance, cholinesterase, which is an enzyme that inactivates acetylcholine. The inhibiting effect of the enzyme is essential to the effective function of the nerve cell, because it terminates the alteration in the cell membrane and thus limits the stimulus. This permits the cell to have a refractory period, or a resting state, during which the conditions necessary for the transmission of the impulse can be restored. The transmission of the impulse is therefore a periodic one, in which an active period is immediately followed by a resting period. Continuous stimulation without a resting period would soon exhaust the cell and render it unable to function at all. However, this is still a very rapid alteration. In large nerve fibers, the refractory period is about 1/2500 of a second, and in such a fiber a maximum of 2500 impulses per second is possible. It is apparent that the impulse is carried very swiftly, even though there are alternating periods of rest.

Any factor in the immediate environment of the nerve cell which alters the permeability of the cell membrane will influence its ability to carry the impulse. A substance that decreases the permeability of the membrane reduces the excitability of the nerve cell, and, of course, if the membrane permeability is increased, the excitability of the cell is increased. A low calcium ion concentration increases cell membrane permeability and thus increases the excitability of the nerve cell. In clinical conditions in which the calcium ion blood level is very low, the individual shows spasm of the muscles so severe that it is described as tetany. On the other hand, a low potassium ion level decreases the membrane potential so that excitability is lessened to the point where the muscles are paralyzed into inaction. The ability of the nerve cell to respond to the stimuli from the external environment is tremendously influenced by the environment that immediately surrounds the cell. Thus, the internal and external environments of the neuron must act together in order to insure effective function.

Since the transmission of the impulse is a progressive one, it is also essential that the system itself be structurally intact. Any disruption in the continuity of the pathway will immediately stop the passage of the impulse. Every neuron has two kinds of fibers associated with it. There are short, branching fibers called *dendrites,* which bring the impulse to the neuron, and long fibers called *axons,* which carry the impulse away from the neuron. The axons may be several feet long, and usually they do not branch extensively, although some branching near their termination point is not uncommon. The axons, because they traverse long areas of the body away from the nerve cell itself, pass through regions where the immediate internal environment may vary considerably. The effect of the concentration of substances dissolved in the tissues through which they pass is minimized by an insulating sheath, called the *myelin sheath,* which apparently protects the membrane itself from the influence of substances in the immediate region. The myelin sheath is not continuous, but is broken at

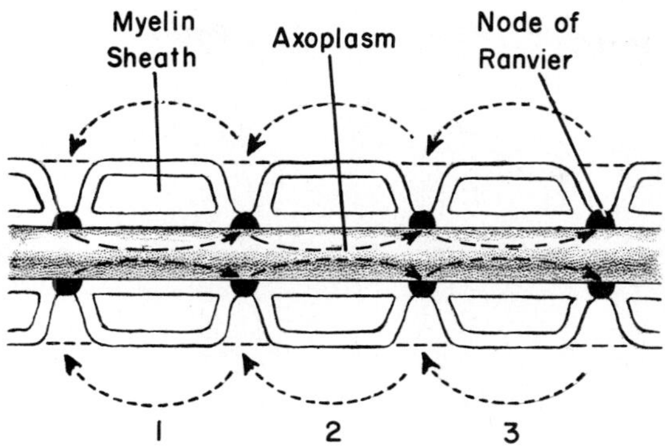

FIGURE 9. Saltatory or "leaping" conduction from one node of Ranvier to the next along myelinated nerve fibers speeds the rate at which the stimulus traverses the nerve fiber. This means of transmission conserves energy as well, so that the process is accomplished rapidly and with minimal loss of the energy resource. (From Guyton, A.C.: *Textbook of Medical Physiology,* 3rd ed. W.B. Saunders Co., Philadelphia, 1966.)

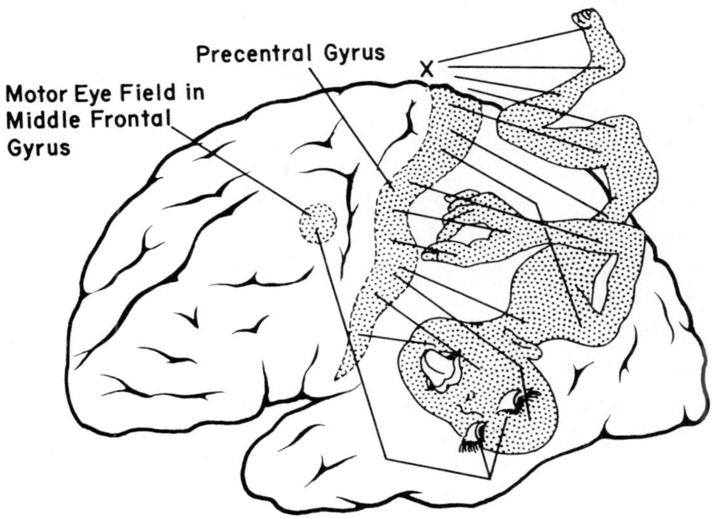

FIGURE 10. The topographical representation of motor control invested in the frontal lobe of the brain emphasizes the relatively discrete motor functions required by some areas of the body, as, for example, the thumb. (From Gatz, A.J.: *Manter's Essentials of Clinical Neuroanatomy and Neurophysiology,* 3rd ed. F.A. Davis Co., Philadelphia, 1966.)

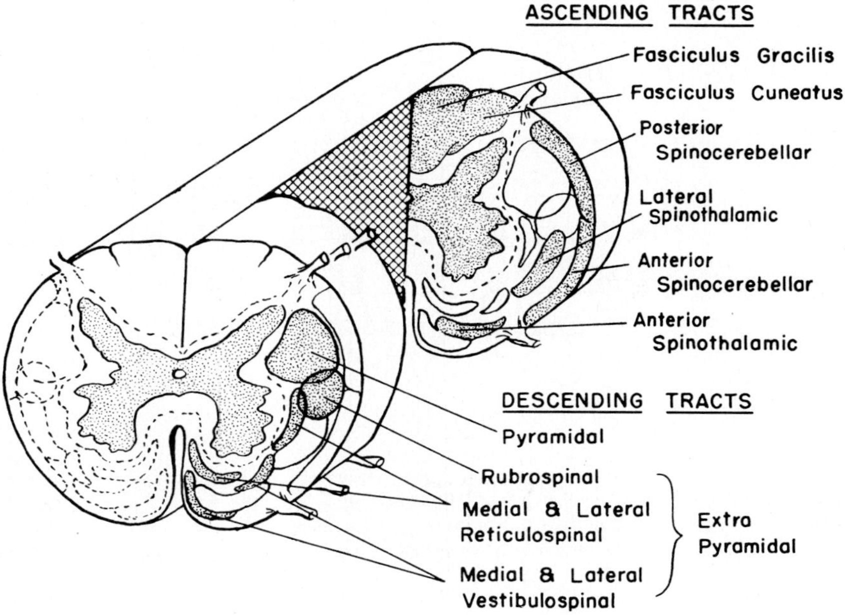

FIGURE 11. The principal tracts of the spinal cord are named in such a way that the first part of the word indicates the origin and the last part the termination of the tract. (From Gatz, A.J.: *Manter's Essentials of Clinical Neuroanatomy and Neurophysiology,* 3rd ed. F.A. Davis Co., Philadelphia, 1966.)

regular intervals by the nodes of Ranvier. It is postulated that the impulse actually passes through the axon by jumping from one node to the next—a process known as saltatory (leaping) conduction. By this means, the velocity of the conduction of the impulse is increased, and the total energy of the nerve fiber is conserved, since the membrane change occurs only at the nodal points. The velocity of the passage of the impulse is proportionate to the size of the nerve fiber. The larger the fiber, the larger the number of ions released and, therefore, the faster the transmission of the impulse from one node to the next. Thus, there is a difference in the rate of conduction of the impulse, depending upon the size of the nerve fiber and, to a degree, upon the nature of the impulse itself. A very large fiber can carry an impulse at the rate of 70 to 120 meters per second, whereas the slowest fibers may carry an impulse at only ½ to 2 meters per second. Rapid conduction usually results in rapid motor activity; slower conduction is the usual response to prolonged and noncritical forms of stimulation. The impulses that permit the individual seated in a chair to retain his balance are slow and continuing, whereas rapid movement, such as that necessary to leave the lecture room, requires much more rapid discharge of nervous impulses.

The anatomical relationships in the central nervous system are organized in a hierarchy of function which further emphasizes the interdependence of one part on the other. As the system ascends, the number of possible synapses and alternative routes increases, so that damage to a lower region causes a highly specific loss of function related to the very discrete role it plays in the total system. The nomenclature of the nervous system tracts may be confusing because many tracts were named before their relationship to the entire system was well understood. In 1955, a standard nomenclature was adopted which simplifies understanding of the anatomical relationships in the nervous system. For example, the pyramidal tract became the corticospinal tract. The first part of the name specifies the origin of the tract, and the second part tells where it terminates. With the standard nomenclature, all tracts can be similarly identified as to their origin and ending. When an interruption in a tract occurs anywhere between the cortex of the brain and the motor neurons in the spinal cord, the resulting lesion is said to be an upper motor neuron lesion. A disruption between the motor neurons in the spinal cord and the effector organs is a lower motor neuron lesion. The symptoms that are clinically apparent are indices of the site of damage. An upper motor neuron lesion, for example, produces a spastic paralysis. This is because the reflex arcs are not damaged, and they continue to stimulate the hypertonic state of the muscles involved. However, the opposing action of the higher centers on those same muscles is cut off by the lesion; as a result, the tonic balance is upset, and the muscles become tightly contracted. A lower motor neuron lesion, on the other hand, often involves a disruption of the reflex arc at the level of the spinal cord; in this case the paralysis of the muscles is a flaccid (flabby) one. The specific interference with muscle function helps to pinpoint the site of the lesion. The accurate observations of the patient can contribute important information to the physician because they help him to localize the lesion. Such observations also influence nursing care, not only by a determination of the patient's general needs, but also by awareness of special dimensions of care necessitated by loss of sensory abilities.

Nervous system integration affects the organism in all of its activities, so it is not surprising that the protective devices that insure its continuous function are, in a sense, ruthless ones. The brain tissue has priority over every other tissue in the body for the continuing supply of oxygen and nutrients. And it is significant that the *only* tissue in the body which is not under nervous control is the cerebral tissue. The oxygen supply to the brain is so vital that the regulatory mechanism that maintains it is one that reacts to the oxygen supply itself. This feedback mechanism, or autoregulation, responds promptly to minute variations in the carbon dioxide blood levels in its own vessels. An excess of carbon dioxide results in a prompt vasodilatation of the cerebral vessels to insure a faster flow of blood to the brain. The brain tissue is very responsive to alteration in the carbon dioxide blood level: for instance, breathing air with a concentration of carbon dioxide of only 6% increases the cerebral blood flow by almost 75%.

It is remarkable how consistently the rate of metabolism, and therefore the oxygen utilization of the brain, remains at the same level, even under widely varying conditions. Approximately 3.5 ml. of oxygen per 100 gm. of brain tissue is supplied per minute by this mechanism during sleep, muscular activity, or even intense mental activity. Quite obviously, successful oxygenation of the brain is closely tied to its vascularization: the vessels must be patent. Furthermore, the anatomical configuration of the cerebral vessels is such as to allow for shunting into collateral vessels when there is interference in a cerebral vessel. The two major arterial channels to the brain are the carotid circulation and the basilar-vertebral circulation, and they form the circle of Willis at the base of the brain. Theoretically, this allows for shunting when occlusion occurs in one or the other, but one researcher has found that the circle of Willis is anomalous in 47% of the human population, and to such a degree that its ability to shunt the circulation is deficient or totally lacking.

Nevertheless, the brain will receive its oxygen supply at the expense of every other tissue in the body, a priority in nature that emphasizes the integrative function of this tissue. The cerebral tissues, both the brain and the spinal cord, are the only tissues in the body (with the single exception of the bone marrow—and this has biological wisdom too) that are entirely enclosed in bony cages. Although they are actually floating gently in a fluid medium that absorbs the shock of the body's movements, the bony structure of the skull and the vertebral column create an extremely limiting environment for these tissues. Any factor which tends to cause swelling in the tissues within their bony cage creates grave danger to their well-being, because the bone restricts the increase in size that occurs when a tissue becomes swollen, and this, in turn, sends the pressure back upon the affected tissues.

In spite of its tremendous importance to the living organism, however, cell division in the central nervous system ceases entirely shortly after birth. This means that all of the individual cellular units of the nervous system—the neurons—that the adult will ever have are present when he is born. Individual cells will continue to grow and enlarge until puberty, but once a nerve cell is destroyed, it cannot be replaced by a new one. The normal attrition, or death of nerve cells throughout life, accounts for many of the changes that accompany aging. The older individual has fewer nerve cells, and thus his reaction time is slowed, his eyesight and hearing may fail somewhat, and, in general, many body activities function at a lower level of efficiency.

The urgency of maintaining the viability of cerebral tissue is actually measured in minutes, for the brain can withstand an oxygen deficiency for only three to five minutes before irreparable damage occurs to neurons. Once the cell has died, it can never be restored. Therefore, any factor whatsoever that limits oxygen supply, either to the organism as a whole or to the nervous system tissues specifically, must be removed within three to five minutes, or the permanent destruction of cells takes place, and the individual's ability to function is lost.

The unification of body activity mediated by the nervous system is reflected in the integrated function of the system itself. No part of the central nervous system can function independently. The nerve processes constitute the communicating pathways from one portion of the nervous system to the next, and any interference along those channels prevents the passage of the message beyond the point of injury. Experience indicates that there can be, to a degree, a substitution of activity in the cortex, which is the highest center of all. Some kinds of loss, in fact, can be compensated for by relearning. But this is by no means generally true.

Some types of environmental stimuli pose immediate and grave danger to the individual so that there must be a means of response that is equally rapid. Such a rapid and almost instantaneous reaction is characteristic of the reflex arc. The reflex is a relatively fixed pattern of nerve response, resulting in behavior that is similar, regardless of the stimulus. Stepping on a sharp object causes the individual to immediately withdraw his foot. The withdrawal response is a reflex one and happens with great rapidity. The sensation of pain, however, even though it seems to be a simultaneous event, actually occurs more slowly. The pain is not the cause of the reflex removal of the foot, but the interpretation placed upon the experience by the higher centers. Even this apparently simple activity is a complex one, however. One foot cannot be withdrawn unless there is a simultaneous readjustment of the body weight onto the other foot so that the individual does not fall down. There are, then, both an excitation, resulting in the removal of one foot, and an inhibition, resulting in a shifting of body weight to the other foot, in this relatively simple behavior. Excitation and inhibition are interacting phenomena, so that there are opposing forces operating on the same muscle groups which allow muscles to relax or contract in accordance with a necessary body movement. The constant readiness of the organism to move through its environment is a result of the coordinated activity of its nervous system. The reflex arc, which bypasses the organizer and sends an automatic response from the level of the spinal cord, assures quick movement. But the nervous system as a whole provides the means for ascertaining the characteristics of the environment and equips the individual with the means to make decisions as to how he can best promote his own safety and comfort.

The Autonomic Nervous System

Most of the activity of the central nervous system is designed to promote the organism's safety in its environment, and therefore it is largely concerned with skeletal-muscle innervation. The total function of the body would, however, be poorly served if the individual had an equal degree of choice in the performance of many life-sustaining activities. Heart and respiratory action, metabolic control, and all of the essential activities that maintain the internal environment are beyond conscious control. The autonomic (*auto,* self; *nomos,* law) nervous system regulates internal homeostasis, but it does so often in direct response to stimuli from the external environment. The efferent fibers that are part of the central nervous system travel directly from the spinal cord to their destination in the effector tissue. However, some efferent fibers do not directly innervate the effector tissue. Instead they pass, at some point in their course, through a *ganglion,* or a collection of neurons found outside of the central nervous system.

The ganglion, composed of many neurons, alters the impulse that passes into it, because the single impulse activates *many* cells. If only one cell is activated, the stimulus is very direct and precise, whereas, if many cells are activated at once, the impulse is diffused, spread, and shared, its effect being therefore multiplied in direct proportion to the number of cells activated. In this sense, a ganglion becomes an *amplifier,* remarkably increasing the effect of the single impulse which entered it. All of the efferent fibers of the autonomic nervous system enter a ganglion, but the point at which this amplification occurs has a remarkable influence on how the tissues respond.

The fibers of the autonomic nervous system that arise from the thoracic and lumbar segments of the spinal cord enter a ganglion immediately after they leave the spinal cord. Many fibers then leave the ganglion to go to the organs innervated. Therefore, the thoracolumbar autonomic nerves have very short preganglionic fibers and very long postganglionic fibers. But, even more important, the passage immediately into the ganglion means that the impulse is immediately amplified; thus, it is not strange that the thoracolumbar division of the autonomic nervous system produces

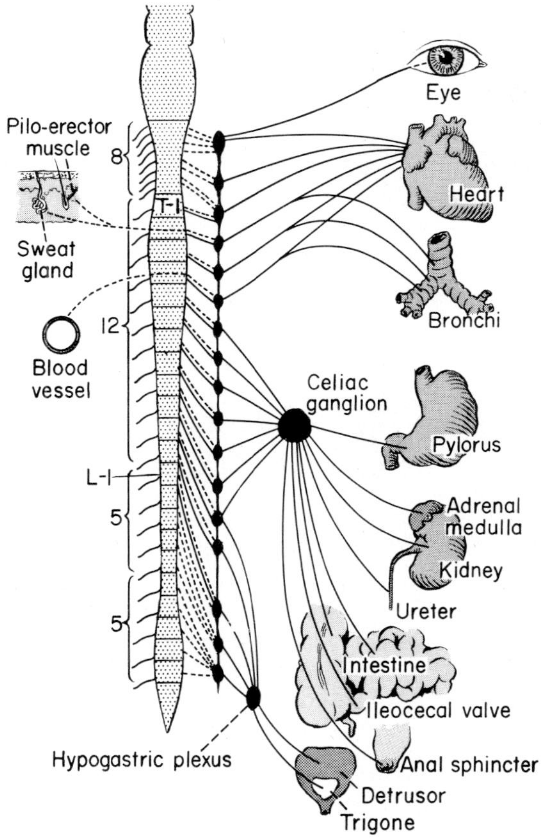

FIGURE 12. The sympathetic (thoracolumbar) nervous system. The "fight or flight" response of the entire organism is aroused by stimulation of this portion of the autonomic nervous system. (From Guyton, A.C.: *Textbook of Medical Physiology*, 3rd ed. W.B. Saunders Co., Philadelphia, 1966.)

a simultaneous response in many tissues and organs in a diffuse but coordinated way. The thoracolumbar nerves are often called the sympathetic nervous system, and it is this system that is capable of creating a widespread response of many organs to a single stimulus. Stimulation of the sympathetic nervous system, in fact, produces an organismic response called the "fight or flight" reaction. To enable the individual either to protect himself from immediate danger or to escape from it, the sympathetic reaction causes an increased rate and output of the heart, and an increased respiratory rate. The pupil of the eye becomes dilated because of lessened tone in the ciliary muscle, and this increases the ability of the eye to accommodate to distance. Although there are increases in mental alertness and in perspiration, there is a decrease in gastrointestinal motility and constriction of the gastrointestinal sphincters, since the individual on the verge of fight or flight does not need digestive function. The entire reaction is a physiological panic reaction. It must be emphasized that this is an involuntary reaction. Even though modern man only rarely finds it necessary to fight or flee, the panic reaction of sympathetic stimulation is still with him. All kinds of threats can elicit the response, and sometimes the threats need only be imagined, but the physiological reaction will occur whether the danger is real or not.

Other fibers of the autonomic nervous system arise in the cranial and sacral segments of the spinal cord. The cranial-sacral division is also

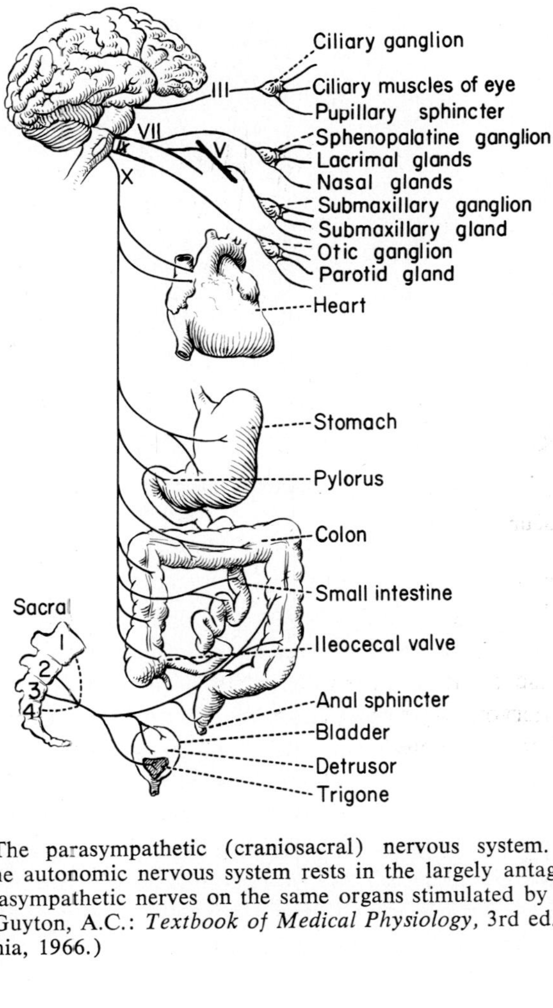

FIGURE 13. The parasympathetic (craniosacral) nervous system. The "control" exercised by the autonomic nervous system rests in the largely antagonistic innervation of the parasympathetic nerves on the same organs stimulated by the sympathetic fibers. (From Guyton, A.C.: *Textbook of Medical Physiology,* 3rd ed. W.B. Saunders Co., Philadelphia, 1966.)

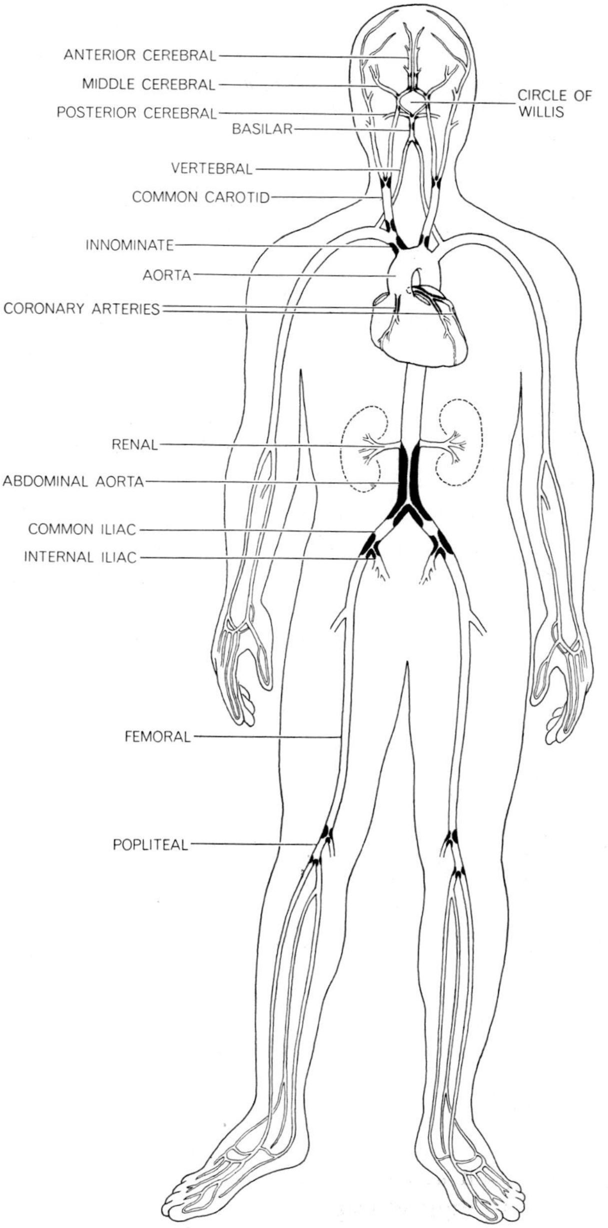

FIGURE 14. Atherosclerotic vessel changes tend to favor sites where the arteries branch. Vessel changes or blood clots obstructing the vessels to the head cause cerebral vascular accidents or "strokes." (From Spain, D.: "Atherosclerosis." Copyright© 1966 by *Scientific American, Inc.* All rights reserved.)

called the parasympathetic nervous system. The fibers of the cranial-sacral division also enter ganglia, but not until the fiber itself has reached the effector organ. The ganglia of this portion of the autonomic nervous system are, in fact, often imbedded in the effector organ itself. The parasympathetic fibers have long preganglionic fibers and short postganglionic fibers. Stimulation of the parasympathetic nerves, therefore, produces a discrete and definitive stimulation of a specific organ.

The discrete and precise effect of the parasympathetic nerves provides for homeostatic control in vital organs because their influence on the organs is generally antagonistic to that of the sympathetic nerves. Therefore, the parasympathetic innervation is capable of slowing the heart rate and thus decreasing cardiac output. These nerves constrict the bronchi, increase gastrointestinal motility, and relax the sphincters of the gastrointestinal tract. They constrict the pupil of the eye and thus enhance near vision by causing a contraction of the ciliary muscle. The opposing influence of the two portions of the autonomic nervous system serves to keep the organs at a level of activity within the homeostatic range or to maintain a "tonus" that predisposes to readiness to respond to many influences but well within physiological limits of safety.

The Pathophysiology of Cerebral Vascular Insult

An intact and functional nervous system is essential in an alert and perceiving individual. Any loss of conscious awareness, that is, any degree of loss from transient dizziness to complete unconsciousness, indicates nervous system interference. The loss of contact with the environment that accompanies cerebral insult, regardless of its cause, immediately prescribes a variety of nursing responsibilities, some of which may be of an extremely urgent nature. Whenever an individual is unable to respond to his external environment, the nurse anticipates and responds for him.

Although many episodes of loss of consciousness are transient with complete recovery afterwards, some are indicative of a serious and lasting alteration in the economy of the nervous system structure and function. The significance of the serious syndromes affecting the nervous system is reflected in the tremendous social and economic issues created by an elderly population in whom the incidence of "strokes" is high. A concerted research and treatment program at the federal government level is testimony to recognition of the widespread tragedy and dislocation that result from insult to the cerebral tissues.

The most common cause of cerebral accidents is an interference with the circulation of blood to the brain. Interference with the supply of oxygen and nutrients to even a portion of the cerebral tissues creates an im-

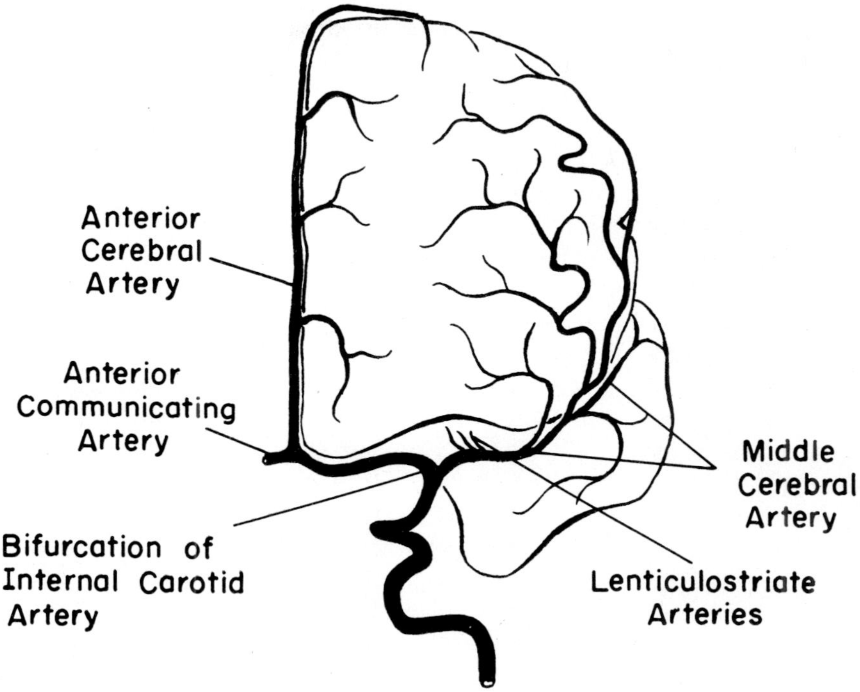

FIGURE 15. Anterior view of the anterior and middle cerebral arteries of the left hemisphere of the brain. (From Gatz, A.J.: *Manter's Essentials of Clinical Neuroanatomy and Neurophysiology,* 3rd ed. F.A. Davis Co., Philadelphia, 1966.)

mediate threat that some of the cells will die and with them the abilities of the individual to perform the activities that these cells direct. Almost all of the information that describes how body function is related to specific areas of the brain has come from pathological changes in the brain. Observation of the loss of functional capacity related to specific areas of brain damage has, over the years, allowed the functional areas of the brain to be mapped. Thus it is often possible to pinpoint the area of destruction by an accurate description of the loss of function in the individual. This is an essential nursing function, and one which contributes in a substantial way to the physician's assessment of the damage and to his therapeutic plan.

There are, of course, several ways in which circulation to the cerebral tissues can be compromised. Most commonly, a small blood clot floating in the circulation finally reaches a vessel that is too small for it to traverse. This is called an *embolus,* and once it becomes lodged in a vessel all of the channel past the clot becomes useless; no blood can flow past the occlusion. Occlusion can also result when there is a build-up of material in the wall of the vessel, gradually making the opening smaller and smaller, and finally closing it off so that no blood can flow past that point. This is called a *thrombus*. Sometimes circulatory interference may result because a small vessel in the brain ruptures, and the resultant hemorrhaging creates a local area of pressure that successfully prevents the flow of blood in the region of the hemorrhage. An infection, with the swelling that accompanies it, may also be responsible for developing pressure that prevents the distention of vessels with blood.

Regardless of the initiating cause, the result is an interference with the oxygenation of brain tissue, and this is clinically evident as a loss of function in some degree by the individual suffering the insult. The most apparent symptom, following the loss of consciousness, is a skeletal-muscular disability: parts of the body become partially or totally paralyzed. The paralysis characteristically involves one half of the body; when it does so, it is called hemiplegia. The affected half of the body is usually the side *opposite* the affected portion of the brain, because many of the motor nerves from the brain lie within the pyramidal tract, and this collection of fibers crosses over from one hemisphere to the other at the midbrain. A cerebral accident on the left side of the brain thus causes right-sided paralysis, whereas a right-sided injury to the brain results in a left-sided paralysis. The significance of the paralyzed side to the individual, while always disastrous, may be enhanced if the affected side is also the dominant side. A right-handed individual will be more severely handicapped if the hemiplegia is also on the right side. In addition, the cerebral centers which control speech and language abilities, in general, seem to be in the left hemisphere, so that a right-sided hemiplegia is often accompanied by severe speech impairment. It must be emphasized that there is no single "speech center" but several areas, probably in both hemispheres, that together make it possible for an individual to use language as communication. The common act of speaking and understanding the spoken word—or the written word, for that matter—results from the coordinated efforts of many cerebral areas. Loss of the ability to speak is called aphasia, and it is a frequent symptom of cerebral vascular injury.

When the individual has a paralysis of one side of the body, all of the muscle groups on that side are affected. The arm and leg are obviously useless, but in addition there may be a noticeable sagging of facial muscles, along with a muscular failure that seriously interferes with swallowing, breathing, and speaking. Interference with the thoracic muscles involved in respiratory movement may create serious problems that involve all of the body's vital functions. And frequently the voluntary control of elimination is affected as well.

The loss of motor abilities, while easily apparent in most individuals, is only a portion of the effects of cerebral injury. There is often a concurrent loss of sensory abilities. The individual loses the ability to *feel* and respond to heat and cold. There may even be a loss of the important sensory function of recognizing pain. Attending the sensory impairment, there is an inevitable proprioceptive loss. The individual can no longer be aware of his position in space. The affected limbs send him no messages that record their presence, and the very essential perceptual awareness of "body image" is thereby destroyed.

The most severe kinds of cerebral injury involve vital centers in the brain that control respiration, cardiac action, and metabolic effectiveness. Such damage, of course, creates immediate emergency demands which are life-threatening. In clinical areas, all degrees of disability are seen in individuals who are victims of a cerebral vascular accident. In each instance, assessment of that individual's status will determine the nature of the nursing care he must receive.

Establishing Priorities of Care

Survival Needs

The old rule of "first things first" has special meaning in the planning of nursing care. Some patient needs are of such vital urgency that they take immediate precedence over all other obligations. These demands are aptly described as "survival needs," because meeting them promptly and correctly determines whether or not the patient will survive the danger in which they place him.

Survival needs are *physiologically determined.* They reflect priorities in the body's economy with which there can be little tampering or temporizing. There is a distinct time limit in the ability of the human body to withstand an oxygen deficit. That time limit is established physiologically by the limited tolerance of nerve tissue to hypoxia. Within 3 to 5 minutes, irreversible damage to brain tissue occurs in a limited oxygen environment, and therefore 3 to 5 minutes is the time span within which corrective measures must become effective. This accounts for the extreme emergency which everyone recognizes in the individual who is drowning or in danger of smoke or gas inhalation. The same aura of decisive, swift action exists when, for any reason, the individual is threatened with interference with his respiratory exchange. Nursing responsibility to maintain a clear and patent airway is a first priority which can never be compromised in any way. Often such responsibility includes anticipation of the possibility that interference may occur, and therefore it is prophylactic as well as therapeutic. Keeping the airway free of mechanical obstruction, including the patient's own secretions as well as oral foods and fluids, is relatively simple in the alert and conscious individual. He can muster his own defense. But whenever there is interference with the person's ability to keep his own airway clear, the nurse assumes the responsibility of doing it for him. This may be as simple as positioning him in bed so that his airway remains patent, or it may be as complex as removing the offending secretions by mechanical means such as suctioning; in severe instances, it also involves the administration of oxygen. The maintenance of a patent airway is a frequent and serious problem in the nursing care of a patient who has sustained a cerebral vascular insult. It is equally urgent, of course, in the care of any patient who is stuporous or unconscious from any cause whatsoever.

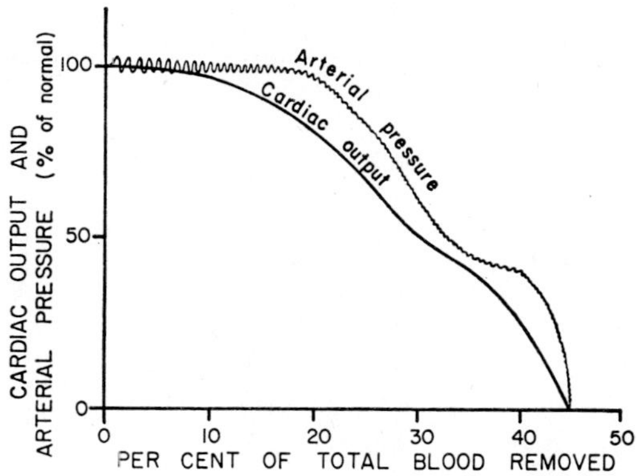

FIGURE 16. The effect of hemorrhage on cardiac output and arterial pressure. Quick intervention to prevent continuing blood loss is urgent. (From Guyton, A.C.: *Textbook of Medical Physiology,* 3rd ed. W.B. Saunders Co., Philadelphia, 1966.)

The danger of blood loss through disruption of the intact circulatory system is a survival threat often equal in urgency to maintenance of a patent airway. The blood circulates through the closed system under pressure, and the loss of a substantial volume of blood through hemorrhaging causes a loss of pressure in the system, which threatens the viability of all body tissues. An episode of acute bleeding must be met by urgent measures that include the closing of the vessel, if possible, and the immediate replacement of the blood that is lost. Hemorrhaging into the cerebrum is usually restricted by the limit placed on the cerebral tissues by the skull, but sufficient blood loss results in pressure on the vital centers, which quickly results in death. It is not, of course, possible to stop intracranial bleeding unless it is very slow, and even then it is a very difficult task.

The next physiological priority is the maintenance of an adequate fluid and electrolyte balance. The time limit is not a matter of minutes, but it may well be a matter of hours, and adjustments of the homeostatic range do not take place as rapidly as in the re-establishment of oxygen transport. All of the vital cellular activites that are summarized as "metabolism" take place in an aqueous solution characterized by very specific concentrations of vital substances. Metabolic disturbances resulting from many disease processes, and, indeed, from fluid deprivation alone, create dangerous imbalances in vital electrolyte levels. Alterations in the blood level within a very finite range may result not only in death of cells, but also in a failure of essential cells—specifically nerve cells—to continue to function at all. It is the nurse's responsibility to make certain that fluid intake is adequate when the patient is unable to do this for himself. The patient who has had a cerebral insult may be unable to perform even the simple act of reaching for a glass of water, and if, in addition, he has lost his ability to speak, he will not be able to ask for it. Fluid and electrolyte intake may be maintained by the administration of fluids intravenously, but whatever the route of administration, the nurse keeps a careful record of fluid intake and output so that adequate amounts can be prescribed by the physician.

The body's needs for nutrients do not cease when illness strikes, and in fact, may increase because of the efforts directed at eliminating the disease. While nutritional deficiencies create serious problems only over a relatively long period of time, they may considerably interfere with recovery unless they are recognized and treated. The body still requires materials for energy and repair, and illness is hardly an excuse to allow starvation. It is often necessary to delay oral feedings during the critical period, and the cerebral vascular accident patient may have difficulty in masticating and swallowing for a long time after the acute symptoms are relieved. Every effort to facilitate feeding must be made as soon as the patient is able to accept food. The additional problem of anorexia, or loss of appetite, may make this a very difficult nursing problem.

The partially paralyzed, handicapped, or unconscious patient depends on nursing care to protect him from the ordinary and extraordinary hazards that exist in his environment. This may be as simple as preventing the possibility that he will fall out of bed, or as complex as preventing cross-contamination with pathogenic organisms in the hospital environment. The responsibility for physical safety, and with it the well-being, of the unconscious patient is entirely vested in the nurse. The cerebral vascular accident patient, unable to move freely by himself, is subject to all the hazards of immobilization, and almost all of these are preventable by excellent nursing care.

Survival needs may arise in any disease process. Attention to these takes precedence over all other activities. There are many other facets of care, especially for the bedridden patient, but nothing demands more immediate and dedicated effort than the appearance of these life-threatening possibilities. Because of the dramatic limitation in time, the patent airway usually elicits prompt action on the part of the hospital staff. Time is, however, a compelling determinant in establishing and maintaining fluid and electrolyte balance and nutritional adequacy. Too frequently, the urgency of the patient's safety is overlooked until an accident has occurred, but additional injury superimposed on an already serious situation is as threatening to the patient as interference with his respiratory function. The sick individual assigns his welfare to the judgement and consideration of others, and recognizing the potential danger he faces when his survival is threatened is a test of the professional competence of the nurse.

Daily Nursing Care as Rehabilitation

Although rehabilitation nursing is often studied as a separate discipline, in a real sense all nursing care is rehabilitative in intent. The recuperative and reparative processes that characterize recovery from an episode of illness are, in fact, rehabilitative processes. It has become increasingly evident that many of the disabilities which finally require the specialized services of rehabilitation experts are a result of the failure of hospital nurses to prevent such disabilities. In the daily care of patients, the nurse has many opportunities to prevent the development of disabilities, combined with a positive obligation to assist the patient throughout the course of his disease to renewed health and well-being. Some of the most difficult disabilities to treat are the easiest to prevent.

The human organism was designed to remain mobile. It is a fundamental physiological fact that disuse leads to disaster. The unused muscles shrivel and atrophy. The unused joint becomes stiff and immoveable. The incompletely expanded lung loses its ability to expand, and the space is quickly usurped by fluid. Even lack of social interaction ultimately produces an individual so deprived that he is unable to respond to the reality that surrounds him. Bed rest alone is one of the most dangerous hazards that confronts the sick person. Even the biochemistry of the body is altered when immobilization is prolonged. Calcium tends to leave the bones, so that they are increasingly susceptible to fracture. And perfectly normal individuals who are placed on bed rest will demonstrate within three days a marked change in their nitrogen, and therefore their protein, balance. Thus, physical and psychological damage is an ever-present threat when disease creates a need for bed rest. Increasingly, the patient is mobilized as soon as possible. This move towards early ambulation has made surgical procedures of all kinds vastly less hazardous than they were when rest in bed was enforced for long periods of time. This trend is equally apparent in the care of nonsurgical patients. And during those periods of time when the patient's condition absolutely demands that he remain in bed, mobilizing him and thus conserving for him his structural integrity become the nurse's responsibility.

The first rule in the care of the bedridden patient is to change his position as often as he can tolerate it, and certainly every two hours unless there are cogent contraindications. This provides for the use of muscle groups and joints, even if such usage is passive; that is, the actual moving of the patient is accomplished by others without his active participation. Changing position insures that the pressure of his own body weight will not remain on one point of his body surface for an extended period of time. This is particularly important in protection of the bony prominences of the body, and therefore becomes a matter of emphasis in the individual who has little protection from body substance over the bony points of his body. When prolonged pressure is prevented, circulation to the part is improved, and the danger that pressure will interfere with circulation, thus causing death of the tissues at that site, can be prevented. However, changing of position without equal consideration to body posture in the intervals is a fruitless effort. Positioning the individual in bed is guided by three major determinants: anatomical integrity, physiological function at optimal levels possible, and psychosocial requirements of the individual.

Anatomical positioning is guided by the skeletal-muscle structure, and often influenced by the individual patient's specific needs in this area. The individual who can move freely in bed can maintain anatomical positioning, and, in fact, tends to do so. He seldom will lie in one position for very long, and when he settles himself into a position, it will not be one that compromises his comfort. But the individual who can move only with difficulty, because he is weak, or perhaps because he is in pain, may not assume a posture in bed that conserves his anatomical function. And, of course, the partially paralyzed patient is totally incapable of adjusting his own posture without assistance. Such postural conservation includes the position of the feet in relation to the lower leg, for example. The foot tends to drop forward with the patient in a supine position, and this in turn places a stretch on the Achilles tendon. Over a period of time, the foot that is allowed to remain in a dropped position becomes permanently dropped, and extensive rehabilitation and physical therapy may not be able to restore it to a functional posture. The same stretching of the tendons may occur at the wrist unless the hand is properly supported. Sometimes lying on a pillow without shoulder support will result in a separation at the shoulder joint which is painful and difficult to correct.

There are simple nursing measures available to prevent these deformities altogether. A footboard, for example, against which the patient may push his feet will absolutely prevent foot-drop. Of course, placing the board is useless unless the patient is instructed or assisted in its proper use. In addition, a tightly made bed over the patient's feet may appear lovely to the admiring nurse, but it creates a hazard to the patient which hardly warrants such practice. Parenthetically, it is important that the patient's bed be made to allow him comfort and safety. If the end result is less than perfect to the eye, then the patient's interests have probably been held paramount.

Positioning the bed patient to enhance physiological function includes consideration of circulatory effectiveness, respiratory excursion, and the performance of essential body activities, such as elimination. The circulation to the periphery of the body is normally dependent upon the squeezing action of the skeletal muscles. Changing of position requires muscular movement by the patient and thus contributes to his circulatory effectiveness. Pressure sores, or decubitus ulcers, arise when circulation to a part of the body is restricted by pressure of the patient's body weight. Frequent position change can often prevent their appearance. Positioning alone will often assist the patient to maintain a patent airway, as well as permit a free and comfortable expansion of his thoracic cage. Positioning is important when he is ingesting food or fluids and extremely important in the prevention of the aspiration of oral food or fluids as well as his own respiratory excretions. Positioning may become a major issue when the patient must urinate, and particularly for the male patient who has performed this activity all his life in a standing position. The use of the bedpan strikes dread in the hearts of many patients, but they may be positioned so that its use is quite easy. The physiology of the defecation act is based on a squatting posture; if the patient can be assisted to assume a posture similar to this, he may find the use of the hated utensil relatively comfortable. It is always important that the body be properly supported in bed, but the use of under-knee rolls should be discouraged because it further limits the free movement of blood in the venous system of the legs and may hasten the development of thrombi in the leg circulation.

Both anatomical and physiological determinants of position in bed include alterations in posture from side to side, from supine to prone, if there are no contraindications. The use of the head rest in various angles may also provide much comfort to the patient. Except for the very sick patient, positioning also must consider the effect of the patient's position on his ability to socialize with others. The absolutely supine position is one of utter helplessness and defeat. It is nearly impossible to establish the facets of normal interaction with others from this position. The faces of those standing at the bedside are distorted, and the very essential exchange of eye movements is virtually impossible. Unless specifically contraindicated, the head should be elevated enough to allow the individual to make face-to-face contact with other persons. As his convalescence progresses, positioning him so that he can become involved in unfettered social interaction is an essential part of his care.

During the daily care of the patient, and particularly when he is being bathed, mobilization is a major activity. During the bath, all of his joints can be carried through their normal range of motion, with the nurse's help if necessary. When the physician has agreed to it, passive and active exercises may be started. Several isometric exercises require very little energy expenditure by the patient, but are useful in sustaining muscle tone and circulatory efficiency. The nurse must approach every patient with the conscious plan for mobilizing him as much as his condition will allow. Most patients greet the order to leave their beds with joy, even though the effort may be a difficult one. When the patient is ordered out of bed, into a wheel chair, or to begin ambulation, the faithful performance of these mobilizations as often as they are ordered will speed his return to renewed strength. A failure to mobilize him as directed by his physician prolongs his hospitalization and slows his period of recovery. Postural disabilities arising from inadequate nursing care are trophicogenic diseases, i.e., diseases that are nurse-induced. Without prolonging the time required for daily care, trophicogenic disease can and MUST be absolutely eliminated.

Care of the Cerebral Vascular Patient

The Conservation of Energy

There are few clinical entities in which the importance of nursing care as an aspect of the total therapeutic regime is more compelling than in the care of a patient who has had a cerebral vascular accident. In the early hours immediately following the moment of insult, care is often directed at survival needs. Even though the presenting signs and symptoms may be very mild or very severe, the incident itself is a signal of grave potential danger to the individual. Conservation of his energy at this stage of his illness has a two-fold purpose. His entire energy exchange must be allowed to defend him from the dire possibilities of inadequate oxygenation of brain tissue. The limitation of activity that accompanies bed rest in a quiet environment serves to conserve the available oxygen supply so that a maximum concentration can be delivered to the vital tissue. In addition, the immediate period following the injury is a time when assessment of the damage must be made by the physician. Observation of the patient by the nurse constitutes a major contribution to his future welfare. When the insult has been severe, there may be little time for quiet inspection of the patient's needs because all of the therapeutic effort must be directed towards his survival. The period of unconsciousness that usually accompanies the early hours of a cerebral vascular incident is, in itself, an energy-conserving defense by the body. In the supine position, the blood flow to the cerebrum is enhanced, and the work that the heart must perform against gravity in forcing the blood through the circulation is greatly lessened. During the time in which the patient is totally unconscious, all nursing activities are designed to maintain his safety by responding *for* him in the external environment. All of his energy production mechanisms must be focused on survival, and the struggle is dramatized by the urgent demand of the embarrassed cerebral tissue for adequate oxygenation. The therapeutic measures that insure a patent airway and adequate oxygenation serve to create optimal conditions for accomplishing this necessary physiological level. In addition, the maintenance of fluid and electrolyte balance also contributes to nervous system function, and, by stabilizing the internal environment, conserves energy needed to struggle for survival.

The return of consciousness, usually within 72 hours, is frequently accompanied by a radical alteration in the individual's ability to perceive and assess his relationship to his environment. There is often a period of confusion and disorientation, but it must be remembered that the injury to cerebral tissue may, in itself, result in a change in the way in which the individual perceives himself. It is often difficult to determine the precise difference between utter confusion and an altered perception. The moment of insult often comes suddenly, and the awakening from the unconscious state, often accompanied by partial paralysis and sensory aberration in the affected tissues, is an extremely difficult change to understand. His confusion as to where he is and how he got there precedes a gradual awareness of what has happened to him. If cerebral damage has been extensive, it may take many days to help him understand what has happened, and the possibility exists that this may never be entirely accomplished. Frequently, the response to these unanswered, and sometimes unanswerable, questions is a restlessness and irritability that sap the individual of energy he needs for vital processes. If, in addition, there is some loss of speech ability, the communication with the individual that can reassure and calm him may be virtually impossible.

During the convalescent period, the energy conservation is clearly designed to permit the wise expenditure of energy and not to minimize it altogether. The aftermath of a cerebral vascular accident that includes the loss of motor and sensory function in one half of the body creates a

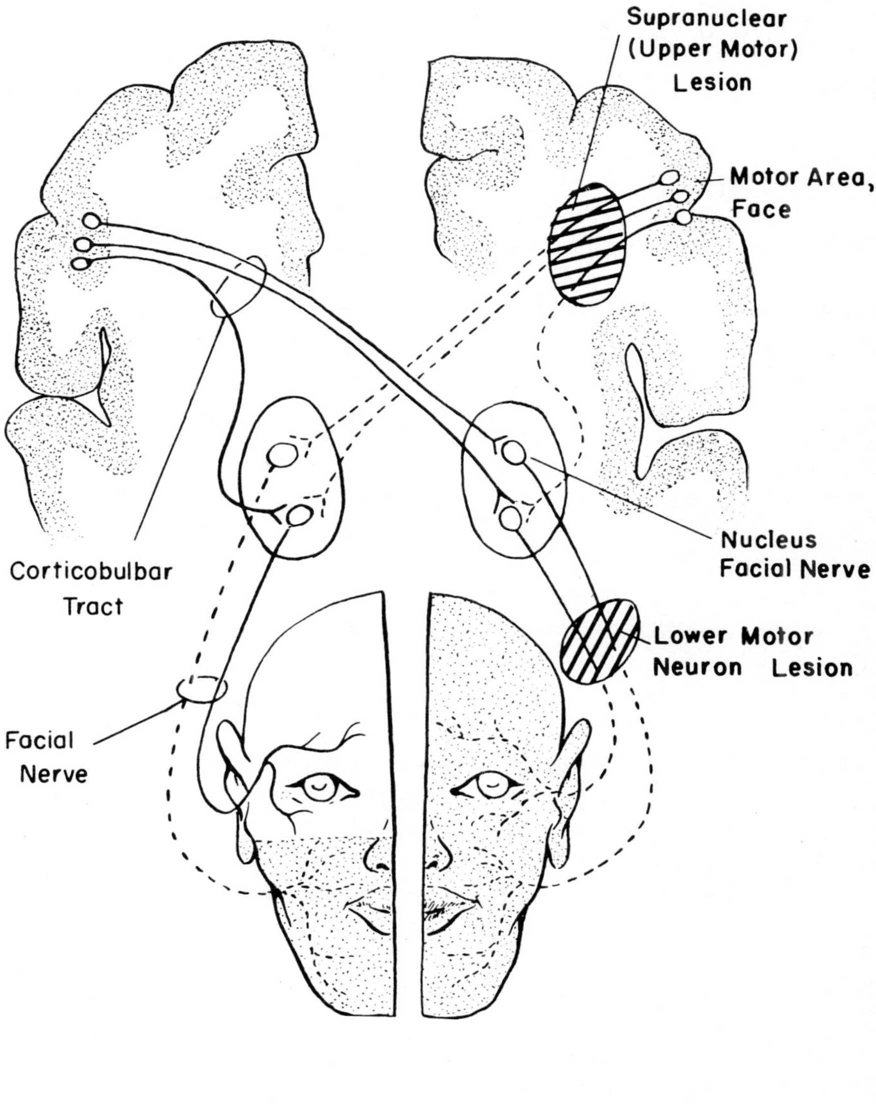

FIGURE 17. A weakness or paralysis of the facial muscles interferes with the individual's ability to chew and swallow his food. Injury to the nervous system involving either an upper or lower motor neuron involves facial innervation. (From Gatz, A.J.: *Manter's Essentials of Clinical Neuroanatomy and Neurophysiology*, 3rd ed. F.A. Davis Co., Philadelphia, 1966.)

decided need to mobilize and ambulate the individual as soon as his condition will permit it. The "keeping-together" function, which is inherent in conservation, is nowhere more apparent or important than in the care of the patient who has had a cerebral accident. The entire pattern of the individual's future life rests in the restoration of function, or, failing that, in the conservation of muscle tone and limb position that will allow function in the future. As soon as his condition permits, the nurse institutes passive range of motion to prevent the loss of further skeletal-muscle action, and subsequently the patient is given physical therapy where he assumes the responsibility for active exercise.

Energy is produced through the metabolic pathways of the body, and they must be supplied with the nutrients necessary for this process. Unless these nutrients are supplied, the body will use its own substance to maintain an energy production level. Even in the aging individual, the supply of proteins to encourage healing is necessary, as well as an adequate source of essentially energy-producing foods, such as carbohydrates. The dietary preferences in older individuals may make it difficult to insure an adequate diet, and if, in addition, there is difficulty in swallowing food because of weakness or paralysis of facial and throat muscles, the issue of nutrition may be a considerable one. The preparation of foods that can be handled by the hemiplegic patient may require considerable attention. And, of course, if the individual is not able to feed himself, his nutritional needs can only be met by careful feeding.

The difficulty of assessing energy utilization is marked when the patient is hemiplegic. The inability to move half of the body makes movement of the functional half more energy-consuming. The individual can be taught to use leverage systems that will minimize the effort required in moving his paralyzed side. The transfer techniques that are part of the rehabilitation procedures are designed to permit safe movement of the individual utilizing leverage systems that will not exhaust him. During the early weeks following a cerebral vascular accident, the patient tires easily, and often, because he is unable to clearly communicate this to the nurse, observation becomes very important in determining his care. The success of finally learning to mobilize himself, even with a one-sided paralysis, depends on his strength, and it is very important that he not become so exhausted with early efforts that he is discouraged. Fatigue can be minimized if his resources are carefully managed, and this is the essential goal of energy conservation.

The Conservation of Structural Integrity

It is often a matter of days or weeks before it is possible to determine what the individual's potential for recovery may be. Nursing care alone, as

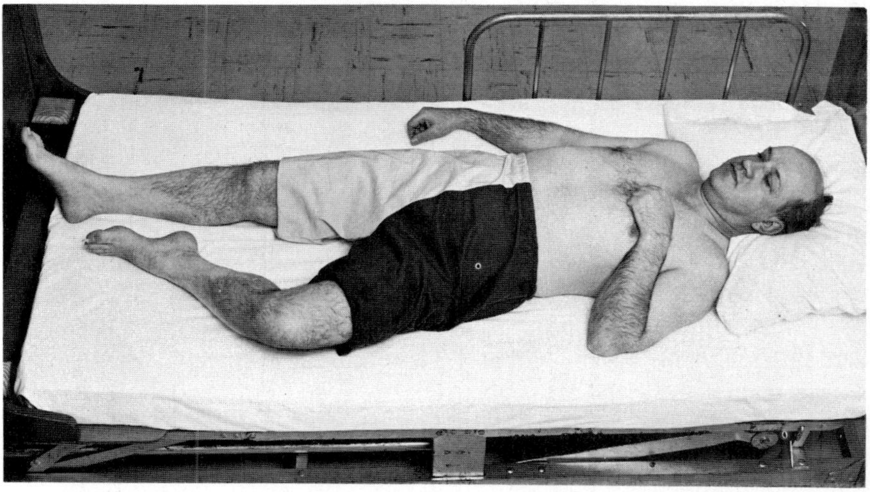

FIGURE 18. The afflicted side of the body, here represented by the dark half of the clothing, responds to the unopposed effect of the reflexes, resulting in "non-functional" positions which leave the cerebral vascular accident victim helplessly crippled unless vigorous nursing care is instituted. (From *A Handbook of Rehabilitative Nursing Techniques in Hemiplegia.* ©American Rehabilitation Foundation, Minneapolis, 1964.)

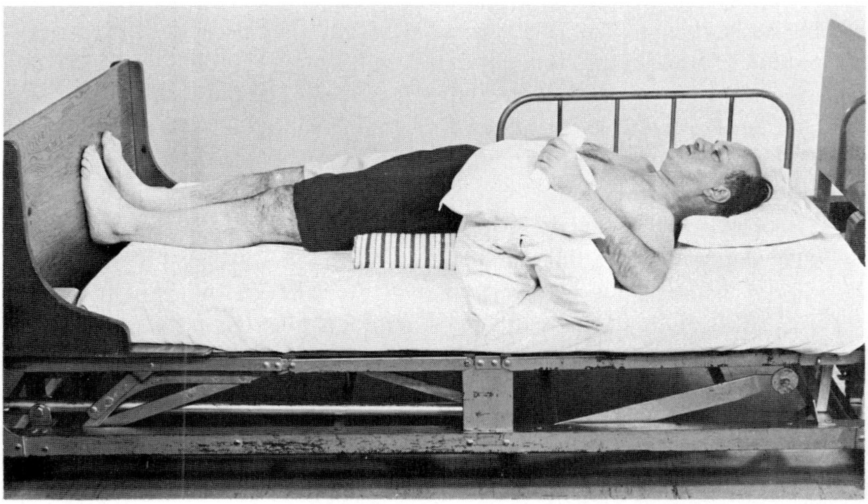

FIGURE 19. Correct anatomical positioning of the cerebral vascular accident patient in the supine position prevents the development of freezing contractures which will limit his rehabilitative potential. The afflicted side is represented by the black half of the subject's clothing. All limbs are supported in a functional position. (From *A Handbook of Rehabilitative Nursing Techniques in Hemiplegia.* ©American Rehabilitation Foundation, Minneapolis, 1964.)

in every disease process, cannot alter an outcome that is determined by the pathology itself. If the cerebral injury results in a residual paralysis, no amount of nursing care can restore the individual to his pre-insult condition. But nursing care CAN elicit the maximum use left to the patient. There are few nursing situations in which the importance of structural integrity has more importance. In the early stages following cerebral insult, the affected limbs hang heavy and limp with an initial flaccid paralysis that emphasizes the effect of gravity on body posture. Lying in bed, the paralyzed leg rotates away from the midline, its own weight responding to gravity. However, within 72 hours the soft, flabby muscles begin to harden and contract. Although the motor fibers from the cerebrum have been rendered useless, those which "oppose" them, arising in the spinal cord, have not. Gradually, the spinal reflex fibers take over, and without opposition from the cerebral innervation, they cause an increasing spasticity in the affected muscles. The unopposed contraction of the muscles shortens them; as they shorten, they alter the position of the limbs by pulling on the joints. To accommodate the shortened musculature, the joints are bent. Unless this process is actively prevented, the limbs may "freeze" into a contracted position and be totally useless to the individual. A leg contracted at the knee will never extend to support the body's weight. An arm contracted at the elbow and at the shoulder cannot enter a sleeve. And a hand clenched into a fist is absolutely useless. All of this can be prevented, but it requires nursing dedication and effort from the moment of injury to the patient. Range-of-motion exercises will keep the joints mobile, and passive, followed later by active exercises will keep the muscles from complete spastic contraction. Even though the individual may never fully regain the use of his arm and leg, if the leg remains extended, he can be taught to walk again, and an extended arm with a moveable elbow is capable of control. Many physical therapy techniques are available to accomplish these goals for the patient, but the task is immeasurably easier if contraction and spasticity have been prevented. When the patient is able to have physical therapy treatment, it remains the nurse's responsibility to assist him in the performance of exercises and activities prescribed by the therapist.

Structural integrity of the integument is threatened when a patient is immobile, and thus frequent turning and positioning of the cerebral vascular accident patient prevent a breakdown of the skin. Any break in the skin surface is a potential source of infection, and decubiti are particularly difficult to manage, since they result because circulation to the area has been allowed to fail. No injury can heal without adequate circulation, and the patient is spared the demand on his resource for healing if such injuries are prevented by conscientious positioning and mobilization during the

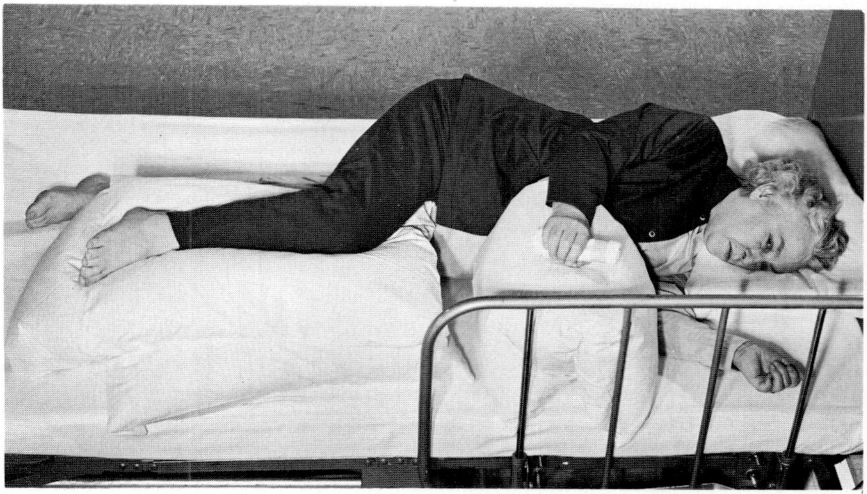

FIGURE 20. Preventive positioning and mobilization are required and are possible in any plane in which the patient is turned. Here, resting on the side, the afflicted side (black clothing) is positioned and supported in a functionally useful way. (From *A Handbook of Rehabilitative Nursing Techniques in Hemiplegia.* ©American Rehabilitation Foundation, Minneapolis, 1964.)

period of his confinement to bed. For the very heavy individual or for one who cannot be sufficiently mobilized because of his condition, the use of sheepskin or air mattresses to prevent pressure areas is necessary. The sooner the patient can be safely allowed out of bed, the better will be his chance for ultimate recovery. Not only are localized areas of pressure prevented, but the additional dangers of pulmonary stasis and infection are also less likely to occur. It must, however, be emphasized that allowing the individual to remain in a single position in a wheelchair for a protracted length of time is as disastrous as failing to mobilize him while he is in bed. The mere fact that he is allowed to be up in a wheelchair is not enough. And his posture in the chair must be as carefully supported as when he is in bed.

The integrity of the skin is often further compromised when the individual has an incontinence of urine and stool. Such events require prompt cleansing as often as necessary to maintain a surface contact for the skin which is dry, smooth, and clean. It is no longer common practice to place a catheter in the urinary bladder and leave it in place for prolonged periods of time to prevent bed wetting. The danger of bladder infection ascending into the kidneys presents a risk with this procedure, which is now widely recognized. Subsequent retraining of bladder function is also considerably hampered when the bladder is kept constantly drained of urine by an indwelling catheter. Sometimes external drainage is provided, although this is much easier for male than for female patients. Any such external arrangement, however, must be regularly changed and the parts of the body thoroughly cleansed every day.

The mobilization of partially paralyzed individuals presents special problems in insuring the patient's safety. Successful standing depends upon a knee which is extended. Some patients will require a knee brace in order to prevent the knee from buckling under them. The hemiplegic patient cannot determine, himself, whether he is in a balanced position; even if he were able to do so, he could not easily maintain his own balance. Whenever he is moved or transferred from his bed to a wheelchair, the nurse must be certain that she can handle him without danger that he will fall, or provide enough help to allow this activity without such danger. His safety from injury must be a concern in the hospital, as well as in the home. The floors must not be waxed so that they will allow him to slip. Grab-rails should be available wherever he requires assistance in changing position. This is important, for example, in the bathroom, and grab-rails should be available both for entrance and exit to the tub and shower, as well as to the toilet. A surface that will provide adequate friction is also important in the tub or shower. Small throw rugs, which slip under his step, should be eliminated from the home, and furniture with sharp corners should never be placed where he could possibly bump into it. The fear of falling is constantly present when the individual is learning how to handle his half-paralyzed body, and a fall that results in injury may make the task of mobilizing him almost impossible.

The structural damage in the cerebral tissues represents a potential threat that the original incident will be followed by subsequent incidents. The alteration in the patency of the cerebral blood vessels usually persists, and the factors that contributed to the original insult may continue to exist. The use of drugs to prevent the coagulation of the blood, and thereby eliminate future thrombic or embolic phenomena, has largely been abandoned in clinical practice because the interference with coagulability often resulted in extensive bleeding into the brain tissue. There have been some efforts to surgically improve the patency of the vessels going to the brain, but only a small percentage of individuals with a cerebral accident are benefited by this kind of intervention. The hypertension that accompanies many cerebral accidents may also be treated with drugs, but this too is not always successful.

The individual who has had a cerebral vascular accident must adapt to a completely altered perception of himself. He has suffered sensory as well as motor loss, and his body image is seriously damaged. He may have difficulty in recognizing that his own arm and leg are actually attached

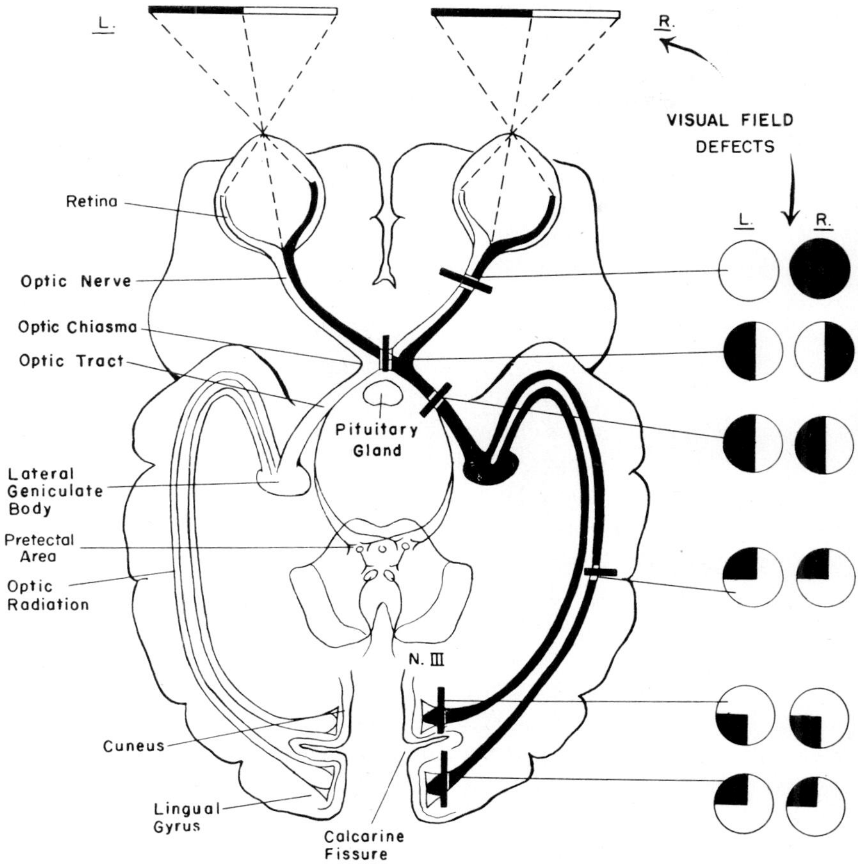

FIGURE 21. Cerebral damage is often accompanied by alteration of the visual fields. Assessment of the individual's visual ability is an important aspect of care, and accommodation must be made to consider such loss in daily nursing care. (From Gatz, A.J.: *Manter's Essentials of Clinical Neuroanatomy and Neurophysiology,* 3rd ed. F.A. Davis Co., Philadelphia, 1966.)

to his body. His sense of balance is entirely altered, and his position sense in both a lying and standing posture is defective. He must learn to perform many simple activities with only one hand, and sometimes this may be an almost unsurmountable task. As common an activity as tying his shoelace or buttoning his shirt may be impossible. Dressing himself may create one disastrous crisis after another unless he is helped to manage these tasks. Wearing slip-on shoes that do not require a tie is a simple solution to one problem. The difficulty of buttoning his clothes may be partially eliminated by substituting zippers where buttons are usually used, or by obtaining an old-fashioned buttonhook to help him in the task. The hemiplegic can be taught self-sufficiency with his altered structure, but it is not a task that is easily accomplished, and often the measure of his impatience with himself is the nurse's confidence in his ability to learn.

The Conservation of Personal Integrity

The degree of alteration of the information coming to an individual who has suffered a cerebral vascular insult is difficult to imagine. He must struggle with the helplessness of his paralysis and loss of body awareness and image, and often his difficulty is increased by aphasia. The nurse quickly learns that it is not always possible to depend upon oral-aural communication to establish contacts with patients. Language barriers of many kinds exist in the clinical practice of nursing. The most obvious, of course, is the patient who speaks another language. There is always the possibility of a translator to bridge this gap. But even when the patient uses the same language as the nurse, there are cultural and ethnic variants in the use of words that will make them mean one thing to a patient and quite another to his nurse. The use of certain words to describe common bodily functions, such as urination and defecation, varies considerably from one subcultural group to another and may have familial patterns of meaning which the nurse can hardly anticipate. The knowledge of colloquial terms is important to the nurse, and it is sometimes necessary to use them even though such usage creates anxiety in the nurse whose own cultural associations are very different. Nurses who care for children quickly learn to use the child's language to describe body functions. It is equally important that this be done for adult patients if communication with them is to be meaningful.

The patient who is in pain, or very weak, or withdrawn and frightened may be reluctant to use language as a means of communication. But the absolute loss of the ability to speak and understand the spoken or written word that accompanies cerebral damage in the cerebral vascular accident patient presents the nurse with frustrating dilemmas. The problem of the aphasic patient rests with his intense desire to communicate through speech, and with the impossibility of doing so when he has lost the function of his speech centers. Aphasia is not the same in all patients. Some patients can understand what the nurse says, even though they are not able to respond except in a garbled way. Some patients do not understand what is said to them. It often requires sensitive and subtle observation of the patient's behavior to determine whether he does, indeed, understand the spoken word. The additional problem of formulating speech with a paralysis of the muscles of the face, tongue, and larynx may make it difficult for the individual to formulate a word so that it can be understood. There are, therefore, at least two ways in which the patient's ability to use language for communication may be impaired. He may be unable to formulate in his mind the thought he wishes to express, and he may be unable to find the proper words with which to express it. This has been called a loss of "inner speech." On the other hand, his inner speech may not be remarkably affected, although the ability to vocalize, which depends upon muscle function, may be prevented by paralysis. In either event, the aphasic individual rarely abandons his wish to speak. He may be able to produce only garbled nonsensical syllables, or the words he chooses may be entirely inappropriate to what he is trying to say. In some individuals, the ability to utter expletives and swear words is all that remains of the faculty of understandable speech.

Many individuals can, however, be taught to speak again. Nothing is ever achieved by shouting at a patient who cannot understand a normal tone of voice. But much is gained towards his ultimate potential for relearning to speak if the nurse does talk to the patient when she is in his presence. Such conversations should be carried out in a normal tone of voice, using simple words repetitively and accompanying them by demonstrations when possible. The sentences should be very short and contain only a single idea. It is tragic that the aphasic patient is so often subjected to the silence of those in his presence because of their frustration in trying to communicate with him. He needs the stimulation of language even though he does not always understand; if he is treated silently, he will never understand.

Communication with the cerebral vascular accident patient may be further compromised by the lability so often demonstrated in the emotional tone of such patients. The patient weeps easily, or readily becomes intensely irritated and frustrated, and then in a few moments appears smiling and happy. The nurse is often tempted to read into this behavior her interpretation of what it means to the patient, but the likelihood is that such speculations are rarely accurate. Lability of emotional tone seems to be part of the organismic reaction of the brain-injured. It has been observed in soldiers who sustained brain injury and is a common experience in the care of patients with cerebral vascular accidents. The individual's own ability to control these reactions is probably very much impaired by the tissue damage itself. Such alteration of mood may, indeed, reflect the individual's dismay and despair, and it is not unusual for patients who have had a cerebral vascular accident to become severely depressed. The only reassurance the patient can have is in the unmistakable signs of progress, and a rehabilitation program that begins as soon as possible after the insult has occurred is the only route to satisfactory readaptation.

With the difficulties presented by inadequate verbal communication, the problem of helping the individual to conserve his personal integrity is not an easy one. Few disease entities demand the kinds of alteration in life-style that arise from a cerebral vascular accident. Every aspect of the individual's daily life must be relearned, and his ability to function as a self-sufficient person is seriously hampered. Even in the face of the rapid mood change so characteristic of such individuals, his personal integrity is fortified if the patient is treated as an adult. He is not an undependable and completely dependent child, and, even though language may not penetrate the barriers of the loss he has suffered, the nurse can communicate respect and concern for him by her approach to him as a responsible adult.

The Conservation of Social Integrity

The rehabilitation process is one which involves not only the patient, his physician, and his nurse, but his family as well. The first tentative steps towards reestablishing his social integrity involve his reaction to the hospital environment itself. An individual who is fearful and anxious will not learn until he has been helped to feel safe and secure. Before a man can learn to walk, he must first learn to stand alone. And every new sign of progress, however small it may seem, is a source of renewed desire to continue. The reflection of his achievement must come from those in the hospital environment who are working with him, but the really meaningful approval must ultimately come from his family and friends. The individual must redefine himself, but, unless the family also recognizes and accepts that redefinition, he cannot regain social integrity.

The damage to the cerebral cells of the patient creates an alteration which influences every individual in his family. They share the fear and despair of the critical hours when the illness first occurs, and the acceptance of the change in the individual must come as slowly and painfully to them as it does to the patient himself. Their apprehension cannot be wiped away, and it is only through gradual education that they can see the rehabilitation goals that are possible for the patient. The family members are often indispensable assistants in the rehabilitation process. The return to family life is one of the strong motivations in rehabilitation of the hemiplegic patient. The goals, however, for both the patient and the family, must be realistic and sensible. A goal which cannot possibly be attained can destroy the entire rehabilitation program. Relearning even the simple acts of daily living requires tremendous effort and devotion on the part of the patient. Families must learn to be patient and to allow the individual to make his own mistakes rather than to attempt to do everything for him.

Often the hemiplegic patient must return to a home where many changes are required in order to assure his safety. The family should understand why small rugs and waxed floors are dangerous for the patient. They will be alarmed at their inability to communicate verbally with the patient and will react to the mood swings with an emotional response of their own. They must understand the nature of the individual's symptoms, and this includes recognition that his ability to feel with his paralyzed limbs is probably limited or absent.

Reference to community agencies which will assist him in the attainment of long-term rehabilitation goals offers the patient and his family another dimension of nursing help. The assistance of a visiting nurse may be made available to the family. Some visiting nurse agencies also have a physical therapist on the staff, and the family members will have to be taught how to help the patient with necessary exercises. Referral for speech therapy, physical therapy, and nursing care can be made while the patient is still hospitalized, so that continuity of care is assured when he is ready for discharge to his home. If it is necessary for the individual to be placed in a nursing home, the family should be helped to select one that will provide decent care. Many urban areas have agencies that supply such information. The problem of cost to the family may loom large, too, in providing adequate care, but the social responsibilities of the community in the care of such patients are increasingly recognized.

The incidence of cerebral vascular accidents in older persons often complicates the long-range rehabilitation goals. The social importance of the aging population in Western societies is limited by the enthusiasm invested in youth. It is not easy just to grow old in a society that cherishes its young, and to be both old and paralyzed is a tragic combination. When the productive years have passed, the tendency to relegate the individual to a social existence without social participation creates pervasive problems for the entire group. Many older persons are not welcomed into the younger family organization, and when the independent aged person becomes dependent through illness, the facilities available to him are very meager and inadequate. It is unfortunate that even the expensive nursing home does not always provide adequate care. With the advent of Medicare and the demand for improved nursing home facilities, there is hope that such agencies will be assisted to provide care for the ill aged. But age alone should not be the deciding factor in the use of rehabilitation techniques. Even in older persons, the joy of life which accompanies well-being is not a goal to be scorned. The future is often measured by the immediacy of the present. Every human being, regardless of his age, deserves the opportunity to find fulfillment in both.

Model II: Body Movement and Positioning

OBJECTIVES

1. To learn the principles which allow the nurse to assist the bed patient in maintaining correct anatomical and physiological body posture, and thereby conserve function.
2. To understand the principles of body mechanics which are conserving of energy and best suited to optimal use of the musculoskeletal structure of the patient and the nurse.
3. To understand the effects of physical forces in relation to the patient's ability to move when confined to bed rest.
4. To understand the effects of physical forces in relation to the patient's ability to move from bed to another conveyance or to ambulation.
5. To recognize the physiological changes resulting from bed rest and to select nursing processes which limit the undesirable sequelae of restricted physical activity.
6. To evaluate the patient's ability to function independently and to assist him as required by his individual physical and emotional needs in a safe, comfortable, and effective way.

ESSENTIAL SCIENCE CONCEPTS

1. Ability to move freely is an essential factor in successful adaptation to the external environment.
   - 1.1 Body function is dependent on maintenance of optimal muscle tone.
     - 1.11 Skeletal-muscular integrity is controlled by an intact central nervous system.
     - 1.12 Muscle volume varies with usage.
       - 1.121 Atrophy results from disuse.
       - 1.122 Hypertrophy results from continued over-usage.
     - 1.13 Adequate circulation to provide nutrition to the skeletal-muscular system is essential.
   - 1.2 Free motion is possible only when the skeletal system and its articulations are intact and functional.
2. The organism is adapted to function in relation to the physical demands of the environment.
   - 2.1 Effects of gravity on the position of the body determine the ease with which movement is accomplished.
     - 2.11 Since the body mass as a whole is attracted toward the earth by gravity, force must be applied by muscles in order to move the body or any part of it (i.e., the muscles perform *work:* W = force × distance).
     - 2.12 A low center of gravity increases the stability of an object.

2.121 The center of gravity is lowest when the body is parallel to the earth (prone or supine).

2.122 A wide base of support lowers the center of gravity and increases balance and stability.

2.13 The circulation of blood is accomplished as work against gravity, and the work increases with change in position from horizontal to vertical.

2.14 Skeletal muscles squeeze venous blood back to the heart against gravity as an essential aspect of circulation.

2.2 Body movements may be analyzed in terms of the principles of mechanics.

2.21 Leverage systems depend on the structure of articulations.

2.211 First class: skull on axis.

2.212 Second class: standing on tiptoes.

2.213 Third class: brachialis muscle at elbow.

2.214 End-loaded compound lever.

2.2141 Two long bones, nearly in line, connected by a joint.

2.2142 Great mechanical advantage, e.g., little energy expended in standing upright.

2.22 Frictional forces limit and restrain movement.

2.221 Minimization of contact between two surfaces limits influence of friction between them.

2.2211 Wheeled vehicles for transporting.

2.2212 Rolling movements rather than sliding.

2.222 Smooth surfaces offer less resistance than rough or sticky surfaces.

3. Restriction of physical activity results in structural and functional changes in the body.

3.1 Skeletal-muscular function is maintained only through use.

3.11 Disuse results in fibrous changes in articulating systems.

3.12 Loss of muscle tone and substance through disuse creates weakness and consequent limitation of ability to move.

3.2 Cardiovascular function is compromised during bed rest.

3.21 Orthostatic adaptations are weakened.

3.22 Peripheral circulation decreases.

3.221 Pressure areas over bony prominences produce local ischemia and subsequent tissue necrosis.

3.222 Venous stasis predisposes to blood clotting and thrombotic phenomena.

3.3 Metabolic shifts occur as a result of limited activity.

3.31 Increased nitrogen excretion reflects loss of body protein and negative nitrogen balance.

3.32 Increased calcium excretion reflects loss of calcium from long bones.

3.321 Weight-bearing provides stimulus which retains Ca^{++} ion in the matrix of long bones.
3.322 Ca^{++} ion depletion of long bones decreases the hardness of these structures, resulting in osteoporosis.
3.323 Increased Ca^{++} ion in the urine predisposes to formation of kidney and bladder calculi.

4. Postural maintenance during restriction of activity preserves structural integrity.
4.1 Anatomical positioning insures continued muscular-skeletal function of the body.
4.11 Range-of-motion and passive exercises maintain integrity of articulating structures.
4.12 Gravity causes structural changes of foot and wrist unless counteracted.
4.13 Maintenance of muscle tone requires muscle use by the patient within the limits of his tolerances.
4.2 Physiological positioning enhances vital functions during bedrest.
4.21 Maintenance of patent airway.
4.22 Freedom for maximal respiratory excursions.
4.23 Maintenance of peripheral circulation, especially over bony prominences
4.24 Facilitation of digestive functions.

5. Ability to move freely is essential to feelings of competence, independence, and worth.
5.1 Physical well-being is impossible in the presence of weakness and fatigue.
5.2 Anxiety and fear may hamper physical activity, especially in the presence of pain.
5.3 Placement of necessary articles within safe and comfortable access prevents danger of over-reaching and falling.
5.4 Consideration to allow socialization and interaction with other persons in the environment.

NURSING PROCESS

1. Nursing intervention is designed to conserve structural integrity during periods of bed rest.
1.1 Assessment of individual patient's capability of activity.
1.11 Influence of disease process on activity.
1.111 Diagnostic entities may require rest as part of the therapeutic regime.
1.112 Maintenance of normal function is adjusted to prescribed requirements for rest.
1.1121 Unaffected articulations may be brought through range of motion during normal nursing care.

1.1122 Insure functional posture.
1.11221 Frequent position change in correct anatomical alignment.
1.11222 Firm mattress of adequate length.
1.11223 Use of devices such as footboard, trochanter roll, pillows (including proper positioning of pillow under head).
1.113 Prolonged restriction to bed requires physician's order for passive and/or active exercises to retain muscle tone and mass.
1.12 Structural limitations as a result of the disease process require nursing intervention to assist patient's adaptation to external environment.
1.121 Interference with central nervous system integration must be evaluated by observation of patient's activity and behavior.
1.1211 Paralysis or paresis of muscle groups requires nursing assistance in patient's adaptation to necessary body movement.
1.12111 Shifting position in bed requires nursing assistance and must therefore be anticipated and planned.
1.12112 Performance of usual activities may require assistance and relearning of skills.
1.1212 Loss of proprioceptive sense must be assessed in order to assist patient to maintain balance.
1.1213 Arrangement of necessary articles in the environment is dependent upon limitations in patient's ability to perceive and reach them.
1.1214 Loss of sensory function requires nursing intervention to prevent injury and insure safety.
1.122 Pain from any source results in limitation of motion.
1.1221 Judicious use of pain medications as ordered by the physician.
1.1222 Assisted position change to relieve muscle spasm and tension.
1.1223 Support of surgical incisions during activity which may cause stress on them.
1.1224 Sufficient nursing assistance to move patient securely and with minimal discomfort.
1.123 Immobilization of a part of the body (as in a cast), or amputation of a part, requires adaptation in gross body movements which the nurse must assess when providing care.

1.124 Extreme weakness accompanying nutritional deficiencies (as in cachexia) requires assessment of patient's ability to move.

1.125 Nursing intervention is the only means for adaptation to the external environment in the unconscious patient.

1.1251 All repositioning and movement are dependent on nursing forethought and assistance.

1.1252 Postural integrity is entirely dependent on nursing care.

1.1253 Safety of the individual is the nurse's complete responsibility.

1.12531 Proper use of bedrails.

1.12532 Sufficient help to move patient without jeopardy.

1.2 Assessment of the influence of bed position on the individual patient's physiological function.

1.21 Nursing care must insure a patent airway by proper positioning.

1.211 Adjustment of nursing processes when orthopneic position must be maintained.

1.212 Observation and evaluation of the effects of position on patient's airway.

1.22 Maintenance of adequate circulation to peripheral vessels may be insured by nursing care.

1.221 Prevention of pressure areas by frequent position change.

1.222 Massage over bony prominences as permitted by patient's diagnosis.

1.223 Daily inspection during bathing to determine early signs of pressure areas.

1.224 Passive exercises as approved by the physician to prevent venous stasis.

1.225 Conscientious fulfillment of orders to mobilize patient to enhance restoration of independent activity as soon as possible.

1.23 Proper position to allow safe and comfortable ingestion of food and fluids.

1.231 Adjustment of nursing care to protect patient when there is demonstrable Ca^{++} ion loss from long bones.

1.232 Recognition of debilitating effect of negative nitrogen balance and adjustment of nursing care to aid weakened patient to move.

1.24 Adjustment of nursing care to provide best physiological position for elimination using bed utensils.

2. Utilization of physical principles allows nursing care which is safe and effective.

2.1 When nurse assists patient to move, the leverage system results from the combined action of nurse and patient.
 2.11 Height and strength of the nurse in relation to the weight and position of the patient.
 2.12 Ability of the patient to use his muscular-skeletal system.
 2.13 The degree of weakness, disability, or state of consciousness of the patient.

2.2 Mobilization of the patient is paced to his tolerance.
 2.21 Assistance is offered which allows the patient to function at his own optimal level.
 2.22 Cue words are agreed upon with the patient and used so that the movement is smooth and effective.
 2.23 Evaluate each situation individually, seeking enough help to achieve movement safely.
 2.24 Knowledge of patient's ability to assist and the purpose of the mobilization procedure planned.
  2.241 Is this the first time out of bed?
  2.242 Presence of drainage tubes, IV tubing.
  2.243 Location of recent surgical incision. Is dressing secure?
  2.244 Period of bedrest which precedes mobilization procedure.
  2.245 Planning for bathing, feeding, use of bedpan, or other processes which should be done first.
 2.25 Observation of patient during and following mobilization to assess his response to activity.

2.3 Minimizing of frictional contact to eliminate injury.
 2.31 Teach patient to move in bed so that friction burns are avoided.
  2.311 Rolling motion is easier than sliding.
  2.312 Use of large muscles rather than small.
  2.313 Body weight should not be supported on elbows when shifting position.
  2.314 Provision for mechanical assistance as required.
   2.3141 Raised bedrails for support.
   2.3142 Trapeze or strap to foot of bed.
 2.32 Reduce friction during moving and positioning when the nurse assists the patient to move.
  2.321 Minimize surface contact whenever possible.
   2.3211 Place arms on chest when turning.
   2.3212 Flex knees so that sole of foot is flat on mattress.
   2.3213 Roll, rather than slide, whenever possible.
  2.322 Provide smooth, dry bed surface.
   2.3221 Maintain optimal skin condition, with use of fine talc for back rub.
   2.3222 Tight, wrinkle-free bed linens.
  2.323 Insure safety by braking or stabilizing wheeled vehicles during mobilization of patient.

3. Successful mobilization has a psychological, as well as a physical, goal.
   3.1 Safe movement grants security which will decrease apprehension when next effort must be made.
      3.11 Provision for as much assistance as is required for the individual situation.
      3.12 Thorough explanation of the process to the patient.
      3.13 Necessary preparations made before procedure is performed.
         3.131 Padding of wheelchairs.
         3.132 Adequate linens to cover patient at all times to maintain propriety and comfort.
         3.133 Footrest on wheelchair in up position whenever patient is being transferred into or out of it.
         3.134 Patient clothed properly, including robe and slippers as required.
   3.2 Patient's ability to tolerate the activity is never exceeded.
   3.3 Provide opportunity for socialization and change of scenery if possible.
   3.4 Remain with the patient until it is certain that he is secure, safe, and comfortable.

Vocabulary

afferent
airway
anoxia
aphasia
autonomic
autoregulation
axon
collateral
comatose
cranial-sacral
dendrite
efferent
electrolyte imbalance
embolus
ganglia
hemiplegia
irreversible
membrane permeability
metabolism
myelin sheath
neuron
nutritional balance
paralysis
parasympathetic
paresis
patency
pathophysiology
priorities
prophylactic
proprioceptive
pyramidal
rehabilitation
saltatory conduction
sensory
stimuli
stuporous
sympathetic
symptomatology
synapse
thoracolumbar
thrombus

General Bibliography

BURN, J. HAROLD: The Autonomic Nervous System, ed. 2. F. A. Davis Co. (Blackwell Scientific Publications), Philadelphia, 1963.

GALAMBOS, ROBERT: Nerve and Muscle. An Introduction to Biophysics. Doubleday & Company, Inc., Garden City, N.Y., 1962.

GARDNER, ERNEST: Fundamentals of Neurology, ed. 3. W. B. Saunders Co., Philadelphia, 1958.

GATZ, ARTHUR J.: Manter's Essentials of Clinical Neuroanatomy and Neurophysiology, ed. 3. F. A. Davis Co., Philadelphia, 1966.

HODGINS, ERIC: Episode. Atheneum Press, New York, 1964.

PETERSON, JEAN C., AND OLSEN, ANN P.: Language Problems after a Stroke: A Guide for Communication. American Rehabilitation Foundation, Minneapolis, 1965.

Rehabilitative Nursing Techniques: 1. Bed Positioning and Transfer Procedures. American Rehabilitation Foundation, Minneapolis, 1962.

Strike Back at Stroke. United States Public Health Service, Washington, D.C.

TRUEX, RAYMOND, AND CARPENTER, MALCOLM: Strong and Elwyn's Human Neuroanatomy, ed. 5. Williams and Wilkins Co., Baltimore, 1964.

WHITEHEAD, ALFRED NORTH: Adventure of Ideas. New American Library of World Literature, Inc., 1964.

Articles

BUCK, MCKENZIE W.: Adjustments during recovery from stroke. Amer. J. Nurs. 64:92-95, Oct. 1964.

CHAPMAN, C. B., AND MITCHELL, J. H.: The physiology of exercise. Sci. Amer. 212:88-96, May 1965.

COLLINS, VINCENT J.: Positioning the patient for surgery. AORN J. 55-66, Nov.-Dec. 1966.

DOTY, ROBERT W.: Philosophy and the brain. Perspect. Biol. Med. IX:23-33, Autumn 1965.

ECCLES, SIR JOHN: The synapse. Sci. Amer. 212:56-66, Jan. 1965.

FISHER, ALAN E.: Chemical stimulation of the brain. Sci. Amer. 210:60-68, June 1964.

HUXLEY, H. E.: The mechanism of muscular contraction. Sci. Amer. 213:18-27, Dec. 1965.

KELLY, MARY M.: Exercises for bedfast patients. Amer. J. Nurs. 66:2209-2213, Oct. 1966.

KOTTKE, FREDERIC J., AND BLANCHARD, RUSSEL S.: Bedrest begets bedrest. Nurs. Forum III:56-72, 1964.

NAPIER, JOHN: The antiquity of human walking. Sci. Amer. 216:56-66, April 1967.

NARROW, BARBARA W.: Rest is . . . Amer. J. Nurs. 67:1646-1649, Aug. 1967.

OLSEN, EDITH V., ET AL.: The hazards of immobility. Amer. J. Nurs. 67:779-797, April 1967.

PESZCZYNSKI, MIECZYSLAW: Why old people fall. Amer. J. Nurs. 65:86-88, May 1965.

PIGOTT, RICHARD, AND BROCKETT, FLORENCE: Visual neglect. Amer. J. Nurs. 66:101-105, Jan. 1966.

REGINA ELIZABETH, SISTER: Sensory stimulation techniques. Amer. J. Nurs. 66:281-286, Feb. 1966.

SPERRY, R. W.: The great cerebral commissure. Sci. Amer. 210:42-52, Jan. 1964.

ULMANN, MONTAGUE: Disorders of body image after stroke. Amer. J. Nurs. 64:89-91, Oct. 1964.

3 Nursing the Patient with a Failure of Integration Resulting from Hormonal Disturbance

The Endocrine System Integrates the Biochemical Processes of Metabolism

The direction and coordination of all body processes by the nervous system is accomplished through the investment of nervous control in other integrating systems. The cellular work is biochemical, and, since it involves many kinds of cells, the total economy of the body is dependent upon a communication system between cells which serves their independent interests while it unifies the activities of the organism. The endocrine system is a system of intercellular biochemical communication. The endocrines are "ductless glands" which secrete substances that are picked up by the circulating blood and are thus carried to distant tissues where they exert an influence on the function of those tissues. The substances manufactured by the endocrine glands are called *hormones,* and they provoke a physiological effect in the "target" tissues to which they are directed.

These remarkable substances carry a "message" which governs the activity of the target cells: it either stirs them to increased action, or indicates that their activity must be dampened. Hormones regulate growth, influence healing, prepare the organism to withstand threat, mediate the cyclic changes in the sexual organs, and are powerful determinants of blood concentrations of essential substances, as well as regulators of the body's water. In fact, every vital function essential and pertinent to the development and continuing well-being of the individual is susceptible to the mediating effect of hormones. Interference with hormonal balance (homeostasis) results in drastic alterations in the body's economy, and a disturbance in the effective activity of one hormone produces an imbalance in the entire endocrine system because their regulatory functions are so intimately interwoven.

The nervous control of the endocrines is directed by the hypothalamus, which regulates the behavior of the "master gland," also called the

HORMONE	SOURCE	CHEMICAL NATURE	FUNCTION
Ecdysone	Insect Prothoracic Gland 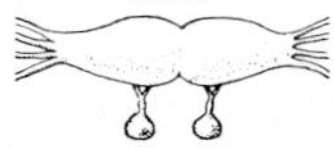	Steroid	Causes molting, initiation of adult development and puparium formation.
Glucocorticoids (Cortisone)	Adrenal Cortex 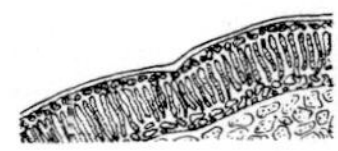	Steroid	Causes glycogen synthesis in liver. Causes redistribution of fat throughout organism. Alters nitrogen balance. Causes complete revision of white blood cell type frequencies. Is required for muscle function. Alters central nervous system excitation threshold. Affects connective tissue differentiation. Promotes healing. Induces appearance of new enzymes in liver. Affects almost all tissues.
Insulin	Pancreas (Islets of Langerhans) 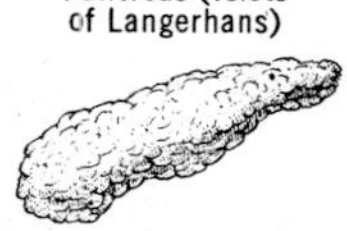	Polypeptide	Affects entry rate of carbohydrates, amino acids, cations and fatty acids into cells. Promotes protein synthesis. Affects glycogen synthetic activity. Stimulates fat synthesis. Stimulates acid mucopolysaccharide synthesis. Affects almost all tissues.
Estrogen	Ovary 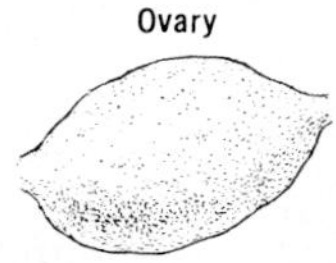	Steroid	Promotes appearance of secondary sexual characteristics. Increases synthesis of contractile and other proteins in uterus. Increases synthesis of yolk proteins in fowl liver. Increases synthesis of polysaccharides. Affects rates of glycolysis, respiration and substrate uptake into cells. Probably affects almost all tissues.
Aldosterone	Adrenal Cortex 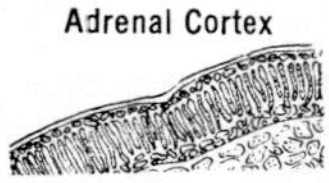	Steroid	Controls sodium and potassium excretion and cation flux across many internal body membranes.
Pituitary ACTH	Anterior Pituitary 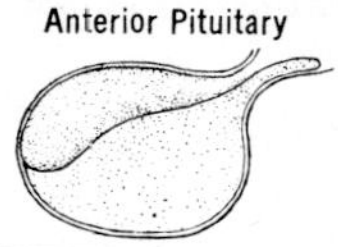	Polypeptide	Stimulates glucorcorticoid synthesis by adrenal cortex. Stimulates adrenal protein synthesis and glucose uptake. Inhibits protein synthesis in adipose tissue. Stimulates fat breakdown.
Pituitary GH	Anterior Pituitary 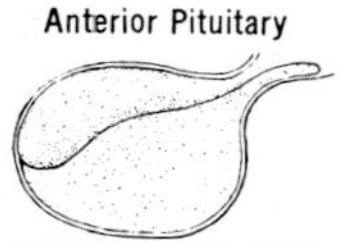	Protein	Stimulates all anabolic processes. Affects nitrogen balance, water balance, growth rate and all aspects of protein metabolism. Stimulates amino acid uptake and acid mucopolysaccharide synthesis. Affects fat metabolism. Probably affects all tissues.
Thyroxin	Thyroid 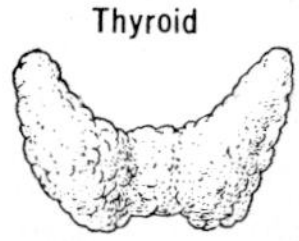	Thyronine Derivative	Affects metabolic rate, growth, water and ion excretion. Promotes protein synthesis. Is required for normal muscle function. Affects carbohydrate levels, transport and synthesis. Probably affects all tissues.

FIGURE 22. Biochemical regulators, or hormones, perform many essential functions, and their individual tasks depend on the interaction which results from their combined effects on body well-being. (From Davidson, E.H.: "Hormones and Genes"

pituitary or the hypophysis. The pituitary comprises at least two anatomically distinct glands, the anterior and posterior, which produce very different hormones. Those elaborated in the anterior pituitary gland (adenohypophysis) have the special task of carrying the message to other endocrine glands. All of the hormones of the anterior pituitary have the suffix *-tropic* (turning) and a stem which indicates the gland they govern. For example, adrenocorticotropic hormone (familiarly known as ACTH) has the specific role of regulating the output of the adrenal cortex. Some hormones act directly on the tissues themselves, and, in fact, their effect may arise from the action of the hormone on many different kinds of tissue. In any event, the governing ability of the hormones is accomplished by an intricate autoregulating system.

As is true of most of the autoregulating systems in physiology, hormonal integration is the result of a negative feedback. Its function is entirely analagous to the familiar negative feedback that regulates the temperature in a room by thermostatic control. When the room temperature falls below the value set on the thermostat, the heating system is stimulated into operation, and it will continue to supply heat until the thermostat setting is reached. At that point, the heating system is turned off. The gland that produces the hormone is stimulated into activity when the supply is deficient to produce the necessary physiological effect. Production continues until that effect has been achieved, and this, in turn, is the mechanism that shuts off the production of the hormone. The rate of secretion of hormones, therefore, is directly dependent upon the need for the hormones by the body cells.

Unlike the furnace that is thermostatically controlled, however, the glands which manufacture hormones demonstrate structural changes in response to the unusual demands that may be placed upon them. Because of disease processes, it is sometimes necessary to surgically remove a portion of a gland. When this occurs, the tissue remaining tends to increase in size: it undergoes "hyperplasia." Even without surgical removal, unusual demand may result in a "compensatory hyperplasia." For example, in certain kidney diseases, large concentrations of Ca^{++} are lost in the urine, and the body's effort to compensate for this loss results in a hyperplasia of the parathyroid glands, the regulators of the body's Ca^{++} blood level. Many hormones are administered as medications, and sometimes a continuous excess of the hormone stimulates a compensatory "atrophy" in the gland which normally produces that hormone. If the stimulation is prolonged, either by drug administration or in disease processes which cause excessive production of the hormone, a condition of irreparable "exhaustion atrophy" may result. Once this has occurred, the body is no longer able to produce the required hormone. Although the full story is far from understood, it is likely that exhaustion atrophy of the beta cells of the islands of Langerhans in the pancreas is part of the pathological picture of youth-onset diabetes.

The relative urgency of the hormonal supply varies considerably with the physiological effect that it governs. All hormones are essential, but alteration of supply of some hormones may place the individual into immediate jeopardy. The hormones of the adrenal cortex fall into two major categories of function. The mineralocorticoids are hormones which regulate the fluid and electrolyte balance of the body, and a failure of these substances is life-threatening to the individual within three to seven days. On the other hand, the glucocorticoids, while important to the individual's welfare, are not as likely to create an urgent life-threatening problem to the organism. The glucocorticoids share with other hormones the governing of the body's utilization of nutrients. The influence of these substances on the formation of glucose, specifically from noncarbohydrate substances such as amino acids and fatty acids, represents a part of a complex hormonal interaction in glucose metabolism which also involves insulin, glucagon, growth, and thyroid hormones. The specific role of glucocorticoids in the creation of glucose from noncarbohydrate precursors is part of the organism's defense against stress. Since glucose is the important currency of energy exchange, the mechanism that permits the individual to manufacture his own when he needs it is an obvious protective device. The glucocorticoids have the effect of raising the blood sugar level and are sometimes called "diabetogenic."

But the hormones of the adrenal cortex influence another essential body response, quite apart from their effect on the electrolyte and glucose levels. The body's usual defense against any kind of insult, microbial, chemical, or physical, is an inflammatory reaction which has the two-fold task of fighting the invader and preparing the assaulted tissues for subsequent healing. The mechanisms of the action of the adrenocortical hormones are not understood, but the mineralocorticoids increase the intensity of the inflammatory reaction, whereas the glucocorticoids tend to suppress the inflammatory reaction. The suppression of the body's defense against invaders may or may not be a useful mechanism. The inflammatory reaction involves a definitive structural change in the tissues affected, and it is characteristic that the body tends to limit and localize an inflammatory reaction to the least tissue involvement possible. By inhibiting the structural changes of inflammation in those tissues not directly involved in the invasion of the noxious agent, the anti-inflammatory behavior of the glucocorticoids conserves the organism's integrity and protects vital functions from the sequelae of inflammatory change. In any event, the role of the adrenocortical hormones in regulating the body's reaction to inflammation indicates that the purpose of hormonal integration is organismic, that is, designed to promote the individual's well-being, even in the face of localized assault.

It is apparent that hormonal integration makes a major contribution to the ability of the organism to heal, and healing itself is a process which emphasizes the interdependence of many body functions. Normal healing cannot take place without normal metabolism. It is dependent upon the supply of nutrients, including protein for cell reconstruction, the necessary chemical mediators, including the hormones, and a circulatory system capable of transmitting to the site of injury the components that are able to fight the noxious invader. The aim of all medical and nursing care is to promote healing, and this can be accomplished only through meticulous attention to all the variables that influence the healing process.

Every healing process, regardless of its nature, occurs over a period of time. The success of the ultimate healing depends in large measure on what happens to the individual during that time. The nurse is the person on the health team who shares the most time with the patient, and thus no worker can influence the success of the healing process more than the nurse. Nursing processes of every kind are dedicated to the promotion of healing. They emphasize cleanliness to prevent or limit infection, the maintenance of the integrity of the skin, the provision of adequate nourishment and fluids, the provision of an environment of regulated rest, and the responsibility for carrying out the medical regime as prescribed by the physician.

Personal Hygiene Ministrations Support the Healing Process

There is probably no aspect of patient care more central to the nursing function than that which involves personal hygiene of the patient. The burden of nursing responsibility involved in the tasks of cleanliness is so relevant to the care of every patient that the routinizing of these tasks has rendered them almost meaningless to the goals of therapy. The necessity to provide bathing facilities for every patient every day has become an end in itself, and the essential purposes, related to the individual's therapeutic plan, have tended to be lost in the incessant repetition of tasks. In fact, the goal of "getting the job done" has obscured the importance of this kind of nursing ministration and its implications for the patient's recovery from illness.

Cleanliness did not become "next to godliness" until the nineteenth century. It arose as a quasi-philosophical doctrine out of the valiant efforts of the Sanitarians to promote some control over the despicable conditions of the emerging urban centers. And perhaps no single group of people has invested it with more emotional overtones than nurses. For some nurses, at least, if the patient has been bathed, he has been nursed. He is much more apt to be—however properly scrubbed—sadly neglected, if that is the entire dimension of his care.

The cleanliness of the body has many implications beyond the performance of simple hygienic acts. Social attitudes are rooted in cultural determinants, and every individual interprets personal cleanliness in the light of his own family experience. In a world of advertising extravaganza, the deodorized, sweetly scented, powdered, cologned, sprayed, and antiseptic modern man is promised every social reward from ebullient good health to a free choice of an equally perfumed and perfect mate. There is a wistfulness in the universal admiration of small, dirty boys, but the unshaven male is hardly welcome even in the privacy of his own home.

Ablution of the body has not always focused on the socioeconomic pressure to handsomely support the manufacturers of soaps, detergents, and the paraphernalia of personal grooming. Some of the earliest records of the bathing mores emphasize that such activities had solemn religious and spiritual meaning, and as a result the act of bathing was restricted to holy men. Ritual ablution has a long history. The fifteenth chapter of Leviticus is entirely devoted to a cleansing of the body as a prerequisite to cleansing of the soul. The partial or total immersion in water, or even its ceremonial equivalent, remains a part of religious ritual in the modern world. This very early association of cleanliness of the body with its spiritual welfare had a paradoxical influence on the hygienic purpose in bathing. The ancient Greeks and Romans built palatial bathhouses, which became centers of social activity where the cult of physical well-being, associated with sensuality, was of prime importance.

Bathing was a communal affair, and few homes were supplied with the facilities for private indulging. During the early Christian days in Rome, the idle and self-centered behavior of the bathers, coupled with a rather free moral code, stirred a reaction that finally made bathing in the nude a mortal sin. It is instructive that the Italian word for bath, *bagnio,* is also a colloquial word meaning "brothel." During the Middle Ages, the cults of asceticism, with their emphasis on mortification, recognized, as suitable penance, a holy indifference to washing. It is said of Queen Elizabeth I that she was a fastidious woman, bathing once a month whether she needed a bath or not! But in the days of knights and ladies, it is probable that only the royalty had the facilities for such indulgence. The rest of the populace had to depend on the public bathhouses, and the pious man was forced to decide between the personal contamination of his body and the threatened contamination of his soul in the immoral atmosphere of the public baths. Not only the good church fathers frowned on bathing, but the medieval physician heartily concurred, and for a while the truly devout were enjoined to cover themselves in flannel gowns while bathing to avoid the mortal sin of nudity in the tub, even when they were alone.

The enameled bathtub has become the symbol of Western civilization, but it was not until 1851 that this essential furnishing was installed in the White House. At first a private tub—especially one with running water—was a status symbol, much as the late-model automobile is in the twentieth century. In some large cities even in the United States, public bathhouses are still operating.

The "Saturday night bath" became a cherished American folkway. But some of the doubt that shadowed the practice of bathing persists even today in folk ideas so often heard from patients. There is a widespread belief that it is dangerous to bathe when one is ill, and especially if there exists any chance that the bathed individual will be subjected to a "draft" either during, or for some time following, his bath. It is equally common belief that bathing or swimming during the menses is fraught with great danger to the individual.

The modern emphasis on bathing possesses moral implications too, because it is the absolute minimum of entrée to social acceptability in a society that insists on deodorants. In some circles, the relative merits of the soaking tub bath versus the shower are argued with a passion that seems to deny the simple hygienic reasons for cleansing the body. And, of course, absolute privacy during the bath is inviolate. Bathing now is condoned for purposes other than mere cleanliness. Relaxation and relief of fatigue are justifiable excuses for bathing. Physical well-being, as well as personal cleanliness, is a suitable result of a bath, and "therapeutic baths," incuding those in natural springs, have a decided social status.

It has long been a nursing dictum that every patient must be bathed every day of his hospitalization. The hospital tradition even specifies that this must occur in the morning, even though, for many individuals, the lifetime habit has placed the bath in the evening before they retire. It is rare, indeed, that the patient is allowed a choice, even when he is able to attend to the bath without assistance. The ritual of nursing practice that includes a linen change and a fresh bed during the morning hours create unrest in the nurse whose patient enters that bed without having first washed himself completely. Actually, the practice of personal cleanliness as a principle of asepsis is perfectly sound. The hospital ward exposes the individual to microorganisms which may cause him injury, and the cleanliness of the patient and his immediate environment is a vital factor controlling the microbiological populations in the hospital.

The patient who remains in bed, furthermore, should receive the refreshment and comfort of cleanliness. But the time that is devoted to bathing the patient is purposeful for more than cleanliness alone. It is an

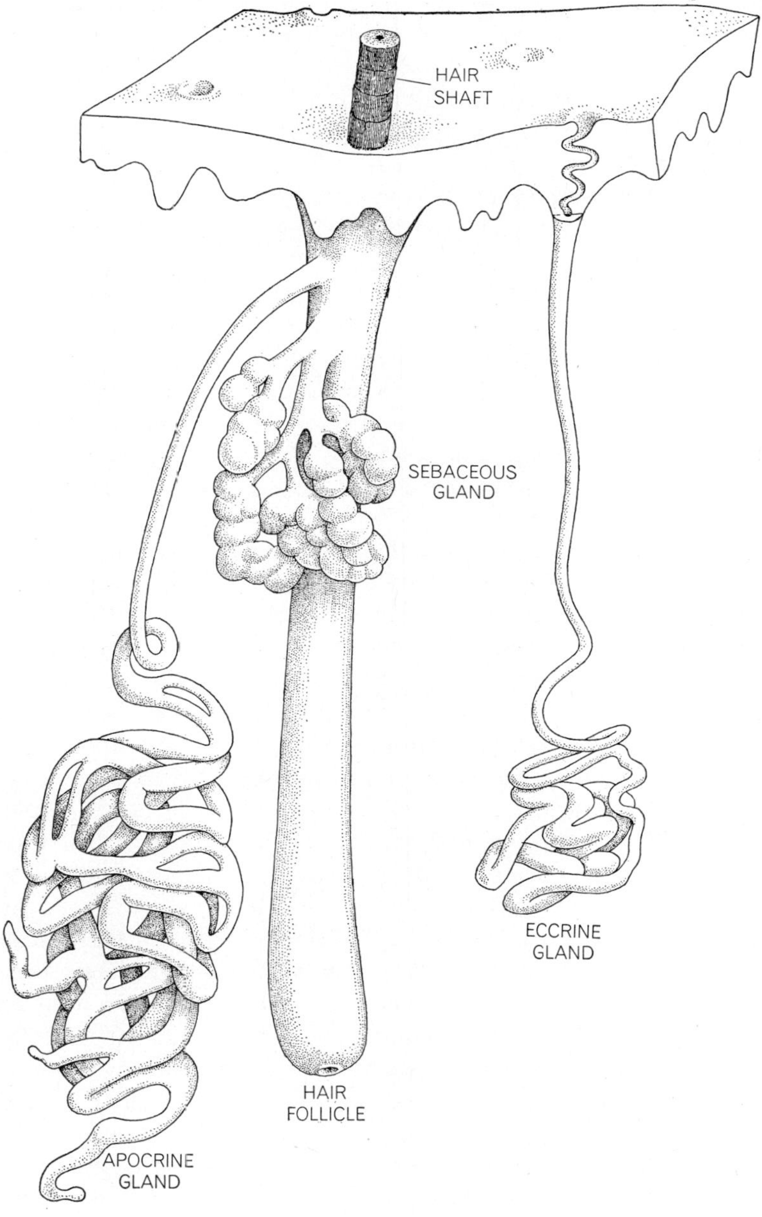

FIGURE 23. Schematic representation of the glands of the skin. The apocrine glands secrete a milky, odorous fluid and, together with the sebaceous glands, produce the body's odors. (From Montagna, W.: "The Skin." Copyright ©1965 by *Scientific American, Inc.* All rights reserved.)

activity which most individuals prefer to do for themselves. Being bathed by another person is a regression to childhood, and for most adults it is accompanied by embarrassment and reluctance, no matter how skillfully the nurse tries to prevent this reaction. As the individual becomes able to perform this duty for himself, he can be permitted a gradual increase of effort and participation, which not only offers him the needed physical exertion, but also alleviates his feelings of helplessness. When he is unable to help himself, the nurse has the opportunity to demonstrate her interest and concern for him as an individual by recognizing and respecting the limitations his condition places on his participation, and his emotional tone in response to his plight.

The daily bath allows the nurse time to make observations that will be useful in the patient's continuing care. His physical and emotional needs can be satisfied and assessed, and information can be gathered which will guide further care. This is a time of specific concern by the nurse for the individual patient—it is *his* time with *his* nurse—and the fundamental nurse-patient interaction can mature and become meaningful for each of them. It is sometimes perfectly reasonable, and in fact even essential, that the bathing process be limited or even eliminated when the patient's condition demands such a decision. When a bath or partial bath can bring comfort and well-being, it is a profitable nursing activity, but it should be equally apparent that such activity should never be so rigidly enforced that it substitutes a nursing ritual for a patient's nursing need.

The provision for the personal hygiene of all patients is a foundation upon which the specialized hygienic needs of some patients rest. The frequency with which such nursing activities are performed may dilute and fail to emphasize the fact that, for some individuals, their hygienic habits vitally influence the course of their disease. In general, any pathophysiological factor that interferes with healing places upon the individual the stringent need to prevent injury, however slight, because even an insignificant injury predisposes the individual to grave danger. Such a possibility creates the need to teach hygiene practices which will preclude the injury of commission or omission. This need adds still another dimension to the nurse's responsibility when she actively provides care, and requires successful communication to the patient, by word and deed, of safe methods of practicing personal hygiene.

Care of the Patient with Diabetes Mellitus

Failure of Biochemical Integration Threatens Healing

The pancreas, although the site of production of essential digestive enzymes, is also a gland of "internal secretion," that is, an endocrine gland.

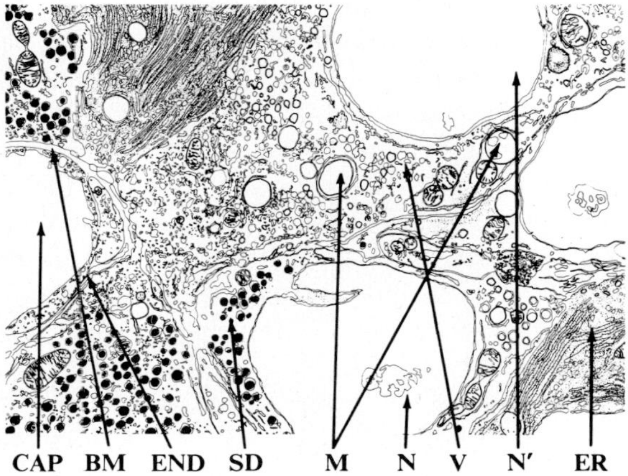

FIGURE 24. Artist's conception of an island of Langerhans (electron micrograph 10,000x). The beta cells elaborate insulin. Alpha cells probably secrete glucagon. *CAP*, capillary; *BM*, basement membrane; *END*, Endothelium; *SD*, secretion droplets; *M*, mitochondria; *N*, nucleus of alpha cell; *V*, vesicles; *N′*, nucleus of beta cells; *ER*, endoplasmic reticulum. (From Galloway, J.A.: *Diabetes Mellitus*, 7th ed. Eli Lilly and Company, 1967.)

The tissue described as the islands of Langerhans elaborates at least two hormones. The alpha cells produce a substance called glucagon. Its physiological effect is poorly understood, but it apparently influences the breakdown of glycogen in the liver to form glucose, and thus increases blood glucose levels. The second hormone, insulin, has been used therapeutically for many years, but its mechanism of action is also incompletely mapped. It is, however, clinically evident that insulin affects the utilization of glucose by the body tissues, and its net effect is to cause a decrease in the blood glucose levels.

The mechanisms that regulate the supply of glucose in the tissues are very complex, involving the active participation of several hormones, as previously indicated, as well as the function of several organs. The homeostatic range of glucose in the blood is regulated by a series of negative feedback mechanisms. Normally, the blood glucose level ranges from 80 to 120 mg%, and, though this may seem a wide range, it indicates a concentration that ranges only from 0.08% to 0.12%. The mechanisms that can maintain glucose within this finite concentration are remarkable indeed.

As the blood flows through the portal system into the liver, it brings with it the glucose prepared by the digestive process for absorption. The liver, directed by hormones, is capable of removing the glucose from the blood and storing it in the form of glycogen. When the blood glucose level begins to fall, the stored glycogen is broken down and released as glucose by the liver into the circulating blood. The blood glucose level normally varies considerably (within the homeostatic range) as body function alters the rate of glucose utilization. It is highest after the ingestion of a meal and lowest when food has not been taken for an extended period of time. Exercise and all types of physical activity use up glucose as, indeed, does stress. In the normal individual, however, the homeostatic range of blood glucose is maintained even during starvation. This can be accomplished because noncarbohydrate fractions can be converted into glycogen when necessary, and the glycogen is subsequently released as glucose to maintain a constant supply of this essential substance for energy production in the body.

The utilization of noncarbohydrate precursors in the production of glycogen emphasizes that proteins and fats are essential in the biochemistry of glucose in the body. All of the nutrients supplied to the body may enter the cycle of events that ultimately produces the energy for all body activities. Any disruption in glucose metabolism necessarily creates disturbance in protein and fat metabolism as well. In fact, it has become increasingly evident that diabetes, often called the "sugar disease" by the layman, is a disease that involves disturbance in the metabolism of all nutrients. The disease was first described by Celsus in the first century and was named "diabetes" by Aretaeus in the same century. The word means "going through," and the additional description of "mellitus," or sweetness, designates the clinical entity which produces copious and unusual amounts of sweet urine. Celsus could not have known that the excessive production of sweet urine was accompanied by a very high blood glucose level. It ranges well above 120 mg%, and may often be recorded as three or four times that amount. The increase in urinary output is caused by the loss of glucose, ordinarily conserved, through the kidney, and the excess fluid is lost because it holds the glucose in solution. This, in turn, creates a marked fluid loss, and the individual is excessively thirsty, drinking unusual amounts of fluids. The loss of glucose in the urine and the excess amounts in the blood are indicative of the failure of the body cells to receive glucose; in the presence of this excessive but inaccessible supply of glucose, the cells are literally starving. This creates the third classic symptom of diabetes: excessive hunger. The following are often called the classical symptoms of the diabetic: polyuria, or excess urine production; polydypsia, or excessive thirst; and polyphagia, or excessive hunger.

The close relationship of carbohydrate, fat, and protein in the metabolic pathways arises because, in the degradation of nutrients for the production of energy, any of these three basic nutrients may enter the cycle of events that ultimately produces the body's energy. A failure of glucose supply results in an incomplete cycle of events, with the result that midproducts of the metabolic cycle are increased in the blood. These midproducts, or partial products of incomplete metabolism, are primarily acid in nature, and their accumulation in the blood upsets the delicate homeostasis of the blood pH. This further embarrasses the metabolic order of the body, and the acid substances produce a condition of "acidosis," frequently accompanied by coma. (The "midproducts" are chemically ketones, and diabetic acidosis is often called "ketosis.")

Until 1922, diabetes was a disease that could not be treated. In that year, Banting and Best successfully tested insulin, and for the first time the diabetic patient could be offered a future. Although it has been widely advertised as such, the life of the diabetic did not become "normal" in the sense of that of the nondiabetic. As long as he lived, his supply of the hormone, insulin, had to be replenished every single day. In conjunction with dietary control, he could be offered a chance to live a social life, and to enjoy relative well-being and comfort, provided that he stayed strictly within his dietary restriction and never failed to take his daily injection of insulin. For the first time in any generation, the diabetics in the population then lived to become married and establish families. But insulin is a protein, and therefore could be administered only by injection, since it was digested if taken by the oral route. The search for a drug that would perform as insulin did, but which could be taken orally, was begun years ago. In recent years, some oral hypoglycemic drugs have been made available, but the original hope that they would prove to be substitutes for insulin has not been realized. Those individuals requiring insulin continued to require it, and the oral drugs were useful only in a limited number of individuals who either did not use insulin at all, or who used such small dosages of it that they might have been "controlled" on diet alone.

The clinical symptoms of diabetes cover a wide range from very mild to very severe, and it had long been apparent that there were at least two basic patterns in diabetes. The most severe cases, as judged by the ease and frequency with which acidosis could develop, were generally very young individuals, often children. They were lean, with very little body fat. In very young children, there was evidence of interference with growth, and they displayed frequent and dramatic symptoms of diabetic acidosis and coma. They were extremely difficult to control, even with insulin and a carefully weighed and regulated diet.

The milder form of diabetes, that is, that in which acidosis was very rare and even then not severe, usually began in an adult past the age of 40. Such individuals were almost always obese, and usually their symptoms could be controlled rather easily with diet regulation alone. On rare occasions, a severe form of diabetes was seen in an older person. These contrasting clinical criteria suggested to many investigators that they were not dealing with a single clinical entity even though all of the patients shared the signs of a failure of glucose utilization. Refined biochemical and laboratory techniques have recently added information which may, indeed, indicate that there are at least two kinds of diabetics. These techniques made it possible for the first time to measure the amount of insulin in the plasma. This assay indicated that, in the young, lean, severe diabetic, there is absolutely no evidence of plasma insulin at all. On the other hand, in the older, obese diabetic with relatively mild symptoms, the plasma insulin levels are normal or very near normal. There is some evidence that the young, severe diabetic has an "exhaustion atrophy" of the beta cells of the islands of Langerhans, whereas the same tissue in the older diabetic seems to retain its functional ability.

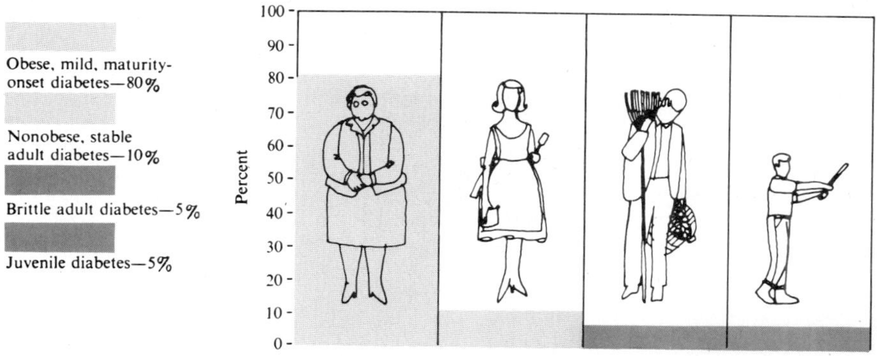

FIGURE 25. The characteristics of age and body structure, as well as severity of symptoms, suggest that there are many kinds of diabetics and at least two forms of *diabetes.* The mild form characteristic of older, obese individuals is the most common, but the severe form afflicts young persons and thus presents a special urgency for understanding. (From Galloway, J.A.: *Diabetes Mellitus,* 7th ed. Eli Lilly and Company, 1967.)

There are many descriptive titles used to differentiate between the two kinds of diabetics, although no specific usage has been agreed upon. The severe young diabetic is called juvenile, or brittle, or youth-onset, or insulin-dependent, or ketosis-prone (acidosis). The older, mild diabetic is called maturity-onset, non-insulin-dependent, stable, or non-ketosis-prone. In any event, as research into the nature of this serious disease goes on, there is every expectation that increasing information will help to define the disease. No specific cause for diabetes has ever been illuminated. It is widely believed to be an inherited disease and is described as carried by a recessive gene. Modern research in genetics may clarify the cause, but the practitioner of today is no more able to understand and prevent diabetes than was Celsus.

Table 1: Ketosis-Resistant (Adult-Onset) Diabetes Compared with Ketosis-Prone (Juvenile) Diabetes

	KETOSIS-RESISTANT	KETOSIS-PRONE
Age of onset	Frequently over 35	Usually, but not always, during childhood or puberty*
Type of onset	Usually gradual	Abrupt
Family history of diabetes	Commonly positive	Frequently positive
Nutritional status at time of onset	Obesity usually present	Usually undernourished
Symptoms	May be none	Polydipsia, polyphagia, and polyuria
Hepatomegaly	Uncommon	Rather common
Stability	Blood sugar fluctuations are less marked	Blood sugar fluctuates widely in response to small change in insulin dose, exercise, and infection
Control of diabetes	Easy, especially if patient adheres to proper diet	Difficult
Ketosis	Uncommon except in the presence of unusual stress or moderate-to-severe sepsis	Frequent, especially if treatment program is insufficient in food and/or insulin
Plasma insulin (endogenous)	Plasma insulin response may be (1) adequate but delayed so that postprandial hypoglycemia may be present when diabetes is discovered or (2) diminished but not absent	Negligible to zero
Vascular complications of diabetes and degenerative changes	Frequent	Infrequent until diabetes has been present for perhaps 5 years
Diet	If diet is utilized fully hypoglycemic therapy may not be needed	Mandatory in all patients
Insulin	Necessary for 20 to 30% of patients	Necessary for all patients
Oral agents	Efficacious	Rarely efficacious

*This age level is arbitrary. Intensive screening programs, especially when glucose tolerance tests of "nondiabetic" relatives of diabetics are carried out, are detecting patients who are likely to have ketosis-prone diabetes before disease progresses to the stage of growth-onset diabetes. (From J. A. Galloway: *Diabetes Mellitus*, 7th ed. Eli Lilly and Co., Indianapolis, 1967.)

The modern practitioner, however, must face a reality which Celsus was spared. The therapy available for the diabetic has successfully prolonged his life. The expectation that this would also allow a normal life span has been rudely shaken by the astonishingly high incidence of changes in the patency of the blood vessels of the diabetic individual. Most textbooks continue to describe these changes as "complications" of diabetes. In 1936, Kimmelstiel and Wilson described changes in the vascular supply to the kidneys which produced irreparable and life-threatening symptoms in diabetic subjects. The incidence of retinal damage and consequent blindness in diabetics became alarmingly high. And gradually it was recognized that, even when the diabetic is carefully controlled, within twenty years after the initial diagnosis of diabetes is made, 90% of the patients have disabling vascular changes involving the eye, the kidney, the peripheral circulation, or the coronary circulation. This sad fact has suuggested to some clinicians that the changes in the vessels are not complications of diabetes at all, but concomitants of the disease, that is, they represent the natural progression of the disease process itself. Years of experience with the treatment of the diabetic patient, all of them rich in the expectation that control and prolongation of life also meant cessation of progress of the disease, make it extremely difficult for physicians and nurses to accept the blunt statistics that demand recognition of the shortcomings and inadequacies of diabetic therapy. Too many young victims of heart attacks are found to be diabetics who were never diagnosed. And the incidence of diabetes in the population seems to be increasing, in part, at least, because the diabetics are now able to live to bear families and thus to perpetuate the gene which carries the seeds of their disability. Many public health agencies have instituted widespread

Table 2: Metabolic and Vascular Changes in Various Stages of Diabetes

	CARBOHYDRATE TOLERANCE			INSULIN-LIKE	
DIABETIC STAGE	FASTING BLOOD SUGAR	GLUCOSE TOLERANCE	CORTISONE-GLUCOSE TOLERANCE	ACTIVITY AND SYNALBUMIN ANTAGONIST	VASCULAR CHANGES
Prediabetes	Normal	Normal	Normal	May be increased	+
Subclinical	Normal	Normal (abnormal during pregnancy)	Abnormal	Increased	+
Latent	Normal or increased	Abnormal	Test not necessary	Increased	++
Overt	Increased	Test not necessary	Test not necessary	Increased	+++

(From J. A. Galloway: *Diabetes Mellitus*, 7th ed. Eli Lilly and Co., Indianapolis, 1967.)

Table 3: Percent of Patients with Vascular Complications among 1,072 Juvenile Diabetics* Followed More Than Twenty Years, by Age and by Duration of Diabetes

YEARS	ALBUMIN (%)	ELEVATED BLOOD PRESSURE (%)	RETINITIS (%)	RETINITIS PROLIF-ERANS (%)	CALCIFIED ARTERIES (%)
Age					
0-9	0	0	0	0	0
10-19	4.2	1.8	4.8	0	6.5
20-29	18.5	16.7	63.2	28.7	45.5
30-39	34.7	40.3	84.4	53.1	83.3
40-49	37.0	51.9	88.0	58.4	95.0
Duration of Diabetes					
0-4	0.8	0.5	0	0	0
5-9	1.5	1.2	2.5	0	1.7
10-14	7.0	4.5	19.0	3.0	14.0
15-19	18.0	15.0	59.0	18.0	44.0
20-24	41.0	32.0	82.0	47.0	73.0
25-29	39.0	44.0	88.0	46.0	88.0
30-34	44.0	53.0	93.0	59.0	94.0
35-39	63.0	70.0	—	—	—

*These comprise 28.7 percent of the 3,732 juvenile cases treated at the Joslin Clinic up to August 1, 1955. (From J. A. Galloway: *Diabetes Mellitus*, 7th ed. Eli Lilly and Co., Indianapolis, 1967.)

detection campaigns, in an effort to find hidden diabetics certain to be in the population and to offer them whatever amelioration is possible with present therapeutic techniques.

It is absolutely essential that the nurse accept the reality of the problems of the diabetic patient in order to provide him with proper care. No service in the hospital excludes diabetes, because the diabetic may require hospitalization for many health problems not directly related to his diabetic condition but invariably complicated bl its presnece. The combination of hormonal imbalance, metabolic aberration, and the interference with the free flow of blood through the small vessels of the circulatory system contribute to a clinical fact which surrounds the care of every diabetic patient, no matter how mild or severe his disease may be. The diabetic does not hael easily, quickly, or normally. This makes every scratch a threat and the prevention of infection a matter of profund importance. Furthermore, the superimposing of another disease process, and especially an infection, stirs a marked increase in the metabolic disturbance in the diabetic. A common cold or the flu is mildly disabling and uncomfortable for any individual, but it threatens the diabetic with acidosis and with the possibility of a life-threatening alteration in his entire body metabolism. The inability to heal normally, coupled with probable slowing of peripheral circulation, creates the necessity for extremely cautious hygiene. This is particularly emphasized in the care of the feet and legs. An infected corn on the small toe of a diabetic, which resists healing and becomes infected, may produce a death of the tissues of the feet that ultimately requires the amputation of his leg. Almost every instance of diabetic gangrene that terminates in amputation begins with a tiny injury which other persons could ignore. The diabetic not only may not ignore such damage, but his entire life pattern must be dedicated to preventing it.

In an exaggerated form, the diabetic patient emphasizes the important goals of providing for the personal hygiene needs of the individual. Teaching the patient proper self-care, observing accurately his response to treatment, and assessing his needs, so that a sensible nursing care plan is possible, become an essential part of the *medical treatment* itself in the care of the diabetic patient. No aspect of his life can go without inspection. The physiological demands on his blood glucose level involve his food intake, his physical activity, and his emotional response; all of these are weighed by the physician in determining the replacement of insulin in order to establish glucose homeostasis. His own autoregulation, so dependable and certain in the normal individual, must now be supervised for the rest of his life by his physician. The diabetic himself must know and understand this. The life he lives is not a normal life, but it can be a satisfactory adaptation, and, within the realistic restrictions of his disease, he may achieve genuine well-being.

The Conservation of Energy

The work of life is essentially a constantly flowing exchange of energy. All of the energy production in the body results from biochemical change, mediated through extraordinary pathways in precise steps, all guided by specific enzymes, and utilizing as their raw materials the modified products of ingested food. Ninety-nine per cent of carbohydrate foods is ultimately converted into energy, in processes that involve measured and controlled biochemical reactions, each related to the one that preceded it and "cyclic" because some of the biochemical components are re-formed to be used again and again. The body's own capacity to conserve its energy resources is remarkable, but the successful completion of the cycle depends, as do all chemical reactions, on an adequate supply of the necessary substances at the specific time they are needed to enter into the evolving patterns of change. Less than a cup of sugar weighs 180 grams, but the completed oxidation of an equal amount of glucose yields 686,000 calories.

This is accomplished slowly and in response to the needs of the tissues, so that the energy is produced and utilized in discrete quantities as required. Like a cautious banker, the oxidative processes spend some energy and save some for future use. The ready availability of glucose is essential, and, when carbohydrates are not available in the cells for this purpose, proteins and fats are changed into fractions which allow them to enter the cycles of energy production. The energy needs of the tissues must be served, no matter what the cost may be. Nerve tissue demands a constant supply of the energy provided by glucose metabolism. When protein and fat are substituted in the biochemical pathways, they often are taken at the sacrifice of other body needs. The body substance itself will be used, as is clinically apparent in individuals who have obviously lost weight.

The major physiological problem of the diabetic patient is the inability to utilize glucose in the biochemical cycles that create energy. The biochemical irony posed by the fact that excessive glucose is left in the circulating blood and that it is even spilled over into the urine and excreted is dramatically apparent in cellular starvation resulting from the failure to move glucose across the cell membrane. The cells starve in the midst of plenty, but, unless the glucose can enter the cell and there engage in the mechanisms of energy production, its presence in the flowing bloodstream is useless to the cell. Although bathed in high concentrations of glucose, the cell must use its own substance to survive.

There is clinical evidence of this dislocation of the body chemistry in all diabetics. The youth-onset diabetic has a lean body structure, evidence of the use of protein and fats for energy production instead of for tissue growth and maintenance. The maturity-onset diabetic, while usually an obese individual, almost always reports weight loss as one of his presenting symptoms, and often in the face of an excessive appetite for some time before he comes for treatment. No matter how balanced and sensible the food intake may have been in the diabetic before treatment is instituted, he comes to treatment suffering in some degree from starvation. Associated with weight loss, or a failure to gain weight, is the frequent complaint of easy fatigue and limited physical activity. The exhaustion that quickly attends the ordinary daily activities of the individual invariably creates behavior changes too. Anxiety and irritability are aroused in the individual who is unable to perform even the minimum of the daily demands on him without extreme tiredness and weakness. And, since every individual functions within a social group, these responses may become exaggerated because other family members find it difficult to understand how anyone could eat large quantities of food and still complain of weakness.

The therapeutic goal in the treatment of the diabetic is to move the glucose accumulating in his blood stream across the cell membrane to the energy production cycles within the cell. Quite obviously, this apparently simple maneuver is fraught with difficulties. Glucose metabolism is dependent upon a number of autoregulatory factors in the normal physiology of the body. The intrinsic factors involve the coordinated relationships of several hormones, including insulin. The extrinsic factors depend on food intake, as well as physical and emotional activity of the individual. A therapeutic plan which attempts to control these interacting variables must, of necessity, prescribe for each of them as well as for their mutual response to each other. The individuality of the diabetic requires that the establishment of an insulin-diet-activity pattern must be a highly individualized prescription. The young accountant who works at a desk all day will not have the same requirement as a young teen-ager whose physical activity has a "rock 'n' roll" beat, and neither of these shares the problems of the elderly grandmother who may, in addition, have a touch of arthritis. The very apparent differences in age, sex, and life style are further compounded by the varying severity of the disease itself. But for every diabetic, the essential issues of energy conservation are summarized in the triad that attempts to impose upon the organism a regulatory function, which, in the normal individual, is accomplished by its own feedbacks. In a sense, diabetic therapy imposes another servomechanism—this one arising outside the organism—into the control of the individual's energy capability.

This, of course, places a very urgent responsibility on those who assume the care of the diabetic. The determination of the precise combination of the three major aspects of diabetes therapy is the doctor's responsibility, and achieving a satisfactory balance is not always a simple task. If the disease is newly discovered, or if previous control has been upset, the process of re-establishing effective control is usually accomplished in the hospital. The purpose of hospitalization is to permit observation and assessment of the individual's response to treatment throughout the day and night, and this essential task is a nursing obligation. Since the treatment itself is designed to restore energy utilization, the evaluation of the individual's response to treatment is a continuing determination of his energy expense and resource.

The administration of insulin, or oral hypoglycemic drugs, compensates for the body's own failure to mobilize glucose across the cell membranes. Imposing this function on the organism through an externally determined quantity of insulin cannot be accomplished with the built-in protective controls that characterize the autoregulation of the supply of insulin. The issue of too little or too much thus becomes a matter for medical decision, based, in every instance, upon observation of the patient's response to the dosage administered. If the dosage is not sufficient, always in relation to food intake and activity, then the signs of continuing

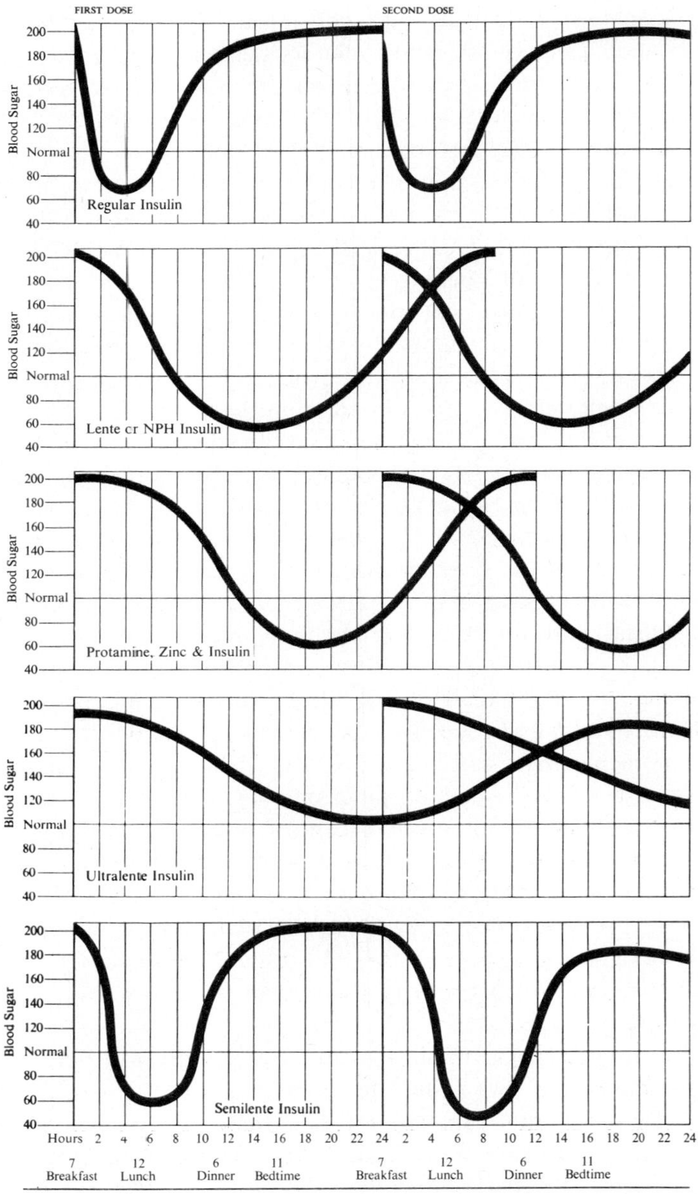

FIGURE 26. Comparative time activities of the various kinds of insulin. Anticipation of periods of hypoglycemia depends on knowledge of the time span of the type of insulin the patient is receiving. The patient, as well as the nurse, should know these activities in order to properly adjust food intake and exercise. (From Galloway, J.A.: *Diabetes Mellitus,* 7th ed. Eli Lilly and Company, 1967.)

<table>
<tr><th rowspan="2"></th><th rowspan="2">DIABETIC COMA</th><th colspan="2">HYPOGLYCEMIC REACTIONS</th></tr>
<tr><th>REGULAR INSULIN</th><th>MODIFIED INSULIN OR ORAL AGENTS</th></tr>
<tr><td colspan="4">Clinical Features</td></tr>
<tr><td>Onset</td><td>Slow—days</td><td>Sudden—minutes</td><td>Gradual—hours</td></tr>
<tr><td>Causes</td><td>Ignorance
Neglect of therapy
Intercurrent disease or infection</td><td colspan="2">Overdosage
Omission or delay of meals
Excessive exercise before meals</td></tr>
<tr><td rowspan="2">Symptoms</td><td rowspan="2">Thirst
Headache
Nausea
Vomiting
Abdominal pain
Dim vision
Constipation
Dyspnea</td><td>"Inward nervousness"
Hunger
Sweating</td><td>Fatigue
Headache
Nausea
Sweating (sometimes absent)
Dizziness</td></tr>
<tr><td colspan="2">Weakness
Diplopia
Blurred vision
Paresthesia
Psychopathic behavior
Stupor
Convulsions</td></tr>
<tr><td rowspan="3">Signs</td><td rowspan="3">Florid face
Air hunger (Kussmaul's respiration)
Finally, respiratory paralysis
Dehydration (dry skin)
Rapid pulse
Soft eyeballs
Normal or absent reflexes
Acetone breath</td><td colspan="2">Pallor
Shallow respiration</td></tr>
<tr><td>Sweating
Normal pulse</td><td>Skin may be dry
Pulse not characteristic</td></tr>
<tr><td colspan="2">Eyeballs normal
Babinski's reflex often present</td></tr>
<tr><td colspan="4">Chemical Features</td></tr>
<tr><td>Urine
Glucose</td><td>Positive</td><td colspan="2">Usually absent, especially in second voided specimen</td></tr>
<tr><td>Acetone</td><td>Positive</td><td colspan="2">Negative</td></tr>
<tr><td>Diacetic acid</td><td>Positive</td><td colspan="2">Negative</td></tr>
<tr><td>Blood
Glucose</td><td>> 250 mg./100 ml. ordinarily</td><td colspan="2">60 mg. or less/100 ml.</td></tr>
<tr><td>CO_2 combining power</td><td><20 volumes/100 ml.</td><td colspan="2">Usually normal</td></tr>
<tr><td>Leukocytosis</td><td>Present; may be very high</td><td colspan="2"></td></tr>
<tr><td>Response to treatment</td><td>Slow</td><td>Rapid; occasionally delayed</td><td>May be delayed</td></tr>
</table>

FIGURE 27. Differential diagnosis of diabetic coma and hypoglycemic reaction. (From Galloway, J.A.: *Diabetes Mellitus,* 7th ed. Eli Lilly and Company, 1967.)

failure of energy production will persist. On the other hand, if the dosage is too large, in relation to the food intake and activity, the rapid mobilization of glucose out of the blood and into the cells, and thereby into the energy-producing mechanisms, produces equally grave symptoms of imbalance. Every diabetic individual who must have insulin supplied is faced with the possibility of over-utilization of glucose, and with the development of symptoms of hypoglycemia. Too little glucose immediately available is as disastrous to the nervous tissue when that limitation arises from this source as from any other restriction resulting in glucose deprivation. The symptoms of excess insulin activity reflect the influence of glucose metabo-

THOSE INCREASING NEED FOR INSULIN	THOSE DECREASING NEED FOR INSULIN
Gain in weight	Reduction in weight (therapeutic)
Increased diet	Reduced caloric intake
Cessation of exercise	Increased physical exercise
Pregnancy	Termination of pregnancy
Thyroid therapy	Termination of thyroid therapy
Epinephrine therapy	Termination of epinephrine therapy
Corticoid therapy	Termination of corticoid therapy
Deep-roentgen-ray therapy	Termination of deep-roentgen-ray therapy
Withdrawal of oral hypoglycemic agents	Oral blood-sugar-lowering agents
Hyperthyroidism	Correction of hyperthyroidism
Sepsis	Correction of sepsis
Acute infections	Correction of acute infections
Fever	Correction of fever
Ketosis	Correction of ketosis
Ultraviolet-ray burns	Correction of burns

FIGURE 28. Many factors alter the need for insulin, so that even a well-controlled individual may from time to time need adjustment in his dosage. (From Galloway, J.A.: *Diabetes Mellitus,* 7th ed. Eli Lilly and Company, 1967.)

lism on nerve tissue. The earliest signs may be subtle behavior changes including vague feelings of anxiety in the patient, which progress with alarming rapidity to increasing nervous system involvement, including disoriented behavior, and culminating in coma and shock. Untreated, such shock leads to death. The treatment is relatively simple and the effects miraculous: glucose must be supplied to the organism in as concentrated a form as possible and as quickly as possible. It is for this reason that an insulin-dependent diabetic, forbidden the free use of candy in his diet, should carry hard candy on his person in order to prevent the development of insulin shock when the first recognizable signs develop. The nurse must acquire the sensitivity to recognize, in the diabetic patient receiving insulin, the subtle, beginning changes in his behavior that are a prelude to the serious symptoms of insulin shock and hypoglycemia. This is, in a very positive sense, an evaluation of his energy exchange, and it constitutes an important aspect of the conservation of energy in the diabetic patient. On most hospital wards where diabetics are treated, a quick and always available supply of orange juice, often fortified with glucose, is used when the signs of insulin shock begin to develop.

Dietary balance is another aspect of the control which therapy aims to achieve in the diabetic patient. The diet of the diabetic is not directed at the limitation of carbohydrates, although this is the interpretation often put upon it by the layman. An intake of food substances which supply all necessary nutrients, including protein, fat, and carbohydrate, is designed for the individual. A growing child requires an adequate protein intake, and this is just as true for the diabetic child. It may, in fact, be even more urgent. The determination of the amounts of different nutrients depends on the individual and all the variables that make him unique from his fellows. Diet alone is often sufficient control in maturity-onset diabetics, but when diet must be regulated in relationship to insulin dosage, it presents a regulatory issue three times a day: every meal influences the successful achievement of control. In the jargon of the hospital, the diabetic patient must consume enough of his diet to "cover" his insulin. This requires that the nurse know what foods, and exactly how much of each, a diabetic individual has actually taken at a meal. Furthermore, any factors that interfere with food intake must be reported at once to the physician so that the insulin dosage can be adjusted, A patient who has been vomiting, or who is nauseated and refuses to eat, or perhaps one who is anorexic and simply unable to eat his meals, will require an adjustment to compensate for his insulin dosage. Many individuals object to hospital food in any event, and the new diabetic will be especially unhappy with his diet restriction. A refusal to eat the food served him may require substitution, but this must be carefully calculated to compensate for the planned diet he was supposed to consume. In general, the individual who is receiving insulin must also consume sufficient food so that he will not become hypoglycemic because of a failure to ingest adequate glucose. The total food intake for a 24-hour period includes snacks or between-meal feedings, and these must be calculated as part of the physician's diet prescription. The distribution of food servings over the 24-hour period is related to the individual's previous meal patterns, his daily activity, and the kind of insulin he is receiving. Preparations of insulin vary according to the time at which the insulin activity reaches its peak in the body, and the patient must receive food accordingly, so that the peak periods are adequately "covered" by a glucose supply.

The third major consideration in regulating the diabetic's glucose metabolism is the physical activity in which he might be engaged. Any kind of muscular exercise increases the rate of glucose metabolism. This is equally true of periods of increased emotional response including anxiety, worry, and fear, all of which may be expected in the hospitalized individual. The expenditure of energy that accompanies restlessness and discomfort may also produce a measurable drain on the energy resource of the individual patient. Nursing activities are available that help to minimize the effects of physical and emotional stress during hospitalization, but it is very rare that nursing care alone can exclude them altogether. Evaluation of these effects on the patient must, however, be a constant nursing function. The patient who is confined to bed requires substantially less food than one who is free to move about at will. And the hospitalized patient may require less food, even if he is freely mobile, than he will need when he resumes his regular activities at home and work.

Before the diabetic is adequately controlled, the disease threatens fluid and electrolyte balance, and diuresis is a common symptom. The re-establishment of fluid and electrolyte balance is one of the important first steps in therapy; it is often accomplished as the control is improved over glucose metabolism. In severe cases, the fluid and electrolytes may be supplied by vein until glucose metabolism has been improved. Because the fluid exchange reflects the therapeutic progress, measurement of fluid intake and output provides vital information about the patient. In addition, progress may be guided in part by testing the urine for the presence of glucose and the intermediate metabolic substances, ketones, which indicate whether or not the metabolic patterns are being re-established. There are a variety of quick methods for determining the presence of sugar in the urine, but the specimen must be a freshly voided one. The testing of the urine provides the nurse—as well as the physician—with information concerning the patient's glucose metabolism within the time immediately preceding the collection of the specimen. When the testing is repeated before each meal, the nurse has a clear picture of the effectiveness of therapy and with it some idea of the individual's energy resources. It must be emphasized that definitive decisions concerning the success of control in many diabetics cannot be based on urine testing alone. Frequent testing of the glucose levels in the blood is also required. This involves blood samples drawn when the patient has not had food for 12 hours and *before* he receives his insulin. When his breakfast is delayed to permit the technician to draw a blood sample, his insulin is also delayed until it has been done. But the food should be served very promptly after the insulin is administered.

The conservation of energy in the care of the diabetic patient requires the attainment of that delicate balance between his unique ability to remain within the homeostatic range of glucose utilization and the details of the treatment outlined for him. The nurse cannot evaluate one aspect of his medical regime without measuring it against the other factors that influence it. The successful control of the diabetic is always threatened in the presence of other disease processes and creates additional problems in providing for his care. The diabetic who must undergo surgery will require specific attention to his needs as a diabetic, but the particular stresses of the surgical procedure will modify the usual pattern of control. The diabetic depends upon adequate control for the vital energy exchange that allows him to function in a social and meaningful way. Every day of his life, he faces the threatening sequelae of a failure to regulate his energy mechanisms. The disease itself threatens him with the danger of ketosis and coma, and, if he needs insulin replacement, he must face the possibility of shock if the control is disrupted. When he is entrusted to the care of a nurse, that daily confrontation is shared, but only the most perceptive and cautious observation can offer him the safety of control which is his only hope for a satisfying life.

The Conservation of Structural Integrity

The frequency of occlusive changes in the small vessels of the circulatory system in the diabetic and the difficulty in healing, which is characteristic of this disease, establish the nursing goals in the care of the diabetic individual. Interference with circulation to the distant periphery of the body, as well as vessel changes that predispose to kidney, eye, and cardiac damage, represent a constant threat to the structural integrity of those parts of the body and, indeed, to the organism as a whole. As has been previously indicated, it is impossible to absolutely exclude the danger of these damaging changes, but effective control often slows them down. Nursing intervention can identify the early signs of change and thus help to focus attention and treatment on them. In addition, any superimposed disease process in a diabetic may alter the metabolic balance previously achieved, so that he must be protected from infection of all kinds and guided in self-care that will aid in preventing the development of secondary disease entities.

The presence of peripheral vascular changes is often accompanied by insult to nerve tissues with a consequent peripheral neuritis; such changes also signal the possiblity of changes in the central nervous system. Nerve damage may result in loss of sensation, including alterations in vibratory sense, position sense, and even the reception of heat, cold, and pain stimuli. When nerve damage does exist, the individual may well injure himself and not even be aware that it has happened.

Table 4: Possible Factors Contributing to Infection in the Diabetic Patient

Hyperglycemia
Defective antibody formation
Decreased complement
Decreased bactericidal power of the blood, presumably secondary to defective phagocytosis by the granulocytes
Defective properdin system
Decreased liver glycogen
Decreased skin glycogen
Interference of ketone bodies with the bactericidal action of lactic acid
Excessive steroid secretion by the adrenals
Dehydration and malnutrition secondary to a catabolic state precipitated by insulin deficiency
Neuropathy
Deficient blood supply (due to microangiopathy and large-vessel disease)

(From J. A. Galloway: *Diabetes Mellitus*, 7th ed. Eli Lilly & Co., Indianapolis, 1967.)

The potential disaster that awaits a diabetic who sustains any kind of foot injury has served to encourage an extremely cautious prophylactic plan for foot hygiene in every diabetic patient. The diabetic is instructed to visit a capable chiropodist for nail-trimming and is enjoined against ever performing any kind of cutting procedure on his feet. Uncomfortable bunions, calluses, and corns should be avoided, if possible, by shoes and stockings which are well fitted and kept in good condition. If such conditions should arise, the diabetic is once more advised to visit a qualified foot specialist for treatment. In fact, the nurse should never perform nail care for a diabetic patient without first receiving approval and a formal order from the physician. The diabetic is instructed to wash his feet carefully and to dry them thoroughly, including between the toes. He may use a bland oil to keep the skin soft, but he should never use "corn pads" or other drugs which cause sloughing of tissue. He is warned never to go barefoot in order to prevent accidental injury to his feet. And he should be told that, if his feet always seem cold, he must report this promptly to the physician. Sometimes during a bath, the nurse will notice that the patient's feet feel very cold to the touch. He may have become so accustomed to this that he is barely aware of it, but it represents the possibility that the circulation is already impaired, and the physician should be notified of this fact. The presence of an injury on the feet should also be promptly reported, as should "athlete's foot" or any persistent and chronic area of inflammation that does not heal. It is far easier to encourage proper foot hygiene than to help an amputee face a crippled future.

While emphasis is placed on foot care, personal hygiene habits that maintain the integrity and health of his skin are also vital to the diabetic patient. He must be cautioned not to use soaps that are drying and irritating to his skin and to exercise careful asepsis if he does sustain an injury anywhere on his body. In the elderly diabetic, pruritus, or intense itching, of the genital and rectal area may be a persistent and annoying problem. Usually this improves when the diabetic condition is under control, but once more cleanliness and the use of prescribed medications on the local area must be emphasized. His clothing should fit comfortably, but not bind; it, too, should be clean in order to limit irritation and possible infection.

Oral hygiene serves to maintain the integrity of the mucosal surface of the mouth, and the prevention of dental caries is important to eliminate potential sources of infection. In older persons who wear dentures, the appliances should be kept clean and in good condition, without rough or irritating surfaces that might damage the gums.

The diabetic must remain under medical supervision all of his life. It is essential that he understand that he must report to the physician certain complaints that he may not feel warrant a doctor's attention. Changes in his visual ability may occur so gradually that he is not aware of them until they disable him to some degree, but they should be reported promptly. An examination of his retina will be part of a regular physical, but changing visual acuity may occur, and this is a sign of impending difficulty. As commonplace an experience as an upset stomach is another symptom which must be reported to the physician; if the diabetic who is receiving insulin is unable to retain his food, this is immediately reported to the doctor. Frequently nausea and vomiting are early symptoms of ketosis, and the physician must differentiate between a transient cause of gastrointestinal difficulty and the possibility of more serious events. No diabetic can afford the luxury of self-treatment and self-diagnosis. It is often easier for the physician to re-establish control if the patient brings

	URINE SUGAR	URINE KETONES AND DIACETIC ACID	BLOOD SUGAR	BLOOD CO_2	PLASMA OR SERUM ACETONE
Diabetic coma	++++*	++++*	High	Low	++++ in at least the undiluted specimen
Hyperglycemic coma†	++++	0	High	Normal or slightly low	0 or minimal
Hypoglycemia	0 or +‡	0 or +‡	Low	Normal	0 or minimal
Lowered seizure threshold	0 or +	0	Low, normal, or high	Normal	0 or +
Cerebrovascular accident	0 or +	0	Often high	Normal	0
Uremia	0 or +	0	High or low	Decreased	0 or + §
Lactic acid acidosis	0 or +	0	High or low	Decreased	0 or + §
Other causes of anion gap, such as salicylate intoxication	0 or +	0	High or low	Decreased	0 or + §

*May be absent in markedly oliguric patients.
†Usually in older patients. Often associated with hypernatremia and hyperosmolarity.
‡Urine present in bladder for a number of hours may contain sugar as a result of earlier hyperglycemia. In addition, ketones (but usually *not* diacetic acid) may be present.
§Positive results may be found in association with uncontrolled diabetes but not of the degree found with ketoacidosis.

FIGURE 29. States of unconsciousness must be differentiated, and a distinction must be made between the two widely different conditions which can result in coma in the diabetic patient. (From Galloway, J.A.: *Diabetus Mellitus,* 7th ed. Eli Lilly and Company, 1967.)

him his early complaints and avoids the danger of an emergency admission to the hospital when he is already seriously acidotic.

The care of the patient who is in diabetic coma demands the same intervention to preserve structural integrity as that required in the care of any unconscious patient. But there is, in the diabetic, the additional concern to prevent pressure areas because of the added difficulty presented by his impaired healing ability. Mobilization, frequent position change, maintenance of a patent airway, and evaluation of changing levels of consciousness are added to the nurse's responsibility to regulate fluid and electrolyte administration, and to observe the effects of insulin and glucose given by infusion.

If it is necessary to catheterize a patient in order to obtain a urine specimen that may be tested for sugar and acetone, the aseptic technique must be scrupulous to avoid introducing infection into the bladder and to avoid the possibility that such infection may involve the kidney as well. The postoperative diabetic patient must be given every assistance in the healing of his surgical wound, and this is dependent upon maintaining control of his glucose metabolism and absolute protection from infection of the wound. The diabetic receiving insulin must have at least one injection a day, sometimes two or three. This, too, must be done with extreme aseptic skill. In fact, any procedure which must encroach on the normal defensive integrity of the skin must be meticulous to avoid the danger of introducing infection. This is true, of course, in the nursing care of *all* patients. The very critical issues in the diabetic simply underscore its importance. Every infection, even a highly localized one, results in a destruction of some tissues, and this is equivalent to a threat to structural integrity. When the physician sees a patient with a severe infection, he investigates for the possibility of concurrent diabetes. The notoriety associated with slow and difficult healing encourages a proper caution in the care of the diabetic. Ultimately healing does takes place, but it can be accomplished only when all of the environmental factors—internal and external—are under sufficient control. Nursing intervention is influential in achieving satisfactory healing, and it must be designed to enhance and speed the process by affording the individual every protective skill available to the nurse in the practice of her art. Personal hygiene care can never be a "routine" if the nurse recognizes that it is an essential dimension of the entire therapeutic plan for the patient.

The Conservation of Personal Integrity

The diabetic can never escape the daily confrontation with his disease. Every morsel of food influences his welfare. Every physical activity and every emotional experience must be evaluated according to their effect on his well-being. In a world shared with unfriendly microorganisms, he must somehow live so that he avoids the dangers they pose for him. If he is insulin-dependent, no day can start without an injection; even if he is not, he must avoid the ordinary bumps and scratches which others can ignore. He is different. He knows he is. And how he achieves the adaptation to his disease which permits a full and worthwhile life is often dependent upon the kind of professional guidance he receives.

It cannot be easy to muster a sense of personal integrity when one faces a lifetime of dependence, in some degree, on the counsel and ministrations of others. The diabetic must learn to manage his own disease, within the limits it places upon him and facing the realities of his specific requirements. There is, for him, a kind of integrity that arises out of the courage and insight that such a task requires. However, the success of his efforts rests with the physician, the nurse, and the dietitian or social worker, who together are able to help him understand how he can manage his life safely and with satisfaction.

Assuming he has average mental ability, the details of self-care that he must learn present very little difficulty. The testing of urine with commercially available kits is simple and easily learned. Administering his own insulin and understanding the technique to make it a safe procedure are usually handled very well by the diabetic. The details of personal hygiene and foot care are also rather simple. The problems of dietary control may be somewhat more complex unless the many variables that enter into diet selection have been considered. It should not be a problem, in the modern world, to provide the ordinary satisfaction of obtaining the necessary materials for bodily cleanliness, proper clothing, proper food, and shelter. But even in the midst of plenty, such basic human needs are not always easily obtained. The diabetic diet may not be an inexpensive one. It is useless to prescribe a diet which the individual cannot afford to purchase. Every nutritionist is capable of suggesting alternatives that are within the patient's means. Expense should be one of the factors guiding the prescription of the diet. The patient also comes to the question of dietary restriction fortified with the food selection habits of a lifetime, many of them culturally determined. Ignoring such preferences is almost a guarantee that he will not be able to maintain the diet. Even at its best, the diabetic diet is restrictive and therefore depriving. Food has various meanings for individuals, many of them beyond the apparent logic that a carefully contrived food list can offer. If the satisfactions usually associated with food are denied, then observing the diet may well depend upon the successful substitution of other satisfactions that reinforce the integrity and sense of worth of the individual. No diet prescription can ignore the terribly personal specifications which each individual must have. The diabetic will be on a restricted diet all his life. If he is not allowed to participate in its selection, the likelihood is that he will not be successful in maintaining it.

There is an unfortunate, if understandable, tendency on the part of the professionals concerned with the care of the diabetic patient to project their own frustrations into the patient's problems. The earliest enthusiasm that attended the discovery of the life-saving ability of insulin created the expectation that diabetes could be completely controlled. It was quickly apparent that a "cure" was not available, but the utter failure that was so characteristic of pre-insulin therapy was dramatically altered, as were the hopes of the practitioner who had witnessed nothing but failure in the past. The promise of control, of a "normal" life expectancy, and of a minimizing of the chronic and persistent nature of diabetes became the hallmark of all diabetic education in the lay public. However, the clinical experiences of the past twenty years have clearly indicated that even this is more than the scientists can deliver for many, many diabetic individuals. The powerful motivation in both physicians and nurses that led them to service occupations will not readily bow to the threat of failure. In "controlling" diabetes, the issue of the patient's contribution to his own management looms large indeed. It is not difficult to understand how the professional practitioner, having carefully educated the patient in his care, would react with dismay and disappointment when that same patient returned to the hospital, out of control and very sick. It is now statistically apparent that the diabetic individual can develop serious concomitants of his disease, no matter how conscientiously he has obeyed the instructions he has been given. However, the expectations of both doctors and nurses who work with diabetic patients have encouraged in them a "moralizing" attitude that stimulates a need to scold and reject the returning individual who left them in good condition, but who now lies semi-comatose in the emergency room. The patient may or may not have failed to fulfill the directions given to him. Often, without considering the many influences that conspire against "control," the patient is scolded for failing in his diet and for being remiss in the letter-perfect adherence to his instructions for care. The question of good or bad behavior in the diabetic, or, indeed, in any patient whatsoever, is external to the focus of professional responsibility. It is sometimes difficult to accept the fact that individuals may make decisions involving their own welfare which may well expose them to continuing difficulty. But the fact is that every person has a right to make such decisions, even when the professional practitioner has invested much time and devotion to dissuading him. And when there exists, as there always does for the diabetic, the real possibility that he had reached a time of crisis in spite of his effort to obey implicitly what he has been taught, then the onus of accusation leveled at him under such circumstances is doubly cruel. No professional can expect to successfully control every variable the patient must face, and if, indeed, the recurrent crisis has arisen because the patient did not understand his role in managing his affairs, then the realistic and most honest approach is to start again and try once more to help him to succeed. Threat, disappointment, and accusation have no place in this process.

The diabetic patient must participate in the management of his disease willingly and with knowledge. It takes some time to accept the implications of chronic illness. The diabetic is told that he must carry on his person at all times an identification card, bracelet, or disk stating that he is a diabetic and providing information that permits notification of the responsible parties if he should become ill or sustain an injury. This, in itself, must indicate to him that the fact of his diabetes sets him apart from other persons. He may intellectually accept the protection that such identification affords him, but it is difficult to believe that he can do so without some distress of the spirit. He is admonished to learn to recognize in himself the subtle beginning signs of difficulty, arising either from his insulin dosage or from a metabolic failure accompanying an exacerbation of the disease process. He knows he must watch his diet, but he also must coordinate his physical activity into a balanced pattern of daily life. He is cautioned against unusual stress, even though he is no more able to enjoin such occurrences in his life than is any one else, diabetic or not.

He must be taught. The delicacy of the interacting forces that operate to keep him functional demands that he understand and learn to manipulate them himself. But he must be taught so that he can face his problems confidently. There is always a right time and a wrong time to teach. He must learn, but, to do so, he must understand the language of the lesson. There are countless opportunities in his daily care during hospitalization when he can be taught by example. And every opportunity to teach him how to live with himself must be seized and used profitably. The teacher must also learn to listen to him, because there is no other way to know what he understands. Handing him one of countless pamphlets about diabetes is *not* teaching. Threatening him—either directly or in veiled allusion to the dire consequences of failure—is *not* teaching. Hastily reciting the steps in a technique, without offering him the chance to try it himself, is *not* teaching. Quickly reviewing the doctor's orders, as he stands ready for discharge from the hospital, is *not* teaching. The nurse-patient relationship built on mutual respect and consideration is the basis for all patient teaching; that which is done at his pace, in his language, and with his willing participation is the only kind of teaching that will fortify him for the decisions he must make for himself.

In large measure, the degree of independence and insight which the diabetic can bring to the management of his daily life is beyond the authority of any professional person to prescribe. He must be what he has always been—diabetic or not—and he must be respected for it. Somehow he will develop for himself, out of whatever strengths and resources he possesses as a human being, the guidelines that allow for life as a diabetic. Some will succeed—marvelously. And some will fail. But every diabetic succeeds or fails in direct proportion to his own personal integrity and to the self-respect which others can strengthen and cherish when it is their privilege to help him.

The Conservation of Social Integrity

Most individuals do not face the consuming problems of life alone, and though families and friends do not always understand the issues confronting the diabetic, they are nevertheless involved in them. The presence of a diabetic in the home creates immediate adjustments that concern the living pattern of the entire family. The most obvious encroachment is the dietary adjustment that the diabetic will require. But the additional possibility that he will need insulin injections, urine testing equipment, and frequent visits to the doctor's office will involve the economics of the family as a whole. Quite beyond the dislocation and expense, there is also their personal concern for the afflicted individual and for the role that he plays in the family structure. The family needs the comfort of knowledge, just as the patient does, and educating him to manage his disease really must include the family members as well.

Once again, the individual considerations arise from the constellation of factors that identify the diabetic patient. The preparation of his meals may be the responsibility of another family member. The mother of a diabetic child, or the wife of a diabetic husband, must know in exact detail what the diet prescription is, and how to fulfill it in an accurate, but still palatable, way. This may require separate preparation for him beyond what is necessary for the rest of the family. Shopping for the food and preparing it so that it is suitable for his diet may require extensive relearning on the part of the homemaker. If, in addition, the noon meal is not eaten in the home, then preparation of a suitable lunch, or even calculating into the daily food pattern the foods selected at lunch, will be the responsibility of the person who supervises the patient's diet. Perhaps no social issue is more intense with the child who is diabetic, because his food intake at school and in social gatherings cannot be supervised by the mother. The pressure of conformity in the young teen-ager makes it very difficult to substitute for the hamburgers and French fries which seem to make up the staple diet in that age group. In planning the diet for such individuals, the nutritionist often tries to recognize the pressure of such contacts, although no diabetic diet can safely allow potato chips. The older diabetic has other problems with food intake, which also find their roots in his social identity. The tried and tested foods of the ethnic group represent more than physical nourishment, and it is difficult, indeed, to abandon the habits of a lifetime.

Members of the family must also be helped to recognize the early signs of impending difficulty, and to realize, with the patient, the importance of continuing medical supervision. They must be assisted to expect no more—and no less—of the diabetic member than his pathophysiology will permit. They have to accept the fact that he is not able to omit his medication without serious consequence, and that exceptional physical activity and fatigue are harmful to him. They should not be made over-anxious or overzealous in their care for him, but they must be sufficiently alert to help him to live safely.

Table 5: Manifestations of the Complications of Diabetes

Eyes	Retinopathy, cataract formation, glaucoma, and extraocular muscle palsies
Mouth	Gingivitis, increased incidence of dental caries, periodontal disease, and greater resorption of alveolar bone
Pregnancy	Increased incidence of large babies, stillbirths, miscarriages, neonatal deaths, and congenital defects
Nervous system	Motor, sensory, and autonomic neuropathy
Vascular system	Large-vessel disease and microangiopathy
Skin	Xanthoma diabeticorum, necrobiosis lipoidica diabeticorum, furunculosis, mycosis, and pruritus
Kidneys	Diabetic glomerulosclerosis, arteriolar nephrosclerosis, and pyelonephritis

(From J. A. Galloway, *Diabetes Mellitus*, 7th ed. Eli Lilly and Co., Indianapolis, 1967.)

The task of teaching them requires that they be given the same consideration and assistance as the patient. They, too, must understand the language and be given the opportunity to ask questions and express their feelings about the situation. They must learn in circumstances which do not frighten or rush them; the same friendly and concerned interest shown to the patient must also be offered to them. The teacher must permit them to express their concern and apprehension and must listen to their fears without censure. Often a family member is taught to administer the insulin injection, and in any event, even if the patient is to do this for himself, another member of the family should know the procedure and be capable of performing it if necessary. They should also be taught the urine testing technique and should understand as well as the patient the of insulin and the absolute necessity to "cover" it adequately with food, so that meals are never unnecessarily delayed for the diabetic. In short, every aspect of care that the patient himself must understand has to be importance of personal hygiene and foot care. They must know the effects made equally clear to his family.

No physician can, without qualification, promise a diabetic that he can anticipate a life without difficulties. For the young adult, the desire to marry and bear children is not eliminated with a diagnosis of diabetes. The young woman may bear children, but the fact of her diabetes can easily influence the outcome of her pregnancy. Often, the undiagnosed diabetic faces the tragedy of a stillborn infant. The known diabetic woman, with careful prenatal care, has an excellent chance to have a normal infant. If, however, the infant is very heavy at birth, there is an excellent chance that it will develop diabetes during its lifetime. The decision concerning the wisdom of bearing children is one which the diabetic must share with her physician. The mother's pathophysiology is a strong determinant in a successful pregnancy. There are specific techniques available to the obstetrician in the handling of the pregnant diabetic woman, but the real criterion of success depends upon the combined efforts of the obstetrician and of the physician who supervises her care as a diabetic, and upon the individual's ability to participate in her own care. No matter what the statistics may be, the desire to have a family is very rarely measured against the figures in a chart. The best scientific guidance available can not always influence the decisions that human beings make for themselves.

Diabetes is a chronic disease, capable of completely altering the life pattern of the individual and his family. Living with it is always a burden. The nurse can offer the diabetic patient the skilled care he must have during illness, and the knowledge that will guide him to the optimal well-being possible for him.

Model III: Ministration of Personal Hygiene Needs

OBJECTIVES

1. To recognize in the individual patient the physiological, pathological, behavioral, and social determinants which influence his personal hygiene needs.
2. To maintain a clean environment in the hospital setting by provision of cleanliness for individual patients.
3. To evaluate the individual patient's ability and need to help himself by adjusting nursing care so that it is consonant with his specific requirements.
4. To utilize the period of daily patient contact for sound observation of individual patient progress and of his response to therapy and nursing care.
5. To provide an opportunity for the mature development of nurse-patient relationships in the interests of improved patient care.
6. To recognize the effect of the artifacts of personal hygiene and their influence on the maintenance of the integrity of the body surfaces in contact with the external environment.
7. To understand the influence of hygienic practices on the patient's well-being, so that teaching of hygiene methods can be tailored to the individual's need and ability to understand.

ESSENTIAL SCIENCE CONCEPTS

1. The integument is the organ of contact with the external environment.
    1.1 The intact skin and mucosa protect the organism from encroachment by microorganisms.
        1.11 Body surface is normally occupied by bacterial flora, including potentially pathogenic organisms.
        1.12 Many nonpathogens normally resident on the skin surface can become pathogenic if proper conditions are created.
        1.13 The body surface represents the first line of defense against infection.
            1.131 Cilia and mucosal sheet "sweep" contaminants off of mucosal surfaces for excretion.
            1.132 Rapid renewal of epithelial cells closes microscopic breaks in body surface.
            1.133 Environmental contaminants may include irritants which stimulate an inflammatory reaction on the body surface.
        1.14 A break in the integrity of the body surface requires mobilization of defense response that requires energy expenditure by the individual.
    1.2 The integument is a vital organ in the adaptation of the individual to variations in the external environment.
        1.21 Physical forces may threaten the integrity of the body surface.

1.211 Contact of body surface with other surfaces creates frictional forces.

1.2111 Skin contact with bed linens represents extensive surface area susceptible to frictional forces.

1.21111 Texture of linens increases or decreases frictional effect.

1.21112 Dryness or moisture of contact areas influences frictional effect.

1.21113 Health of skin tissues influences frictional effect.

1.2112 Skin surfaces in contact with other skin surfaces represent potential source of friction damage.

1.212 Local pressure compromises circulation and may result in death of tissue.

1.22 Regulation of body temperature requires controlled evaporation of water from body surface.

1.221 Heat of vaporization produces cooling since required heat energy is supplied by the surface area from which evaporation takes place.

1.2211 Heat of vaporization of water is the amount of heat (540 calories) required to change 1 gram of liquid water to vapor.

1.2212 High vapor pressure of alcohol compounds produces rapid cooling of body surface.

1.2213 Rate of evaporation is related to environmental conditions.

1.22131 Humidity of room.

1.22132 Air currents and drafts.

1.22133 Vapor pressure of liquid.

1.222 Loss of body heat is mediated by circulation to body surface under nervous control.

1.2221 Heat loss by conduction results when one surface has a different temperature from that of the contacting surface.

1.2222 Rapid heat loss from body surface results in chilling, and shivering represents muscular work to restore warmth by increased circulation.

1.223 Evaporation of perspiration from body surface regulates heat loss.

1.2231 "Insensible" loss responds to variations in environmental temperature and humidity.

1.2232 Diaphoresis may occur with rapid lowering of elevated body temperature.

1.3 The body surface is an essential perceptual system, providing the individual with knowledge of his environment.
  1.31 Sensory nerve endings responding to touch and pressure assist in recognition of position.
  1.32 Response to temperature change and discrimination of hot and cold are accomplished by body surface.
  1.33 Pain perception safeguards the individual from environmental threat.
    1.331 Localized stimuli create a response that varies from mild discomfort to acute distress.
    1.332 Subjective discomfort of pain encourages withdrawal from source.
      1.3321 Localized stimuli may be counteracted by specific treatment or withdrawal.
      1.3322 Behavioral response includes restlessness and apprehension when source cannot be easily eliminated.
    1.333 Internal pain is often referred to areas on body surface.
  1.34 Sensory organs of smell-taste are integral parts of the perceptual apparatus of the oral cavity.
    1.341 Reception of stimuli by taste-smell end-organs presupposes functional nasal passages.
    1.342 Taste receptors function only when solutions of ingested substances are available.

1.4 The lips, mouth, and buccal cavity constitute a specialized body surface in contact with the external environment.
  1.41 Effective toilet by mucosa is dependent upon proper moisture.
  1.42 Teeth and gums offer harbor for microorganisms which are not readily accessible for cleansing.
  1.43 Contaminants are readily introduced by ingesting of food and during inspiration of air.
  1.44 Tissues of lips and mouth (including tongue) are highly sensitive to texture, shape, size, and temperature of local stimuli.

2. The integument reflects the condition of the internal environment.
  2.1 Adequate circulation to the body surface is essential for its nourishment and effective function.
    2.11 Localized impairment of circulation over pressure areas of the body results in death of tissues and decubitus ulcerations.
    2.12 Regional impairment of circulation threatens health of integument as well as other tissues.
      2.121 Control of temperature of immediate environment may exert marked influence on peripheral circulation.
      2.122 Positioning of limbs exerts influence on effectiveness of peripheral circulation.
      2.123 Reduced peripheral circulation predisposes to increased

difficulty in healing of even small injuries on the body surface.

2.2 Systemic disease processes are reflected in alterations of the quality and color of the skin and mucous membranes.

2.21 Alteration in body temperature is reflected on body surface.

2.211 Febrile condition is accompanied by flushing and local heat in some parts of the body, often in conjunction with cold sensation of extremities.

2.212 Low body temperature is usually accompanied by pale appearance with cold feel to skin.

2.22 Metabolic disturbances may be reflected in alteration of skin appearance.

2.221 Yellow discoloration accompanies jaundice.

2.2211 Variation in hue is related to cause and intensity of jaundice.

2.2212 Alteration also occurs in mucosa, as well as in sclera of eyes.

2.2213 Some forms are accompanied by intense itching with consequent danger of infection from scratching.

2.222 Variations in hemoglobin level may be reflected in alteration of skin color.

2.2221 Cyanosis is a late sign of inadequate oxygenation of hemoglobin.

2.2222 Perioral pallor and cyanosis around lips and at finger tips appear before general cyanosis occurs.

2.2223 Pallor usually indicates a vasoconstriction of local vessels at the body surface.

2.223 Alteration of turgidity of skin cells may reflect fluid imbalance.

2.2231 Dehydration is accompanied by loss of turgidity and dryness of skin surface.

2.2232 Edema at body surface increases friability of cells and predisposes to local damage from pressure and friction.

2.23 Allergic reactions, rashes, and skin manifestations are frequent in many disease entities.

2.231 Rashes that are itching and irritable must be treated to eliminate danger of spread of infection by scratching.

2.232 Some rashes are pathognomonic and characteristic of specific disease entities.

2.24 Appearance of the skin surface may be of intense importance to the individual.

2.241 Use of cosmetics to improve appearance is usual social practice.

2.242 Shaving of the male patient has cosmetic, as well as comfort, purpose.

2.243 Well-being is often identified in the appearance of the skin.

2.2431 Anguish of teen-ager with acne.

2.2432 Folk ideas associate skin blemishes with "social" diseases.

2.244 Local skin blemishes represent entry sites for microorganisms.

2.245 Age of individual affects the health and appearance of the skin.

2.25 Appearance of appendages (hair, nails) is often altered during illness.

2.251 Even normal hair loss presents sanitary problem, be-because hair is grossly contaminated.

2.252 Accumulation of dirt under nails provides protection for microorganisms.

2.253 Hair loss may become marked in some disease conditions, and is enhanced by poor hygiene.

2.26 Disease process may be accompanied by unpleasant odors arising from body surface or orifices.

3. The hygienic care of accessible parts of the body surface is related to social and cultural expectations.

3.1 Personal cleanliness has a social goal.

3.11 Scrubbed, deodorized appearance is valued in the social milieu of modern middle-class cultures.

3.12 Social determinants of frequency of bathing and use of cosmetic aids vary from one cultural group to another.

3.2 Personal cleanliness has individualized meaning for every patient.

3.21 Comfort and relaxation of cleanliness may be important to sense of well-being.

3.22 During acute and serious illness, effort to maintain social appearance may be secondary to energy mustered to fight illness.

3.23 The nurse brings her own value systems related to personal hygiene practice to the bedside.

3.231 Censure is often directed at individuals who are perceived as practicing poor personal hygiene.

3.232 Individual's image of himself may include hair style and cosmetic effects that are disquieting to the nurse.

3.3 The technological artifacts in every culture influence its hygienic practice.

3.31 Availability of cleansing devices.

3.311 Cleansing is accomplished by mechanical removal of skin debris and contaminants.

3.312 Soaps and detergents lower surface tension and emulsify fatty substances so that removal is expedited.

3.3121 All soaps tend to be drying to skin surface because of removal of normal skin oils.

3.3122 Soaps are foreign to skin and must be completely removed by adequate rinsing.

3.313 Tools to assist cleansing are designed to expedite frictional removal of surface contaminants.

3.3131 Washcloths and towels have surface allowing for mechanical scrubbing.

3.3132 Brushes are used for teeth, hair, and nails.

3.32 Use of cosmetics, deodorants, powders, and perfumes reflects the age, sex, cultural background, and habits of the individual patient.

4. Dependency on others for performance of personal hygiene presupposes a psychological regression in the adult.

4.1 Social restriction demands privacy during performance of personal hygiene activities.

4.11 Exposure of parts of the body is forbidden so that embarrassment is compounded by guilt.

4.12 Individual's responsibility for his personal cleanliness is related to his concept of "self" and his independence.

4.2 Pathophysiological determinants restrict participation to individual's ability to spend energy in hygienic activities.

4.21 Bathing in bed requires stretching and reaching against gravity in a supine position.

4.22 Use of tub or shower may require assistance in ambulating and mobilizing individual.

4.23 Sequelae of disease process limit active participation.

4.231 Dependency may be associated with anxiety when weakness prevents full participation by individual.

4.232 Safe expense of energy demands that physical need be given precedence over emotional need.

4.233 Restoration of independence is measured against rate of convalescence.

NURSING PROCESS

1. Personal hygiene provisions for the individual create a clean environment in the hospital milieu for all patients.

1.1 Control of the total microbial population is exercised through control of individual patient areas.

1.11 All equipment and materials with which individual comes into contact constitute extensions of area of individual contamination.

1.12 Symbiotic bacterial relationships vary from one individual to another, necessitating restriction of organisms to their willing host.

1.2 Patient safety demands that cross-contamination within the hospital environment be absolutely prevented.

1.21 Microorganisms inhabit all available sites on the body surface, including hair and nails.

1.211 Absolute exclusion of organisms requires extensive technical means, but restriction is accomplished by cleanliness.

1.212 The nurse may become a vector for transmission of disease unless personal techniques are precise and unfailing.

1.22 The hospitalized patient struggles with his own pathophysiology.

1.221 Introduction of superimposed infection or disease interferes with the individual's response to initial problems.

1.222 Prevention of superimposed infection in some disease entities is crucial because of limited healing and defense potential.

1.223 Superimposed, hospital-induced disease prolongs hospitalization and expense, as well as threatening the ultimate well-being of the individual.

2. Personal hygiene activities protect the integrity of the integument and related structures.

2.1 Prevention of injury or insult to the skin preserves its natural defense against encroachment by microorganisms..

2.2 Maintenance of circulation to all areas of body surface assures local nutrition and health of cells.

2.21 Positioning and postural maintenance prevent development of localized pressure areas.

2.22 Massage techniques enhance local circulation.

2.221 Movement in direction of venous flow (towards the heart) stimulates circulation.

2.222 Control of local pressure depends on use of lubricant or powder to limit friction.

2.223 Back rub is effective when area becomes faintly flushed.

2.224 Massage may be restricted when occlusive disease of circulation is present.

2.3 Confinement to bed requires a contact surface area free of irritants, wrinkles, and moisture to minimize local damage to skin suface.

3. Personal hygiene affords the individual patient comfort and well-being.

3.1 Specific attention to personal needs is reassuring and promotes security for the individual patient.

3.2 Physiological effect of cleansing and massage promotes physical well-being.

3.3 Cleanliness of mouth enhances ability and willingness to take foods and fluids.

3.4 "Social acceptability" is assured the individual within the social structure of the hospital ward.

4. Personal hygiene routines allow a structured and planned resumption of independent activity for the individual patient.

4.1 Decision as to type of bath provided is dependent upon the individual patient's physical condition.

4.11 Complete assistance by the nurse is required when individual's illness requires absolute limitation of physical activity.

4.111 Activity paced to patient's tolerance.

4.112 Privacy respected by draping routine.

4.113 Safety of individual rests with nurse.

4.1131 Prevention of chilling by washing of limited areas at a time.

4.1132 Bath water temperature kept at 100 to 105°F.

4.1133 Side rails in place when nurse leaves bedside.

4.1134 Assist with moving patient as required.

4.1135 Stable position of patient when change is required for bathing activities.

4.12 Sufficient assistance to adequately support individual who is being placed in a tub.

4.121 Absolute cleanliness of areas shared by other patients.

4.122 Environmental conditions controlled, including warmth of tub room.

4.123 Tub and bath mats available to minimize danger of slipping on wet surfaces.

4.124 Provision for personal privacy, including use of loin cloths during bathing.

4.125 Sufficient assistance to assure safe entry and removal from tub.

4.126 Patient is never left alone in tub room.

4.13 Repetition of partial bathing throughout the 24-hour period as required by patient's needs.

4.2 Individual is allowed to help himself as his condition warrants.

4.21 Self-help during bathing serves the patient's interests, not the nurse's.

4.211 Individual should not be allowed to do more than he can safely do for himself.

4.212 Materials brought to bedside placed in easy access to the patient to prevent overreaching and danger of falling.

4.22 Returning interest in appearance indicates positive aspects of convalescence.

4.221 Complete grooming, including hair and nail care, provided or supervised by nurse.

4.222 Materials required for shaving male patient made available.

4.223 Cosmetics available for female patient in accord with individual desires.

4.23 Back care and massage offered all patients who are restricted to bed for any length of time.

4.24 Nurse determines whether or not patient has succeeded in performing adequate hygienic care for himself.

4.25 Provision for handwashing and oral hygiene before meals for all patients.

5. Personal hygiene routines allow for meaningful nurse-patient interactions.

5.1 Time of nurse-patient contact allows for adequate and sound observation of patient's response to illness and therapy.

5.11 Opportunity provided to assess patient's personality and response to ward interactions as a basis for assessing his progress.

5.12 Problems which may be referred to other hospital personnel may be elicited.

5.13 Continuity of care from day to day provides only meaningful base for assessing progress.

5.14 Permits personalized attention in an aura of depersonalized routine.

5.2 Communication of information and observations by written and oral statements to other ward personnel assures continuity of care.

5.21 Focus of attention on the specific needs of the individual patient.

5.22 Cooperative effort to meet problems of individual becomes possible.

5.23 Legal record and accumulation of knowledge assured when charting is relevant and pertinent to individual's needs.

Vocabulary

acidosis
adenohypophysis
adrenocorticotrophic
carbohydrates
chemical mediators
complications
concomitants
corticosteroids
diabetes mellitus
diabetogenic
endocrine
glucagon
glucocorticoids
glycogenesis
glycogen
glycogenolysis
hormones
insulin
internal secretion
islands of Langerhans
ketogenic
ketones
ketosis
learning
lipids
master glands
maturity-onset diabetes
mineralocorticoids
peripheral vascular
polydypsia
polyphagia
polyuria
proteins
secretions
servomechanism
target glands
teaching
youth-onset diabetes

General Bibliography

DANOWSKI, T. A.: Diabetes Mellitus. Williams and Wilkins Co., Baltimore, 1957.

JOSLIN, E., ET AL.: Treatment of Diabetes Mellitus. Lea and Febiger, Philadelphia, 1959.

KIRA, ALEXANDER: The Bathroom: Criteria for Design. Bantam Books, New York, 1967.

LEVINE, RACHMIEL: Diabetes Mellitus, Clinical Symposia. Ciba Pharmaceutical Co., Summit, N.J., 1963.

MARKOWITZ, AARON, ED.: Essentials of Dental Health for Nurses, ed. 2. Council on Hospital Dental Services, New Jersey State Dental Society, 1961.

PYKE, D. A., ED.: Disorders of Carbohydrate Metabolism. J. B. Lippincott Co., Philadelphia, 1962.

WILLIAMS, ROBERT H.: Textbook of Endocrinology, ed. 3. W. B. Saunders Co., Philadelphia, 1962.

Articles

CAHN, MILTON M.: The skin from infancy to old age. Amer. J. Nurs. 60:993-996, July 1960.

DAVIDSON, ERIC H.: Hormones and genes. Sci. Amer. 212:36-45, June 1965.

KRYSON, GERMAINE S.: How do we teach four million diabetics? Amer. J. Nurs. 65:105-107, Nov. 1965.

LOCKE, RAYMOND K.: Foot care for diabetics. Amer. J. Nurs. 63:107-110, Nov. 1963.

MARTIN, MARGUERITE: Diabetes mellitus: Current concepts. Amer. J. Nurs. 66:510-514, March 1966.

MARTIN, MARGUERITE: Insulin reactions. Amer. J. Nurs. 67:328-331, Feb. 1967.

MONTAGNA, WILLIAM: The skin. Sci. Amer. 212:56-66, Feb. 1965.

RUSHMER, ROBERT F., ET AL.: The skin. Science 154:343-348, Oct. 1966.

TASSMAN, GUSTAV, ZAYON, GILBERT, AND ZAFRAN, JACK: When patients cannot brush their teeth. Amer. J. Nurs. 63:94-97, Feb. 1963.

TAYLOR, JOHN C.: Decubitus ulcers. Nurs. Sci. 2:293-309, Aug. 1964.

4 Nursing the Patient with a Disturbance of Homeostasis: Fluid and Electrolyte Imbalance

Body Water as an Integrating Factor in the Internal Environment

While the nervous and hormonal systems exercise an integrative function that allows the body to adapt to a wide variety of circumstances, there is another functional system without which no physiological activity would be possible. This is the body water, a vital constituent within cells, and an indispensable constituent of the environment of each and every one of the 100 trillion cells that make up the body structure. Every cell is a dynamic and living system, constantly at work to maintain its specific function in tune with the functions of its neighbors, both far and near. The work of the cell is biochemical and therefore also electrochemical; its orderly function depends upon a milieu wherein a vast multitude of complex chemical reactions must proceed quickly and effectively. One of the truly miraculous facts about life is that extremely complicated chemical reactions take place in a lukewarm, mildly saline, slightly alkaline but complex aqueous solution in a totally dark environment. The chemical exchanges are the stuff of life itself, but none of them could take place without the constancy of a water supply to form the solvent within which the biochemistry of living goes forward.

Water is the remarkable substance which, in a real and poetic sense, makes life itself possible. It has the quality of unusual stability among chemical compounds; without water, life as it is known on earth could never have evolved. A people well supplied with water is fortunate indeed, and great political and social issues are created whenever the supply of water is endangered, restricted, or contested. Water is called a universal solvent, because more substances can be dissolved in it to some degree than in any other solvent known. The stability and unity of the physical properties of water serve as the basis for measurement of the physical properties of all other substances. It is the standard for measurement of mass: 1 gm. = mass of 1 ml. of water at 4°C. It is the unit of measurement of temperature: 0°C = freezing point of water; 100°C = boiling point of water. It is also the basis for the measurement of heat quantity: the amount of heat necessary to raise the temperature of 1 gm. of water 1°C = 1 calorie. And in addition, it is the basis for measurement of thermal capacity and specific heat. The specific heat of water is 1.0, so that the heat capacity of other substances is sometimes called the "water equivalent" of those substances. Water is used to assess the larger environment of the world as a whole, as well as the smaller universe within the confines of the human body.

Water molecules often become involved in complex ways in the chemical reactions which occur when substances are dissolved in it, but in the vast number of chemical reactions, water is not changed. When substances that are dissolved in water are removed from it, the water itself remains unchanged. Water ionizes only slightly under ordinary conditions, and yet the ionization of electrolytes can take place only in an aqueous solution. The chemical reactions involving electrolytes also require an aqueous solution because chemical reaction is virtually zero unless electrolytes are ionized. As a solvent, water is indispensable to life. The chemistry of metabolism depends upon the properties of water, including its ability to hold in solution the substances which are the vital contributors to metabolic activity.

Water as the Medium for Membrane Transport

In considering the fluid requirements of the body, the essential structural design consists of the vast membrane surface of its 100 trillion cells. That membrane is a limiting one, which must retain certain body constituents and never lose them, while allowing free passage in and out of the cell of many other substances. The dynamics of movement of substances across the cellular membrane establish the rules by which body fluid is utilized for the processes of life.

The membrane is limiting, but not entirely so; it is therefore considered to be semipermeable. The exact mechanics of the ability of the membrane to selectively allow passage through its walls is not understood. Theoretical models, however, seem to be substantiated by electron micrographs, although no picture is yet available which clearly establishes the nature of the cell membrane. The membrane is thought to be composed of a complex and architecturally precise arrangement of lipids in a protein matrix. Its thickness is so unbelievably tiny that measuring it requires a scale based on one ten-millionth part of a millimeter—the Angstrom unit. The thickness of the cellular membrane is 70 to 85 Å. This does not seem a formidable distance to traverse, but a water molecule has a

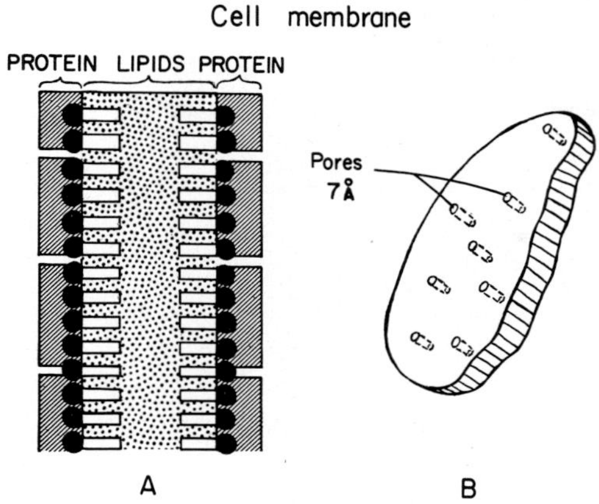

FIGURE 30. (A) The postulated molecular organization of the cell membrane shows the protein and lipid matrix through which all substances must pass to enter or leave the cell. (B) The presence of "pores" in the membrane have never been demonstrated by even the most remarkable electron micrographs, but the cell behaves as if it had such pores. (From Guyton, A.C.: *Textbook of Medical Physiology,* 3rd ed. W.B. Saunders Co., Philadelphia, 1966.)

diameter of 3 Å, while that of a glucose molecule is 8.4 Å. The lipoprotein constituents of the membrane tend to exclude all substances which are not fat-soluble, although it is well known that water and other molecules of its relative size pass freely through the cell membrane, whereas glucose does not. Since small molecules, including water, do pass through the semipermeable membrane, it is postulated that the membrane contains "pores" (although these have not yet been demonstrable by electron micrograph). The pores are probably about 8 Å in diameter, since all molecules larger than this are not freely diffusible through the membrane unless they are fat-soluble. The rapidity with which fat-soluble substances are carried through the membrane is demonstrated by the immediate effectiveness of general anesthetics, most of which are fat-soluble and therefore promptly absorbed through the lipid portion of the cell membrane.

The random passage of water molecules through the pores of the membrane is characteristic of osmosis. All molecules are in constant motion, and it is inevitable that some of the moving water molecules will approach the membrane at the site of a pore so that they will move through the opening. In simple diffusion, i.e., in the absence of any limiting membrane, the distribution of all the molecules in the solution ultimately becomes equalized throughout the solution. If a concentrated solution of salt is poured into a beaker of pure water, diffusion alone explains the fact that the salt molecules are distributed evenly throughout the beaker in a

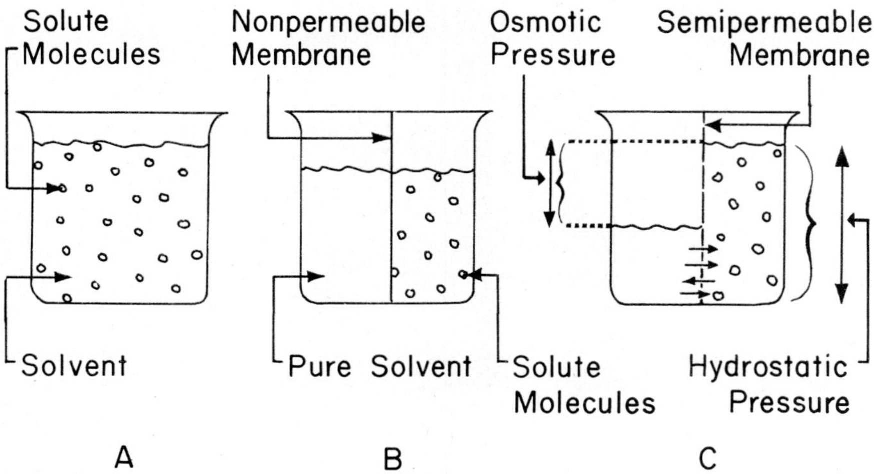

FIGURE 31. Schematic representation of the movement of the molecules dissolved in water. (A) The movement of the solute molecules themselves assures dispersion throughout the solution when no limiting membranes intervene. (B) If an absolutely limiting membrane intervenes, there is no movement of any molecules from one side of the container to the other. (C) When the membrane is semipermeable, water molecules move through the membrane, while the solute molecules do not. A status quo is finally attained when the osmotic pressure and the hydrostatic pressure reach a balance.

very short time. If, however, a limiting (semipermeable) membrane is placed in the beaker, separating the salt solution from the pure water, then the freedom of movement of the water molecules is somewhat restricted. Some water molecules will reach the membrane at a site where a pore will allow passage through it, and some will not. Many more water molecules will hit the membrane on the side where there is only pure water than on the side where the water molecules are sharing the space with the salt particles. Water molecules may pass through the membrane from either side, but, because of the advantage of sheer numbers, and therefore the number of actual contacts with the membrane, more of the water molecules will pass *from* the pure water side into the salt side than in the opposite direction. Eventually an equilibrium will be reached. As the water molecules move to the salt side, the level of the salt solution will rise, and it continues to do so until the hydrostatic pressure (arising from the weight of the column of fluid) is balanced by the osmotic pressure (the difference between the heights of the two fluid columns in the system). The movement of water molecules through the membrane from both sides continues, but the relative pressures create a status quo which maintains the pressure relationships. In osmosis, the direction of movement of water across a limiting membrane is always greatest from the region of lower concentration to the region of higher concentration. Absolute equalization of concentrations cannot occur as long as the membrane does not permit passage of the solute particles. Equalization, therefore, implies the condition which results when the osmotic pressure and hydrostatic pressure are in balance, rather than a sharing of the same number of all kinds of molecules involved in the transaction.

The movement of molecules through a semipermeable membrane is dependent on the number of particles that hit the membrane and on whether or not they are small enough particles to pass through a pore in the membrane. Thus, their *size* limits their passage through the pore, and their *number* determines how many will hit the membrane. Their nature and chemical properties are immaterial. If the particle is small enough to pass through the pores of a semipermeable membrane, it is called "diffusible." If it is too large to pass through, it is called "nondiffusible." But the number of particles in the solution determines the osmotic pressure. If a particle is nondiffusible, its size makes no difference. Both glucose and albumin are too large to pass through the pores of a semipermeable membrane. Their influence on osmosis depends entirely on the number of albumin molecules or the number of glucose molecules in the solution. A simple percentage statement of the strength of a solution, i.e., how much solute in the solvent, does not indicate the number of particles in the solution. A 5% glucose solution, or a 5% albumin solution, simply states that there are 5 parts of each of these substances for every 100 parts of the solution. There is, however, a way to determine how many particles are present, and therefore how much osmotic pressure each of these solutions can exert. The chemist knows that chemical reactivity takes place in *whole units.* In the age of atom-splitting, it is still a fact that a chemical reaction takes place between whole atoms or whole molecules. Therefore, the chemist describes the reactivity of a substance by expressing its molecular weight in grams. The gram molecular weight of glucose is 180 gm., whereas that of albumin is 70,000 gm. But the gram molecular weight of *any* substance contains the same *number* of particles as the gram molecular weight of any other substance. That number is called Avogadro's constant. The gram molecular weight of every substance contains 6.023×10^{23} molecules. The number of particles in 180 gm. of glucose and in 70,000 gm. of albumin is the same; therefore, the osmotic pressure exerted by a gram molecular weight of each of these substances, dissolved in the same volume of water and at the same temperature, will be the same.

Although both glucose and albumin are nonelectrolytes, many substances dissociate into ions when they go into solution. One gram molecular weight of sodium chloride is 58.5 gm. But, in an aqueous solution, sodium chloride dissociates into two particles: a postively charged Na^+ ion and a negatively charged Cl^- ion. A gram molecular weight of this electrolyte, then, provides twice the number of particles that might be expected from its molecular weight alone. The osmotic pressure exerted by a gram molecular weight of NaCl is therefore twice that exerted by a gram molecular weight of either glucose or albumin.

During osmosis, it is the solvent molecules that pass through the semipermeable membrane, and in the body the solvent is always water. Some of the water is always *held* on the side of the membrane that contains the solute. When the solute is a nondiffusible substance, such as albumin, it holds water very effectively. This is a critical mechanism in maintaining the distribution of water in the body. Albumin and other protein substances are found within the cells and within the closed vascular system of the circulation. The ability of these proteins to hold the water in which they are dissolved serves to stabilize the relative volume of water in the cells and in the circulatory system. The body water on the outside of the membranes of the cells and blood vessels (the interstitial water) contains little protein under normal conditions. In fact, the body has an effective means of promptly removing any proteins which might spill into the interstitial body water. The lymphatic system constantly removes protein and returns it to the vascular system. The ability of the proteins to hold water is given a special name: the colloid osmotic pressure, or the oncotic pressure. The oncotic pressure is that osmotic pressure which is created by the retention of water because of its dissolved proteins. In disease conditions in which protein is spilled into the interstitial compartments, a threatening redistribution of body water occurs, and this seriously interferes with metabolic function.

Active Transport: Energy-Utilizing Systems for Membrane Passage

Glucose is too large a molecule to pass through the semipermeable membrane, and yet glucose does enter the cell. In fact, many nondiffusible substances must enter the cell in order to keep it nourished and operative. The precise mechanisms whereby this is accomplished have not been definitively proved. But it is apparent that the passage through the membrane of such substances requires some system which actively (that is, through the use of energy) carries them through the membrane. The expense of energy indicates that a chemical change takes place at the membrane surface. Mediated by enzymes (organic catalysts), the substances are changed into compounds which enter the outer surface of the membrane, pass through the membrane, and change at the inner surface of the membrane to be deposited inside the cell. Thus, a needed substance is carried through the membrane by changing it into a substance that can be dissolved in the lipoprotein matrix, and then, when it is inside, restoring it to its original form for use by the cell. The "carrier" substance is freed of its burden at the inner surface of the membrane and can return once more through the membrane to pick up another "load" at the outer surface for transport into the cell. There is some evidence that insulin is the "carrier" for glucose into the cell. This process, active transport, makes available to the cells substances they cannot receive by osmosis alone, but it is a system requiring energy utilization by the cell. The passive movement of water through the pores does not demand the use of energy by the cell; however, very few substances are small enough to enter and leave the cell in this passive way.

There is a second function of active transport that influences the kinds of substances brought into and out of the cell. Osmosis represents the movement of water molecules across a semipermeable membrane from a site of lowered concentration to one with a higher concentration of the solute. But there is a movement of materials in and out of cells which defies this concentration gradient. The concentration of Na^+ ion outside of the cell is much higher than its concentration inside the cell. Conversely, the concentration of K^+ ion inside the cells is much higher than its concentration outside the cell. The movement of the vitally needed K^+

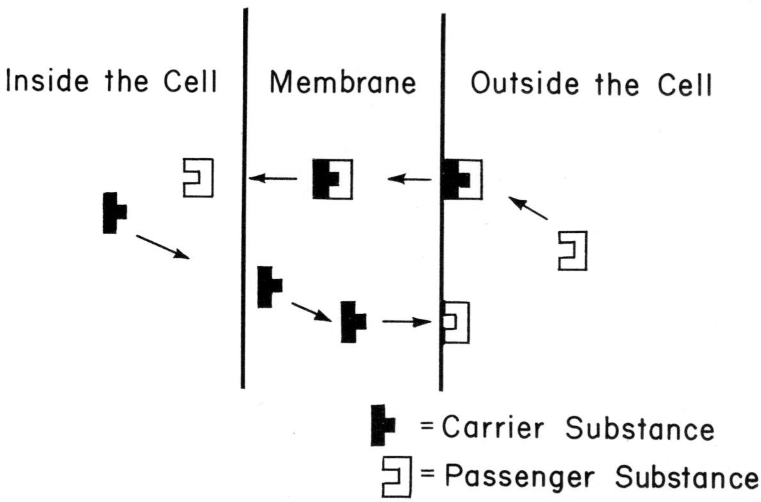

FIGURE 32. Schematic representation of active transport. A "carrier" substance combines with the otherwise nondiffusible particle at the cell membrane, carries the particle through the membrane, and then deposits it within the cell, returning through the membrane to pick up another passenger.

ion into the cell would not be possible by a simple osmotic exchange against the high concentration gradient of the ion already within the cell membrane. However, movement of K^+ ion into the cell and of Na^+ ion out of the cell does, in fact, occur. This interaction requires a complex carrier system involving both ions, against the concentration gradients. This system is sometimes called the sodium pump.

Fluid and Electrolyte Balance: A Single Problem

The fluid needs of the organism cannot be understood without also recognizing the influence of the solutes dissolved in the body water. The movement of water in and out of the cells is entirely dependent upon the concentrations of its dissolved substances. Water and electrolyte balance are therefore dimensions of the same problem. The normal range of concentration of substances within the limits of homeostasis is, in most instances, a very narrow range indeed. Disturbances in the fluid distribution in the body are always accompanied by shifts in electrolyte distribution, and since the homeostatic limits are very precise, such a shift may create symptoms of great urgency in the individual.

Recognition of the range permissible for continuing well-being requires that the biochemical importance of the dissolved substances be understood. The quantification—the question of "how much"—of essential body chemicals is a measure, not only of their concentrations, but also of the availability of these substances to enter into essential physiological processes. Nondiffusible nonelectrolytes such as glucose can be measured by the usual weight-per-volume relationships that describe the concentration of the solute in the solvent. The gram molecular weight of any substance is called a *mol*. Since the gram molecular weight of glucose is 180 gm., one mol of glucose is 180 gm. However, this is a rather large quantity of glucose, and most of the concentrations of substances in the body are actually very small quantities. It is therefore common to use a smaller unit of measure, the millimol, instead. The millimol is 1/1000 of a mol; thus, a millimol of glucose would consist of 180 mg. of the substance. Millimols are the units of measurement for nondiffusible nonelectrolytes in the body fluids. The millimol, of course, represents 1/1000 of the number of particles specified by Avogadro's number and indicates the number of units (or particles) of that substance available to enter into chemical reactions.

Unlike the nondiffusible nonelectrolytes, substances that dissociate into charged ions in solution cannot be measured in millimols, because there are more particles available in the solution, and each particle is capable of entering a chemical reaction. The gram molecular weight of

NaC1 is 23 + 35.5 = 58.5 gm. = 1 mol of NaC1. In solution, however, NaC1 becomes Na^+ ions and $C1^-$ ions. A mol of Na^+ ion is equivalent to 23 gm., whereas a mol of $C1^-$ ion is equivalent to 35.5 gm. Because each of these ions is available to enter chemical reactions in the body, they are, in fact, measured in *equivalents* rather than in mols. The equivalent of the ion is equal to its atomic weight divided by its valence. Since the valence of each of these ions is 1 (positive or negative), each has an equivalent equal to its atomic weight. When the substance is univalent, the equivalent is equal to a mol. Because the quantities in the body are so small, equivalents are also expressed as 1/1000 of a mol, and such a unit is then called a milliequivalent, or mEq. It is therefore correct to say that a mEq. of Na^+ ion is 23 mg. and a mEq. of $C1^-$ ion is 35.5 mg. It is apparent that one milliequivalent of Na^+ ion is available to react with one milliequivalent of $C1^-$ ion, and this is a meaningful description of their chemical potential. It is much more meaningful than to say that there are 23 mg. of Na^+ ion and 35.5 mg. of $C1^-$ ion, because, on the face of the figures alone, this does not immediately indicate a chemical balance of 1:1.

If a laboratory report indicates 140 mEq. of Na^+ ion and 103 mEq. of $C1^-$ ion in the blood, this signifies at once that there are 37 mEq. of Na^+ ion available to react with other negatively charged ions. This same

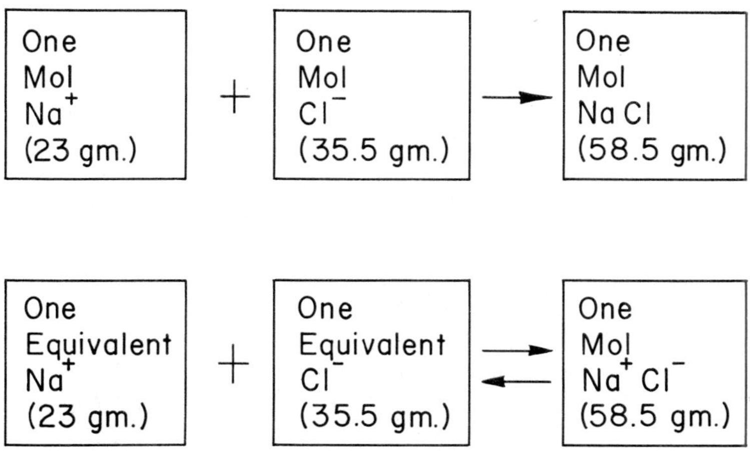

FIGURE 33. Since particles of matter react as *whole* units, one mol of Na^+ ion, although weighing 23 gm., reacts with one mol of $C1^-$ ion which weighs 35.5 gm. An equivalent is thus a description of the whole units available to enter a chemical reaction. In the body, such small amounts are involved that they are described as millimols or milliequivalents, or 1/1000 of the gram molecular weight. Thus, an equivalent of Na^+ ion and an equivalent of $C1^-$ ion form a mol of NaC1, and when this substance dissociates, it yields an equivalent of each of its component substances.

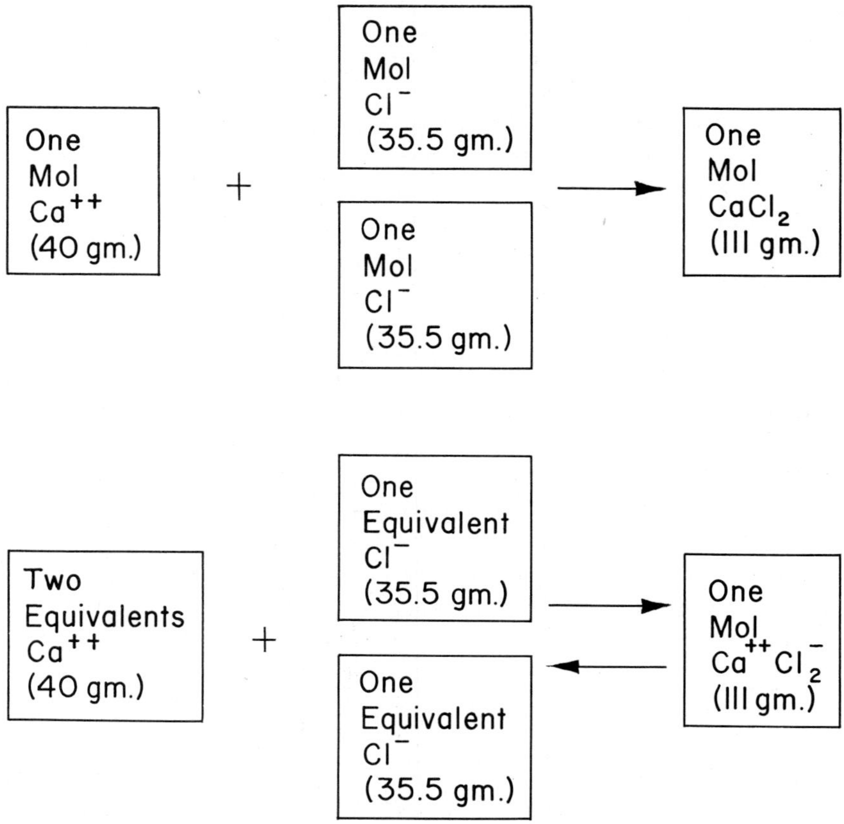

FIGURE 34. A substance with a valence of two, such as Ca^{++} ion, requires two equivalents of a univalent substance, such as Cl^- ion, to form a molecule such as $CaCl_2$. Thus, when $CaCl_2$ dissociates, it provides *two* equivalents of Ca^{++} ion and two equivalents of Cl^- ion. A mol of Ca^{++} ion is therefore equal to two equivalents of Ca^{++}—and an equivalent of Ca^{++} ion weighs 20 gm.

relationship expressed in milligrams would be very misleading, because the equivalents represent 3220 mg. of Na^+ ion and 3456.5 mg. of Cl^- ion.

The use of milliequivalents as measures of electrolyte concentration serves two purposes. It indicates the concentration per unit volume of electrolytes in the body fluids by consideration of the number of particles in solution, thereby reflecting the effect of these substances on the osmotic equilibria in the body. It also indicates the number of ions available to enter into chemical reactions, a factor of tremendous importance, for example, when assessment of acid-base balance of the blood is vital in determining therapy for the patient.

Electrolytes and Acid-Base Balance

One of the wondrous properties of water is that it is composed of H^+ ion and OH^- ion, both associated with the traditional definitions of acids and bases. New knowledge has made this terminology of more academic interest than practical value, but this characteristic of water remains of fundamental importance.

It is improbable that the hydrogen ion, as designated by the symbol H^+, ever exists in that state. As such, it represents an atomic nucleus with a positive charge of one, and this, of course, is the proton. Ionization of pure water under usual conditions is very slight indeed, but, when the biochemist talks about H^+ ion in water, he is understood to mean H_3O^+, the hydronium ion. In any event, the presence of the proton, H^+, has long been the important criterion in the description of acids. By the same token, the hydroxyl ion OH^-, was identified as the essential constituent of bases. From the viewpoint of the biochemist and the biologist, the regulatory mechanisms that establish homeostasis in the internal environment are centered on the concentration of the hydronium ion. The importance of this regulatory function cannot be overemphasized, because the hydronium ion concentration in the body fluids establishes the environment in which all of the biochemical activity of the body takes place. An alteration towards either extreme in the homeostatic range produces dire symptoms which must be reversed if the individual is to survive.

The identification of the hydrogen ion balance is very difficult in living tissues because the ion is rarely, if ever, available in a "free" condition; it is always bound into numerous different compounds, many of them undergoing the change of metabolic processes. The normally acid urine, for example, has a relatively high hydrogen ion concentration, but much more hydrogen ion is excreted in the urine tied up in ammonium salts. Furthermore, the presence of free hydrogen ion presupposes an acid environment, and, except for the gastric juices and the urine, the body tissues are bathed in a slightly alkaline fluid. The extremely minute amounts of free hydrogen in the body fluids present an additional problem in that expressing such amounts in numerical values results in a cumbersome figure.

The very slight ionization of water, for example, results in a hydrogen ion concentration of 1/10,000,000 grams per liter. This may also be written: 1×10^{-7} grams per liter. The concentration of OH^- ion is also 1×10^{-7}. In 1909, Sörenson proposed a less cumbersome method for expressing the hydrogen ion concentration. Using a negative logarithm, the concentration of the hydrogen ion in equivalents per liter is called the pH. A pH of 7 indicates neutrality, because it describes a concentration of hydrogen ions exactly equal to a concentration of hydroxyl ions. A pH of less than 7 indicates the presence of more hydrogen ions than hydroxyl ions and therefore a solution that is acid, whereas a pH above 7 indicates a basic solution because it contains more hydroxyl than hydrogen ions. Thus, as the value of the pH goes down, the hydrogen ion concentration goes up, and vice versa. The pH, in other words, describes an inverse relationship. However, the difficulty in the use of the pH is even more disconcerting, inasmuch as a variation in the value does not indicate the actual change in concentration that is taking place. For example, if the pH of a solution falls from 7.4 to 7.1, the hydrogen ion concentration has actually doubled. The apparent difference of 0.3 in the reading of the pH is therefore deceptive, because the actual change is a remarkable one, even though the measurement reflects only a slight change.

Instead of using pH, some investigators are now expressing hydrogen ion concentration in millimicroequivalents. (The milliequivalent = 1/1000 of an equivalent. The millimicroequivalent is 1/1000 of a milliequivalent, or 1/1,000,000 of an equivalent.) A pH of 7.4 is equal to 40 millimicroequivalents. The normal range of the pH of the blood is from 7.44 to 7.36. By sheer coincidence, the pH of 7.44 is equal to 36 millimicroequivalents and the pH of 7.36 is equal to 44 millimicroequivalents. The range from 36 to 44 millimicroequivalents, however, represents a range of some 20% increase in hydrogen ion concentration, and in the homeostatic balance of the body a 20% difference may be quite significant. This extremely limited concentration of hydrogen ion in the body fluids is maintained at this level by remarkably effective systems. Some of the hydrogen ion is excreted in the urine, and obviously removal of the acid-forming ion will aid in keeping its concentration in the body fluids very low. But, in addition to removal, the body is also capable of neutralizing the hydrogen ion in a number of chemical relationships that are very effective in maintaining this extremely fine balance of hydrogen ion concentration.

The language of science, like all communication of ideas, must change in response to knowledge that clarifies and modifies previous concepts. There is obvious difficulty in dealing with the concepts of acid-base balance, but all of it is related to the evolution of understanding through modern scientific explorations. The acid radical was quickly identified as the hydrogen ion. This, in turn, soon became the hydronium ion (H_3O^+). Some writers refer to it as the hydrion ion. Regardless of how the functional unit is named, all agree that it is structurally a *proton*. Use of this terminology allows understanding of the dynamics of acid-base relationships. A substance which possesses a proton, and can therefore contribute a proton to a chemical reaction, is called a proton-donor. Acids are proton-donors. There is no problem in applying this concept to substances recognizable in other chemical properties as acids. Hydrochloric acid dissociates and donates a proton as follows:

$$HCl \longrightarrow H^+ + Cl^-$$

By the same token, water is also a proton-donor:

$$H_2O \longrightarrow H^+ + OH^-$$

However, some substances that have never been identified as acids and possess none of the "classical" properties of acids are also clearly proton-donors:

$$NH_4^+ \longrightarrow NH_3 + H^+$$

Of course, if a substance can donate a proton, there must be other substances that will accept a proton in a chemical exchange. These proton-acceptors are bases. A proton-donor must possess a proton in order to provide one, whereas a proton-acceptor must have a negative charge in order to accept a proton. In the dissociation of water and ammonium ion, the arrow can (and should) point both ways.

$$H_2O \rightleftarrows H^+ + OH^-$$
$$NH_4^+ \rightleftarrows NH_3 + H^+$$

Written in this way, water is both an acid and a base because it is capable of either donating or accepting a proton. It is therefore called amphoteric. The dissociation of the ammonium ion also demonstrates the donation or acceptance of a proton, and, although the reaction to the left (to form NH_4^+) can occur only with difficulty in the laboratory, it is an essential reaction, mediated by enzymes, in the formation of urine in the body. The ability of a single substance to either donate or accept a proton makes it very talented indeed in a chemical reaction. When the proton must be "freed," i.e., donated, the substance is capable of doing so. And when the proton must be "tied up," i.e., accepted, the substance is equally capable of doing that. This capacity to make a chemical "choice" is the essence of the "buffer." A buffer system, involving two or more substances which interact by exchanging a proton, can control the concentration of protons by freeing them when necessary or tying them into a chemical compound when necessary. The mechanisms that maintain the proton concentration in body fluids are buffer systems.

The body fluid most accessible for study is the blood, and the concentrations of electrolytes that appear in laboratory reports are invariably measurements of blood levels. It is far more difficult to obtain samples of the interstitial or intracellular body fluids, but buffering systems are operative there as well as in the blood. The buffer systems, measured at blood levels, are fast-acting chemical systems that control proton concentrations. They represent a first line of response to alterations in the proton concentrations, and the rapidity of their action assures a fine control that stabilizes the proton levels within the homeostatic range. A radical alteration of proton concentration, however, quickly overwhelms the blood buffer systems. The second line of defense rests with the excretion of carbon dioxide through the respiratory system, which acts as a physiological buffer system, and can actually handle twice as much proton concentration as all of the chemical systems combined, but at a slower rate. The third defense rests with the kidneys, which can excrete the excess proton by a variety of mechanisms, all of them very effective. This process, however, is relatively slow.

The most reactive chemical system in the blood is the bicarbonate system:

$$H_2CO_3 \rightleftarrows H^+ + HCO_3^-$$

Carbonic acid (H_2CO_3) is degraded into CO_2 and water in the completed metabolic process. The bicarbonate system demonstrates how interrelated the control mechanisms are that sustain proton balance, because its efficiency is enhanced by respiratory regulation of CO_2 and kidney regulation of HCO_3^-. In the intact and healthy organism, this interaction is an essential factor in maintaining proton concentration in millimicroequivalents. Its importance is also reflected in clinical measurements of acid-base balance. The measure of Na^+ ion in milliequivalents above and beyond that required to balance $C1^-$ ion in milliequivalents is called the "alkali reserve," because it is assumed that the excess Na^+ ion is available to bind the HCO_3^- ion in the blood.

The phosphate buffer system in the blood is considerably less powerful than the bicarbonate system, but it may be a vital intracellular buffer since the phosphate ion is an essential intracellular ion. The principal elements of the phosphate system are sodium acid phosphate, NaH_2PO_4, which can donate a proton, and disodium phosphate, Na_2HPO_4, which can accept a proton.

The proteins of the blood also act as buffer systems and, because they are so plentiful, they constitute an important system. Proteins are amphoteric inasmuch as they contain the organic acid radical, —COOH, which can donate a proton, and the amine radical, $—NH_2$, which can accept a proton. The protein buffer system is also undoubtedly important inside the cell as well. The most effective buffer action in the blood, however, takes place in the hemoglobin-oxyhemoglobin system. If the bicarbonate system is used as a comparative base, the hemoglobin-oxyhemoglobin system is 6½ times more effective. The effectiveness of this system is related, in part, to the ability of hemoglobin to carry both oxygen and carbon dioxide in loose chemical combination, so that carbon dioxide can be tied up in hemoglobin and transported to the alveoli for excretion by the lungs.

The buffer systems maintain the pH of the blood at a very consistent level of 7.36 to 7.44. Even in disease processes, the alteration consistent with life is very limited. The clinical description of acidosis refers to a lowering of the pH, but it rarely falls as low as 7.0; in fact, this is a limit which is not compatible with life. A severe alkalosis will not exceed a pH of 7.8. An increase in the proton concentration (acidosis) is accompanied by increasing somnolence and finally coma in the individual, reflecting an increasing depression of nervous system activity. Acidosis is seen much more often clinically than alkalosis. It is a frequent problem in the uncontrolled diabetic, for example. The manifestations of clinical alkalosis reflect an increased excitability of the nervous system; thus, the individual displays excessive motor activity and restlessness, and ultimately convulsions. Death usually results from tetany (spasm) of the respiratory muscles.

Distribution of Body Water: The Structure of Electrolyte Balance

Fluid and electrolyte balance does not develop out of a random series of interactions, but from an intricate catalogue of responses based on a very specific structural design. The surface of the limiting membrane of the body cells establishes a boundary line which defines the structural integrity of each cell and the functional relationship to the solutions that always bathe it. Each cell, made turgid by the microscopic drop of fluid captured inside its membrane, must protect its independent function and, at the same time, contribute to the general welfare of the organism. Within the cell membrane is a highly specific solution, characteristic only of the "intracellular compartment." From 45% to 50% of the total body weight of the average adult (70 kg.) is due to the intracellular fluid. This percentage varies with age and sex, as well as with body structure, but the major differences occur in infancy, when only 25% of the body weight is due to intracellular fluid, and in old age, when a decline of as much as 10% of intracellular water is not uncommon.

Although constancy is the rule inside the cell, the extracellular water must be fluid, in the sense of fluidity—or movement. It is the fluid of transmission of the metabolic products essential to the well-being of the cells. Several systems share the extracellular fluid, but the volume that is held within the circulatory system (sometimes called the intravascular compartment) is maintained at an extremely constant 5% of the total body weight in all individuals, regardless of weight, age or size. This persistent volume serves the additional function of maintaining, within the closed circulatory system, a pressure that permits the pulsatile pumping action of the heart to keep the fluid (blood) in motion throughout the system. The 5% of body fluid within the circulatory system refers to the blood plasma, not to the formed elements which are cells, and therefore share the intracellular solution with all other body cells. The circulating blood is obviously a transport system; it is separated by the vascular walls from the water which constitutes the rest of the extracellular compartment, i.e., the interstitial fluid. The fluid outside of the vascular walls and outside of the cell membrane is responsible for 15% of the total body weight. But the interstitial fluid and the intravascular fluid exhibit real resemblance except for the difference in protein concentrations. The intravascular

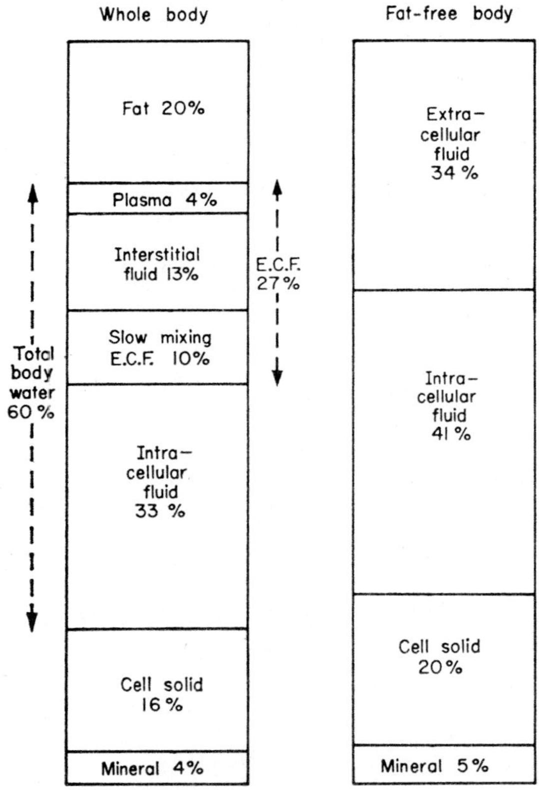

FIGURE 35. The distribution of body water. The fluid composition of the "fat-free" body is less variable, and the usual description of fluid compartments is this type of measurement. I. Fluid = interstitial fluid; ECF = extra-cellular fluid. (From Black, D.A.K.: *Essentials of Fluid Balance,* 4th ed. F.A. Davis Co. [Blackwell Scientific Publications], Philadelphia, 1967.)

FIGURE 36. Balance of the main anions and cations in plasma (extracellular fluid) and in the intracellular fluid. (From Black, D.A.K.: *Essentials of Fluid Balance,* 4th ed. F.A. Davis Co. [Blackwell Scientific Publications], Philadelphia, 1967.)

Table 6: Electrolyte Structure of Plasma and Intracellular Fluid

	PLASMA MEQ./L.	INTRACELLULAR FLUID MEQ./KG. INTRACELLULAR WATER
Cations		
Na^{+}	142	11
K^{+}	4.5	164
Ca^{++}	5	2
Mg^{++}	3	28
Anions		
Cl^{-}	103	—
HCO_3^{-}	27	10
$PO_4^{\equiv}$	2	105
$SO_4^{=}$	1	20
Protein	16	65
Organic acids	6	5

(After Black: *Essentials of Fluid Balance*, 4th ed. F.A. Davis Co. [Blackwell Scientific Publications], Philadelphia, 1967.)

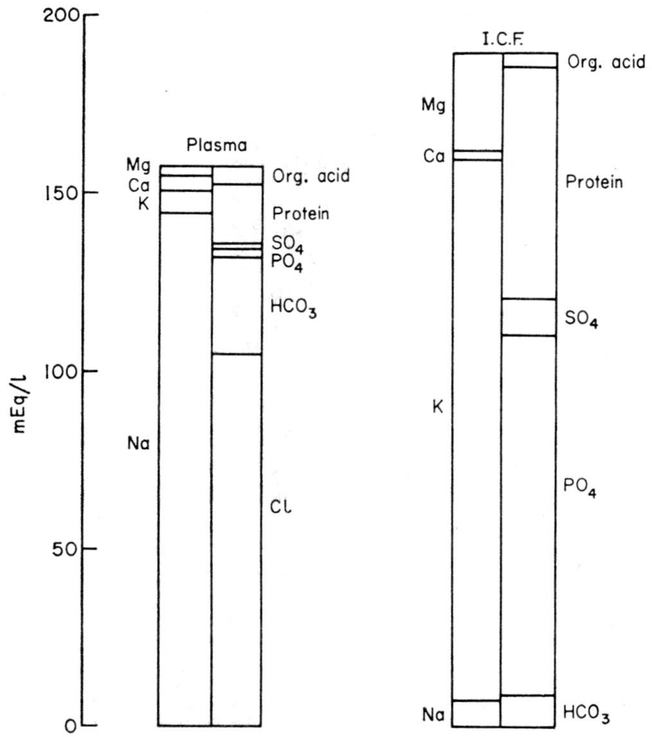

system depends upon its proteins to maintain the colloid osmotic pressure that assures its constant volume, and, of course, there is normally little protein in the interstitial fluid. In most other respects, the concentrations of solutes in the two fluids are very similar. The potential for exchange of materials between the circulatory system and the interstitial compartment is amazing. Most of the exchange takes place at the capillaries, and the supply of these tiny vessels is so extensive that virtually no cell in the body is more than 20 microns away from a capillary. The capillary bed is estimated to have a surface area of 5000 square meters—an area roughly equivalent to one-half of a city block. The capillary walls represent a gigantic sieve, through which occurs a constant exchange of materials both into and out of the circulatory system. The importance of the electrolytes that influence osmosis becomes even more apparent when the path of a single particle is traced, because it must traverse not only the cell membrane, but also the capillary wall. In each instance, the direction it takes depends upon the relative concentration of substances on either side of the retaining structure. When this is multiplied by the astronomical number of exchanges that occur every minute of a lifetime, the homeostasis maintained in health is remarkable indeed.

The relative protein content of intracellular fluid and extracellular fluid, even when the measurement of extracellular protein concentration is determined by using blood plasma, indicates that the major concentration of proteins is within the cell. And the measurement of the electrolytes in the intracellular and extracellular compartments demonstrates, a definitive difference in the nature of these two solutions. The positive ions, or cations (so-called because they migrate to the cathode), and the negative ions, or anions (so-called because they migrate to the anode), must be balanced in both solutions: there must be a positive ion for every negative ion. But the nature of the cations and anions in each compartment is very different.

The essential cation of the extracellular fluid is Na^+ whereas that of the intracellular fluid is K^+. The active transport mechanism that conserves the relationship between these two cations was described previously (see page 133). From Table 1, it is also apparent that Ca^{++} is found in the extracellular fluid in higher concentrations than Mg^{+++}, whereas the reverse is true inside the cell. The Cl^- ion is the most important anion of the extracellular fluid, while the $PO_4^{\equiv}$ and $SO_4^{=}$ are more essential in the intracellular fluid. Thus, the solutions characteristic of each of the major compartments are decidedly different in their make-up. The substances in each are essential to the chemical activity in each, but they are also significant in maintaining the pressure relationships so important to regulating the water content of each compartment. Alteration in the

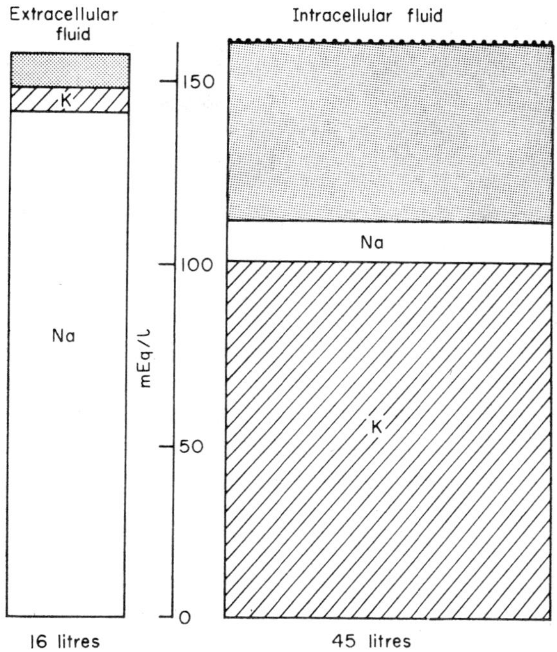

FIGURE 37. The partitioning of Na^+ and K^+ ions in the extracellular and intracellular compartments. (From Black, D.A.K.: *Essentials of Fluid Balance,* 4th ed. F.A. Davis Co. [Blackwell Scientific Publications], Philadelphia, 1967.)

values of any of the major components of either system results in a general alteration in the distribution of water in the body compartments. When this occurs, the central clinical problem is to re-establish the normal patterns of water distribution, and this is a nursing task of major importance.

The fluid and electrolyte system is not self-sustaining. Every day of every individual's life, the essential components—both water and its solutes—must be replenished. The urgency of the need for water supplies by communities of men is a reflection of the urgency of the need for water by individual human beings. The water that represents so much of the substance of a man is *used* by his body and thus must be restored in direct and exact proportion to its use. It fulfills several functions, all vital to his continuing health and well-being:

1. Water is the solvent for the essential constituents of the body. It forms colloidal solutions with proteins, and is the best medium known for ionization of electrolytes.
2. Water provides the transport mechanism for communication and transmission of *materiél* between cells, because it is a fluid and fluids flow, i.e., they move and carry their solutes with them.

3. Water provides the volume of fluid necessary to exert a force per unit surface, i.e., it is essential in the maintenance of pressure relationships within the body.
4. Water is an essential participant in certain chemical exchanges.
5. Water is vital in the maintenance of homeostatic body heat because of its high specific heat and its heat of evaporation.

It has been estimated that the half-life of ingested water is 9 to 11 days. This means that, within this time span, half of the water taken into the body will be excreted, and half of what is left will be excreted in a similar period of time. There is much variation in the individual need for fluid intake, but the criterion of efficient fluid balance is an intake and output of water over a period of time without a significant change in body weight. Since over half of the body weight is water, a rapid weight loss almost always means a loss of body water. In some pathophysiological conditions, the measure of body weight is crucial to the therapeutic plan.

Under normal circumstances, water is supplied by oral ingestion of food and fluids. In a total intake of 2500 ml. of fluid in a 24-hour period, about 1500 ml. is taken as fluid, including water, coffee, tea, milk, and other fluid foods. Another 700 ml. is available in solid foods. And 300 ml. is produced during the metabolic degradation of nutrients. In the same 24-hour period, 1500 ml. of water will be excreted in the form of urine. Another 300 ml. will be lost in the feces. And an additional 700 ml. will be lost by the evaporation of water from the skin and mucous membranes and from the lungs. The loss of fluid by evaporation is called the "insensible loss," because it is rarely apparent to the individual except on very hot and humid days when the evaporation is not swift enough to keep the skin surface dry.

The kidneys are able to conserve water for the body during periods of water deprivation, and the adaptation of the concentration of the urine is an important aspect of fluid balance. But the kidneys must eliminate 35 grams of solids daily—the waste materials of metabolism—and 400 to 500 ml. of water must be excreted in order to hold the solute in solution. Furthermore, even under comfortable environmental conditions, the insensible fluid loss of 700 to 1000 ml. daily continues, and this amount must be replenished and accounted for in fluid balance.

Unusual situations may place an even more drastic drain on the body's fluid supplies. The hot and humid day is one example. The loss of body fluids by vomiting or diarrhea may produce remarkable imbalances, especially in infants and young children, in whom dehydration from this source occurs quickly. The loss of body fluids through these symptoms is compounded by losses of electrolytes normally present in the gastrointestinal tract. Massive loss of body fluids can occur in individuals who are severely burned, and there is always a significant loss when there is exudate or drainage from wounds. This type of fluid loss is accompanied by protein loss as well, and this must be compensated for in the treatment.

The actual loss of fluid from the body, however, is no more serious than a redistribution of fluid in the compartments of the body so that the usual balance between them is sacrificed. In the diabetic, the excess loss of fluid in the urine occurs at the expense of the intracellular compartment. But fluid deprivation of the intracellular compartment may also occur when the total body water, trapped in the interstitial spaces, is vastly increased over its normal volume.

The Pathophysiology of Fluid and Electrolyte Balance

In the absence of unusual demands in the internal or external environment, the individual comfortably maintains fluid and electrolyte balance by the ingestion of food and water. Most of the salt the body requires is readily accessible in the daily diet, and the drinking of relatively small volumes of water throughout the day is sufficient to maintain the body's fluid balance without difficulty. The need for fluid intake is a familiar physiological experience called "thirst," but beyond the fact that it stimulates the individual to seek water, the physiology of thirst is very poorly understood. While there is some evidence that it reflects an increased salt concentration in the body fluids (and therefore a need to dilute them to their normal levels), it is an equally common experience that dryness of the mucous membranes of the mouth is a powerful index of thirst for most people. The influence of these local factors is evident in the administration of some drugs that cause a drying sensation of the oral tissues, even though the individual is adequately supplied with fluids. Such patients will want tiny sips of water; they are obviously relieved by small amounts to moisten the mouth but do not drink amounts that indicate an urgent need for fluids per se.

The function of the body water in maintaining the body temperature is complicated in the human body, because the loss of water by the evaporation of perspiration on the body surface always means a loss of electrolytes as well. A profuse perspiration (called diaphoresis) is frequent in disease processes as well as in response to environmental factors and always threatens the individual with a significant loss of essential salts and water. However, this loss is reflected in little alteration in the concentration of the body water, since the loss of both salts and water serves to deplete the volume, but conserves their isotonicity (same concentration). Both the donkey and the dog respond to extreme environmental conditions of heat by panting. This permits a relatively large fluid evaporation without the attendant salt loss. As a result, there is a considerable concentra-

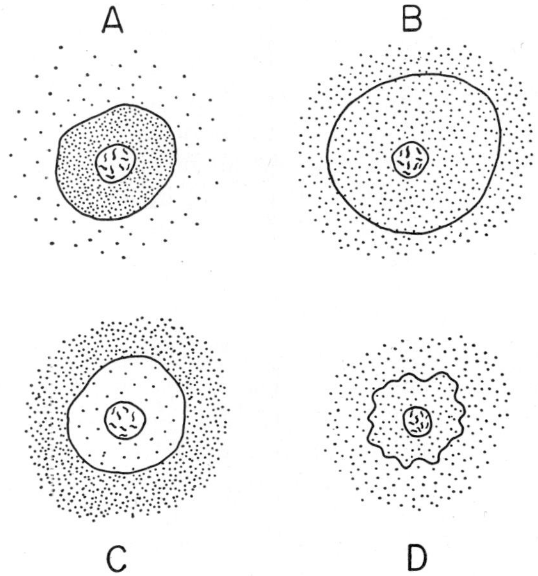

FIGURE 38. The concentration of the solutions inside and outside the cell establishes a dynamic exchange between the two compartments. (A) The concentration inside the cell is much greater than that outside, so that, as equalization occurs (B), the cell becomes markedly enlarged as fluid enters it to dilute the increased concentration within the cell. In (C) the higher concentration is outside the cell, and fluid thus leaves the cell (D) so that the cell shrinks markedly in size. (From Guyton, A.C.: *Textbook of Medical Physiology,* 3rd ed. W.B. Saunders Co., Philadelphia, 1966.)

tion of the body fluid in these animals (hypertonicity = increased concentration). When given fluids, the donkey may drink as much as 12% of his body weight at one time and thus restore the proper concentration in his body water. In the human body, restoration of lost fluids by water alone may actually create symptoms of water excess, because such replacement dilutes the body water (hypotonicity = lowered concentration), and this represents an imbalance, which is accompanied by clinical symptoms. The protection of the isotonicity of body water by this physiological mechanism demands that medical and nursing intervention be designed to enhance the body's own defense. Thus, profuse diaphoresis requires replacement of both the body salt and body water.

It is more evident that fluid and electrolyte balance is threatened in individuals who have obviously sustained a measurable fluid loss than in those for whom such a loss cannot be immediately demonstrated. However, the most common clinical problems related to fluid and electrolyte balance exist in individuals whose loss has consisted of a shifting of

Table 7: Electrolyte Losses in Fluids from Various Parts of the Body

SOURCE	Na^+ (mEq./liter)	K^+ (mEq./liter)	Cl^- (mEq./liter)
Sweat	50	7	40
Stomach	60 (20-116)*	9 (5-32)	100 (50-154)
Bile	148 (130-60)	6 (3-12)	100 (80-120)
Pancreatic juice	140 (110-150)	5 (3-10)	75 (54-95)
Small bowel (suction)	110 (72-148)	5 (2-15)	105 (43-137)
Ileostomy (recent)	129 (105-44)	16 (6-29)	116 (90-136)
Ileostomy (adapted)	46	3	21
Cecostomy	80 (45-115)	15 (11-28)	48 (35-70)
Formed stool	10	10	15
Diarrhea (watery)	50-100	20-40	40-80
Transudates: edema	140	5	115

*The upper figure is an average, while those in parentheses indicate the width of the range. Compiled from the data of Randall, 1952; Cook & Crowley, 1952, and the author. (From Taylor, W. H.: *Fluid Therapy and Disorders of Electrolyte Balance*, rev. ed. F. A. Davis Co. [Blackwell Scientific Publications], Philadelphia, 1967.)

the fluid from one body compartment to another, with a consequent train of events that modify pressure relationships, electrolyte and fluid exchange across membranes, and the control of fluid excretion by the kidneys. In such patients, a genuine thirst and dehydration is present, even though the body tissues are obviously waterlogged. The accumulation of body fluids beyond the normal requirements of the organism is called edema. In a control system as complex as that which maintains fluid and electrolyte balance, interference at any point in the process can result in abnormal accumulations of fluid. An alteration in the permeability of membranes is one obvious source of difficulty, and this does, indeed, occur. A change in colloid osmotic pressure, as reflected by a change in protein concentration, also predisposes to edema formation. Such forms of edema are seen in starvation and in kidney diseases in which there is an uncontrolled loss of protein in the urine. Alterations in kidney function always presuppose a fluid and electrolyte imbalance; some of the most common drugs are capable of influencing radical alteration in kidney function, often as an intended response to treatment for fluid and electrolyte imbalance.

The most frequent incidence of edema accompanies a failure of the heart to adequately pump blood through the circulatory system. The heart muscle, as big as a man's fist, is capable of pumping 5 liters of blood into

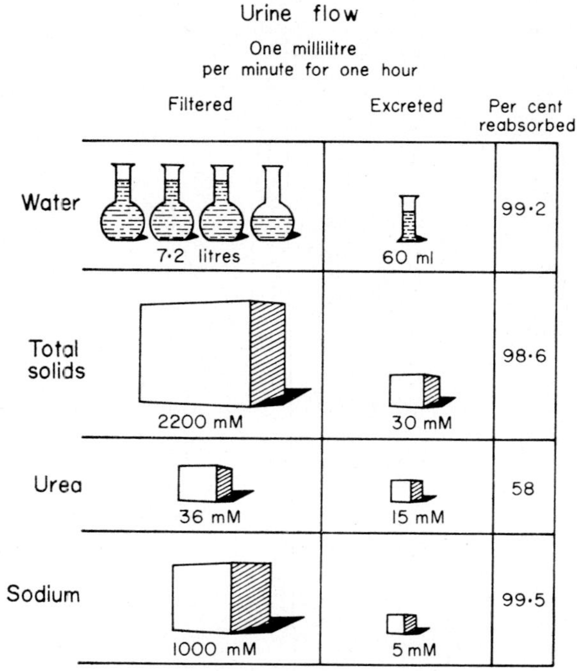

FIGURE 39. The normal control of fluid and electrolyte balance is vested in the kidneys, which filter a large volume of fluids but selectively excrete only that volume which will maintain balance. (From Black, D.A.K.: *Essentials of Fluid Balance,* 4th ed. F.A. Davis Co. [Blackwell Scientific Publications], Philadelphia, 1967.)

the circulation every minute, even when the individual is at complete rest. In the healthy adult, the heart is capable of delivering as much as 20 to 25 liters of blood per minute during vigorous exercise. A trained athlete may have a cardiac output as high as 35 liters per minute. But the heart can succeed in this task only so long as its contractions are strong and occur in a consistently rhythmic pattern. The diseased heart loses its "reserve," or its ability to increase its output in response to demands made upon it by the body cells for oxygen and nutrients (including electrolytes). Damage to any part of the heart decreases its efficiency as a pump, and some structural change in the heart muscle is inevitable when the regulatory factors are altered by disease elsewhere in the body. The interacting regulatory mechanisms are very complex, but essentially they influence the movement of a volume of fluid through a closed system of distensible vessels of varying diameter, with a resultant pressure differential within the vessels that insures an adequate blood supply to all tissues of the body in all of the postures the body may assume. To move the fluid through the system, the heart imparts a force to the blood, which sends it

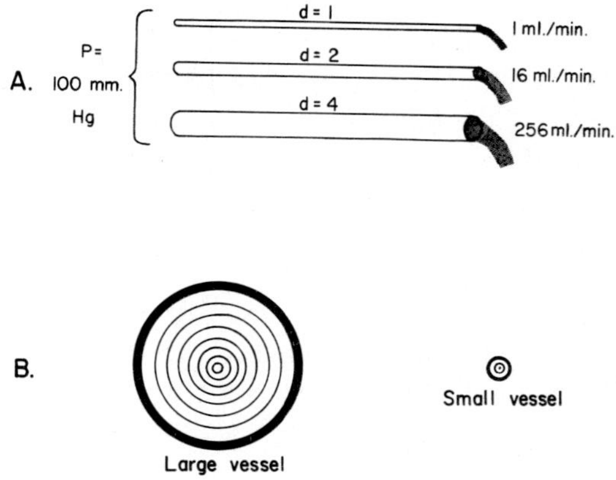

FIGURE 40. (A) Poiseuille's law describes the effect of diameter on the rate of flow. In (B) the concentric rings flow at different velocities so that the fastest flow is furthest from the vessel wall. (From Guyton, A.C.: *Textbook of Medical Physiology,* 3rd ed. W.B. Saunders Co., Philadelphia, 1966.)

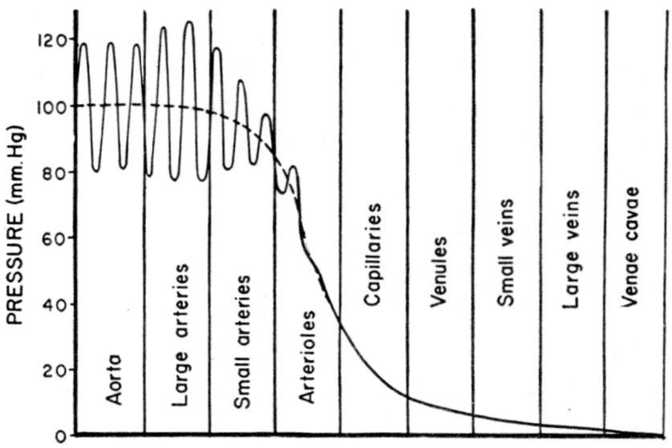

FIGURE 41. The pressure gradient in the circulatory system results in different blood pressures in different portions of the systemic circulation. (From Guyton, A.C.: *Textbook of Medical Physiology,* 3rd ed. W.B. Saunders Co., Philadelphia, 1966.)

moving through the vessels. The greatest force is exerted when the ventricles contract to send the blood on into the arteries, and, since the force per unit area is the pressure, this represents the high point in the pressure within the circulatory system. The ventricles then relax, and as they do, the chambers fill again in preparation for the next pumping action. During this time, the total pressure in the closed system is at its low point. At the point of maximum pumping (contraction of the ventricles), the blood pressure is said to be at systole (a contracting), and at the point of maximum relaxation of the ventricles, it is said to be at diastole (dilatation). In health, the homeostatic range of the two points of pressure within the system is rather constant and is generally measured (with a sphygmonometer) at 120 mm. Hg over 80 mm. Hg, where the first figure is the systolic pressure, and the second is the diastolic pressure. This measurement is usually written as 120/80.

This is, however, a measure of the pressure in the arterial tree. By the time the moving stream of blood has reached the capillary, it is no longer under such pressures. It is difficult to measure the pressure within the capillary, but it ranges from approximately 25 mm. Hg at the arteriole end to about 9 mm. Hg at the venule end. This gradient, coupled with the large number of capillary pores, and in relationship to the concentrations of electrolytes in the interstitial fluid, permits water and solutes to rapidly leave and return to the capillary, thus accomplishing the essential tasks of the circulatory system to carry metabolites to and from the tissues. The movement of water and its dissolved substances is facilitated, because the capillary pores are 80 to 90 Å in diameter, and therefore allow the free passage of all except the large protein molecules. The movement through the pores is a random one, for the most part, and the predominant direction, that is, into or out of the capillary, must depend upon the relative pressure within the capillary and within the interstitial fluid through which it passes. The advantage, normally, rests with movement out of the capillary at the arteriole end and back into it at the venule end, although the pressure differential is only of the order of 7.5 to 8.5 mm. Hg. A mere 10 mm. Hg rise in the capillary pressure increases the flow of fluid *out* of the capillary to 21 times the normal volume. When this occurs, fluid tends to accumulate in the interstitial compartment, and edema occurs.

The measure of arterial blood pressure reflects the total fluid volume, the resistance to the flow of blood created by the friction of vessel walls, the size of the vessels, and the viscosity of blood itself. The homeostatic range is maintained by a complex interaction of nervous and hormonal control. Some gradual elevation of blood pressure occurs with aging, often in response to decreasing distensibility of the arteries. An elevated blood pressure indicates that an excess demand is being made on the heart to pump blood against increased resistance to its flow. Inevitably, this results in structural changes in the heart itself. The cardiac muscle must be nourished and oxygenated by the pumping action of the organ, just as all other tissues must be. When the cardiac output is lessened by increased arterial pressure, the heart enlarges in an effort to improve cardiac output. Unfortunately, enlargement creates increased metabolic demands in the cardiac muscle itself, and, as a result, the enlarged heart is not able to contract strongly enough or completely enough to assume the added burden effectively.

The precise pathogenesis of the redistribution of body water that accompanies the ineffective pumping action of the heart is a matter of continuing clinical debate. One point of view visualizes that the kidney cells falter because the decreased cardiac output results in a decreased blood supply to the kidneys. This results in a retention of Na^+ ion due to decreased excretion of urine. When Na^+ ion is retained, water must also be retained to hold it in solution. The retained fluid elevates the venous pressure, and this, in turn, alters the capillary pressure relationships so that edema occurs. The other point of view emphasizes that incomplete emptying of the ventricles results in an ultimate increase of fluid volume

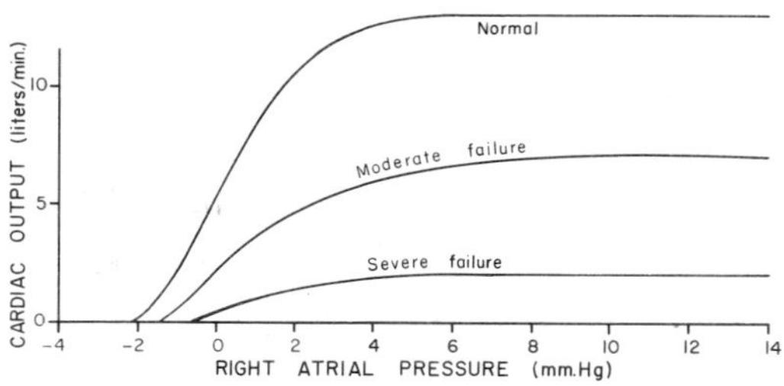

FIGURE 42. Cardiac output curves of the normal, moderately failing, and severely failing heart demonstrate the intimate relationship between blood pressure and the effective pumping action of the heart. (From Guyton, A.C.: *Textbook of Medical Physiology,* 3rd ed. W.B. Saunders Co., Philadelphia, 1966.)

in the venous system, and once more the altered pressure gradient results in fluid and Na^+ ion retention and edema. The likelihood is that some combination of both of these theories is operative in most instances. The important consideration is that the ineffective pumping action of the heart produces a pressure alteration which, in turn, results in a retention of fluids and electrolytes in the interstitial compartment. When this occurs, the heart is said to be decompensated. Often the edema itself, by creating pressure in the capillaries, further compounds the fluid retention. The increased resistance to blood flow through the microcirculation, as well as through the arterial and venous systems, adds to the heart's burden, and its ability to maintain an adequate cardiac output is more and more threatened. All of the body tissues are penalized when this occurs, because none of them, including the heart muscle itself, is receiving a blood supply adequate to provide enough nutrients and oxygen. The danger to the individual rests with the degree of impairment suffered by vital tissues.

Often the earliest sign of beginning decompensation is swelling of the feet and ankles. It is characteristic of cardiac edema that the fluid becomes "dependent," i.e., it tends to accumulate in the lower parts of the body because of the effect of gravity. As decompensation increases, the amount of retained fluid increases, and the level of the edema creeps higher and higher in the body tissues. A massive edema, accompanying extremely severe decompensation, always a very grave index, is called anasarca. But long before the dependent edema has become severe, the threat always exists that an accumulation of edema fluid will interfere with respiratory function. While distinction is often made between "right" and "left" heart failure, the likelihood is that they usually occur simultaneously. The right side of the heart drains the large veins returning from the periphery, so that right heart failure is characterized by peripheral and dependent

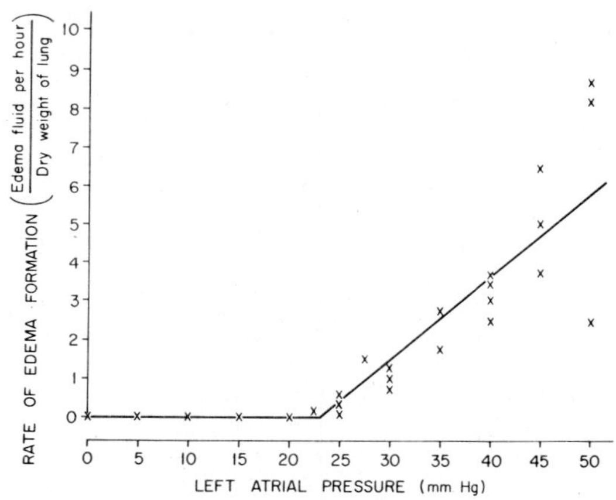

FIGURE 43. When the left atrial pressure and pulmonary capillary pressure are increased, the rate of fluid loss into the lungs is markedly increased, predisposing to the acute condition of pulmonary edema. (From Guyton, A.C.: *Textbook of Medical Physiology*, 3rd ed. W.B. Saunders Co., Philadelphia, 1966.)

edema as described above. The left heart, however, receives blood from the pulmonary circulation, so that ineffective pumping results in a back-up of fluid in the lungs. Left heart failure always involves respiratory effectiveness. In some instances, a persistent, dry cough during the night is the first sign of impending left heart failure, but it is obvious that the retention of fluid in the lungs will quickly interfere with gaseous exchange, and respiratory difficulty is quite common in decompensated heart disease.

It is extremely important that the excess fluid be removed from the body to lessen the work of the heart and to make it possible to nourish and oxygenate the tissues throughout the body. The goal of therapy is the mobilization of the fluids. This can be accomplished by the use of drugs which strengthen the contraction of the heart muscle and other drugs which force the kidney to excrete Na^+ ion, carrying the solvent fluid along. Na^+ ion intake is restricted, since it is this cation of the interstitial fluid that holds the excess fluid. Usually water intake is not restricted, and the edematous cardiac patient often suffers a paradoxical thirst created by dehydration of the intracellular compartment due to the altered concentration of electrolytes in the interstitial fluid. The limitation of urine output in the edematous cardiac patient may be quite severe, and the oliguria (little urine) establishes a retention of waste products in the blood plasma, produced by protein catabolism. This increases the hazard for the individual and complicates the already serious interference with tissue oxygenation and nutrition.

Care of the Patient with Congestive Circulatory Failure

The Conservation of Energy

In the earliest hours of embryonic growth, the pulsating, bright-red tissues that become the heart represent the life-activity itself. That rhythmic movement continues every minute of every day of every year of life, and when it finally ceases, the life of that organism is ended. It is not unusual that a tremendous amount of psychic, as well as physical, dependence rests in the heart's activity for every individual. The deepest emotions are expressed in the language of the heart, and while great joy is "heartfelt," great sorrow produces "heartbreak." When the individual is encouraged, he is "heartened," when he is disappointed, he is "heartsick." The heart is the tissue of life, its usual activity silent and unremarked but possessing the ability to be reassuringly present when the individual has responded to unusual stimuli and discovers in the pounding in his chest that the mobilization has been a thorough one. The intermittent signals of heart action arise when the organism's need to respond is quickened, and the pulsating message is equally intense whether there has been unusual physical activity or simply the sight of a loved person after a long separation. Every living person measures the resource of life in the activity of the small muscle in his left chest. Here rests the rhythm of life itself.

Rhythm implies movement, and movement cannot occur without an energy exchange. No single organ of the body requires an energy exchange as exacting and unremitting as does the cardiac tissue. All of the body's protective capability is directed at the well-being of nervous tissue, and yet a functional pump in the circulatory system is indispensable to this purpose. The heart tissue itself must be nourished and oxygenated, its metabolic wastes must be removed, and unless this is assured, no other physiological function can be fulfilled. The development of congestive circulatory failure immediately suggests cardiac default, and the first issue of therapy is to restore function to the heart by insuring the cardiac cells their maximum supply of essential metabolites. This cannot be achieved independently of the complicating pathophysiology elsewhere in the organism. The faltering heart establishes the conditions which create the retention of body fluids, but the increasing accumulation of body fluids places a growing demand on the heart. This is a positive feedback, rare in normal physiology but often demonstrable in pathophysiology, and it is best described as a "vicious cycle." The cyclic nature of these events emphasizes that all elements must be dealt with clinically, since no single process will rectify the displacement. Until the excess fluid is mobilized, and the fluid and electrolyte balance restored, the heart tissue, in common with all other body tissues, cannot be returned to a safe range of activity.

Since the energy utilization in congestive circulatory failure must be made in confrontation of the alteration of fluid balance throughout the body, it is essential that the individual restrict unnecessary activity to an absolute minimum. There are drugs that will increase the strength of the contractions of the heart, and they are very effective in achieving this. But until the fluid balance is restored, the cardiac output must exceed the minimal demands of a resting metabolism, and therapy must emphasize not only energy conservation, but a positive minimizing of energy expense. Nursing intervention can achieve this based, in every instance, on the individual's specific requirements.

In the upright position, the heart works against gravity, but when the individual is supine, the effects of gravity are evenly distributed and the extra demand on the heart is relieved. For this reason, bedrest aids in the conservation of energy. However, bedrest in itself poses a threat. With a circulation already sluggish and slow, immobilization will speed the probability of stasis of the moving bloodstream, with all the possible sequelae of occlusion or moving clots in the vascular system. Only intensive devotion to positioning and mobilizing the patient in bed can prevent such events. Positioning and mobilization of the bedridden patient can be performed so that the patient spends very little effort in the process, but when his participation is limited, the nurse's participation is increased. The edema-ridden body of the patient in congestive failure is heavy and difficult to move, and the ever-present respiratory embarrassment affords little reserve when effort must be expended. Bed posture is frequently a crucial issue. The difficulty experienced with every breath may make a supine position impossible. The patient who must virtually sit up in order to breathe is said to be "orthopneic," and such individuals are totally incapable of assuming a horizontal position for any period of time, even though recumbency eliminates the heart's work against gravity. Remaining in bed in a relatively upright posture makes position-changing more complex, but it is possible to turn such patients on their sides, providing sufficient support so that they need not spend effort in maintaining the position against gravity themselves. In the supine semi-sitting position, the arms should be supported so that they need not be held against gravity by the individual's own efforts. During bathing and bed-making, the nurse must constantly assess the patient's tolerance even to passive movement. And the physician should prescribe passive exercise (such as isometrics) and permissible degrees of range of motion allowable for the individual.

Patients confined to bed often spend energy in fruitless and unnecessary ways. All necessary items, such as facial tissues, should be within easy reach to eliminate stretching and overextending the patient's effort. He should be assisted with his meals if necessary, and this should include consideration of the ease with which he can chew his food. Foods requiring much chewing and the muscular effort so involved may leave him too tired to eat, long before he has taken sufficient nourishment. He may spend considerably less energy if he is allowed to use a bedside commode rather than a bedpan, even when this requires lifting him in and out of bed for this purpose. Restless and random muscular activity, whether it grows out of discomfort or anxiety, may exact a high toll in energy expense, and therefore such individuals are often mildly sedated even during the day. And finally, when respiratory activity is severely handicapped, the work of breathing itself may be overwhelming and exhausting. The administration of oxygen and the use of drugs to assist respiration aid in minimizing the energy spent in difficult respiration.

Mobilizing and removing the excess fluid in the body bears an energy cost too. The fluid must be excreted by the kidneys, and with assistance of drugs, this results in an extraordinary urine production, often in a rather short time. This priming of urine formation is called "diuresis" and often results in a dramatic weight loss (" a pint is a pound the world around"). The body weight is, in fact, the best index of the effective removal of edema fluid. But the ordeal of diuresis places a great burden on the congestive failure patient. It means frequent use of the urinal. Each time this is attended by physical effort, and it may be complicated by emotional effort as well if there is the least question of obtaining a urinal as often and as promptly as the individual will need it. It is not uncommon for patients to lose as much as 30 pounds in the course of diuretic therapy. The precise measurement of all fluid intake and output is used as a guide to the prescription of drugs and establishment of electrolyte balance by the physician; the importance of accurate and continuous recording of these values cannot be emphasized enough. Often daily weighing of the patient may also be ordered. This may prove a trying ordeal if it involves a great deal of activity; sometimes a special scale is used so that the patient can be weighed in his bed and spared the need to leave it or to stand erect while being weighed. The loss of edema fluid is not the excretion of water alone but of sodium as well. The hormonal influence on kidney function establishes regulation of sodium ion excretion, but the control of potassium ion excretion is not as competent. In any situation in which large volumes of urine are excreted, some potassium loss also occurs, and because the homeostatic range is so finite, measurement and replacement of potassium ion often must accompany diuresis. When drugs are used to improve cardiac function, their influence on potassium loss makes this therapeutic responsibility even more urgent. The potassium ion level markedly influences cardiac function, and a low potassium level may give rise to increased irritability of muscles, including that of the heart. A rapid heart rate (tachycardia) which is arrhythmic is a symptom of low potassium levels, but this is often a symptom of congestive failure as well.

Table 8: Potassium Content of Commonly Available Beverages

	POTASSIUM (MEQ./8 OUNCES)
Grapefruit juice, canned, sweetened	9
Orange juice, fresh	10
Tomato juice, canned	14
Beef broth, canned	2.5
Cola beverage	3
Skim milk	7

(From J. A. Galloway: *Diabetes Mellitus*, 7th ed. Eli Lilly and Co., Indianapolis, 1967.)

During diuresis, therefore, it is urgent that the nurse observe the individual's behavior and report changes promptly. Muscular weakness also accompanies a low potassium level, and distinguishing this from the symptoms already present requires very sensitive observation. As the fluid of edema is lost, and cardiac function becomes more adequate, the individual is gradually guided back to a level of activity that is suitable for him. The restoration of his freedom to move about may encourage him to more activity than is safe, and the nurse must continue to exercise control over his energy expense. His pulse rate during various kinds of activity should be known, and, correspondingly, his respiratory function should be assessed in relation to his activities. Rest periods and assistance must be planned for the individual as long as activity results in evidence of tiring, even though it may be as subtle an indication as a persistent increase of pulse or respiratory rate during moderate exercise.

THE CONSERVATION OF STRUCTURAL INTEGRITY

The appearance of the symptoms of congestive circulatory failure indicates a structural alteration in the heart. The enlarged heart represents the increasingly futile effort to cope with circulatory effectiveness, but any pathology involving cardiac tissues, either congenital or acquired, predisposes to the loss of pumping efficiency and to the development of congestive failure. Even if the decompensated heart can be compensated through treatment, the initial pathology will remain and continue to pose a threat to the individual's well-being. The structural integrity of the heart is compromised before congestive failure occurs, and this situation usually continues even after therapy has proven successful. It is now possible to offer surgical relief for some kinds of cardiac pathology, but this is an alternative not available to all patients. Even when feasible, such a question must be decided individually on the basis of the patient's condition and the elements of risk involved. The acute episode of congestive failure, however, represents the danger of overwhelming demand on the diseased heart and always increases the likelihood of even more structural loss.

The accumulation of incredible amounts of fluid in the interstitial compartment always produces marked alteration in the structural integrity of the entire body. The swelling of the tissues may create gross disfigurement, and the skin is drawn very tightly over those areas that are waterlogged. Pressure in such tissues will often leave a pitting deformity in the skin for many minutes after it is withdrawn. The dependency of the edema, i.e., its tendency to accumulate in response to gravity, is often dramatically apparent in the bed patient, when the distribution of edema fluid is clearly marked on the lower body surface, especially in the legs, buttocks, and genitalia, as well as in the back. The gradual displacement of edema to dependent parts suggests that structural changes can, in a sense, be controlled by nursing intervention. Once more, positioning influences the way in which the pathology is manifested in the individual patient. While the hard swelling typical of cardiac edema is always uncomfortable and threatens circulation in the affected tissues, the transient edema of the genitalia may create acute distress in the male patient, and only slightly less discomfort in the female. The male genitalia should be supported either with a commercial scrotal support or with wide tape to reduce their dependency, and with it the degree of fluid accumulation. Moving such an individual should be done cautiously to prevent injury to the skin surface, particularly of the scrotum, which is quite dependent whether there is edema in the parts or not. The integrity of the skin in edematous tissues can best be protected by frequent cleansing and a dry, powdered surface to reduce frictional contact with the bed linens. The susceptibility of the taut, stretched skin to injury by friction or pressure is markedly increased.

The retention of fluids in peripheral tissues is always evidence that there is retained fluid in the internal organs as well. Wherever edema occurs, the structural integrity of the organ is compromised, and with it the functional ability of the organ. The nausea, anorexia, and bowel dysfunction, including gaseous distention, are probably related to edema in the gastrointestinal tract. There is usually some structural change in the liver, which may be reflected in metabolic efficiency, and cerebral edema may result in lethargy and even disorientation, if it is marked enough. The most apparent restriction of function, however, involves the respiratory tree. The congestive failure patient is usually dyspneic (difficult respirations) and will himself alter his position so as to relieve respiratory distress. Such a change in position is a reflection of the movement of fluid into dependent areas. In the orthopneic position, the weight of the abdominal organs is minimized against the diaphragm, and the individual enjoys a subjective relief in respiratory difficulty. The subjective nature of this relief is real enough for the individual, but there is no measurable improvement in his ability to exchange gases in the lungs as long as the fluid accumulation remains. The respiratory difficulty may become paroxysmal and lead to an acute episode of respiratory embarrassment very similar to asthma. The most alarming respiratory problem, however, is a sudden filling of the lung tissue with fluid, resulting in a critical and emergency situation. This is called pulmonary edema, and it is a complication of congestive failure which should be prevented if it is possible to do so within the limits of the patient's pathophysiology. Pulmonary edema is characterized by a marked inability to breathe and a choking sensation created by a productive cough which yields a large amount of pink, frothy sputum. The individual is literally threatened with drowning in his own secretions. Emergency treatment must be prompt and consists of reducing the total fluid volume in the circulatory system (usually by occlusion of three of the four limbs of the body for specified periods of time) and the administration of oxygen under pressure.

Any respiratory difficulty is fraught with threat and anxiety, and the effective treatment of such symptoms rests in large measure on the security the individual feels in the care he receives. It is in the interest of structural integrity that such care be offered, because the component of emotional influence on respirations is large, even in the normal individual, and successful treatment will be thwarted if the individual's emotional demands are ignored. Many respiratory emergencies in congestive failure patients occur during the night when sleep decreases the cardiac output and respiratory rate; with the cardiac reserve already diminished to almost zero, the physiological change that occurs in sleep alone is enough to precipitate a serious respiratory problem. While the restorative potential of sleep is hardly understood, its function is essential to every individual's life habit, and when rest is the prescription, this includes restful sleep. Fear of the threat of respiratory emergencies during the night robs many a cardiac patient of restful sleep, unless the nursing care anticipates and recognizes its presence and plans for dealing with it. In addition, the restriction of adequate circulation through the lungs provides an open invitation to pulmonary infection. The defense potential of the respiratory tree is hampered by the excess production of sputum, and the presence of fluid provides an excellent medium for the growth of microorganisms. Positioning and adequate cleansing of the respiratory tract are essential to prevent the threat of respiratory infection. It is, of course, equally urgent that no individual with an upper respiratory infection be allowed to come in contact with the patient.

The anorexia that so often accompanies congestive failure interferes with nourishing the patient, and in addition the salt-restricted diet is one which most patients find unpalatable. Restriction of sodium intake is essential to mobilizing the edema fluid, and it is only when this substance is withheld that its presence in ordinary foods becomes apparent. Even milk, which is so often used (but not always wisely) as a substitute for a full diet in the sick, contains too much sodium to allow free use on a sodium-restricted diet. The patient in congestive failure is also undergoing a serious failure of metabolism, and the foodstuffs of recovery, especially the proteins, are important to his eventual healing. The provision, and acceptance, of an adequate diet pose many nursing problems which are solved individually by persistent attention to each patient's personal requirements.

The Conservation of Personal Integrity

The heart is the monitor of living, and a threat to its welfare is a threat to the life of the individual. The freedom to move confidently through the activities of daily living is a measure of the personal integrity of the individual, and there can be no freedom if the cardiac function limits the individual's participation in life. The physiological restriction, created by rapid development of dyspnea and a fatigue and weakness that attend the simplest tasks, exacts a high toll in emotional well-being. That focus which makes the heart the essential organ of physical and emotional health is not lessened, but sharpened, when disease threatens it. It is not surprising that real or imagined disease in the heart stimulates profound behavioral changes, some of which are extreme enough to be classified as serious emotional disease. Not every individual with cardiac damage displays such behavioral symptoms, but it is difficult to believe that any such patient is entirely free of the anxiety stimulated by altered cardiac function. Denial is a frequent defense against serious illness, and the nurse must always be suspicious of the acutely ill individual who manifests no emotional reaction to his plight. The modern behavioral scientist recognizes that some anxiety establishes an emotional tone that is helpful to the individual, particularly when there is a justifiable explanation for it. Such awareness is the basis upon which the patient's participation in his own care can be made sensible and profitable for him. The level of anxiety, however, may be reflected in physiological parameters as well as in the behavior of the individual, and no organ responds more sensitively to emotional stimuli than the heart. Thus, the care of the cardiac-disabled individual must focus on his behavioral tone, not only to offer him the comfort of support, but to fortify his body's response to the process of the disease itself.

It is not often possible to wipe away the anguish of fear that may arise in response to disease, but it should be a definitive goal of all nursing care to provide the security and assurance that is possible for each individual. This is so frequently dependent upon the nurse-patient interaction that it becomes central to all nursing intervention. The symptoms of congestive failure are anxiety-provoking in themselves, and the patient must invest some of his energy in demanding that the professional persons caring for him assume some of the responsibility for responding to the threat. The knowledge, for example, that fluid retention in the lungs may first be made evident by a dry, hacking, nocturnal cough alerts the nurse to early pathophysiological change that can be dealt with easily, compared to the extreme urgency of treating a frank pulmonary edema. The difficulty he experiences during the night hours will be increased if the patient does not have the assurance that the nurse is watching his condition and is available to him without heroic efforts to attract her attention. In fact, night or day, the cardiac patient in distress deserves the continuing attention and presence, if necessary, of a nurse who knows what she is doing and communicates that certainty to him.

The accumulation of edema fluid distorts the body. The limbs are swollen and heavy, and the individual may be unable to wear even a very large size slipper. The involvement of so much of the body is frightening in itself, and the individual may see in the shapeless enlargement an alteration in his image of himself that creates shame and despair. The treatment that must emphasize diuresis increases the frequency with which he must depend on others to help him with these private activities. He may become apologetic and even reluctant to ask for the urinal as often as he will need it, unless he is helped to understand that it is recognized as a necessary part of his care. The attention placed on this body function in itself stimulates embarrassment, and much must depend upon how the nurse behaves in respect to the needs of the patient during diuresis. The dependency created by the fatigue and weakness is also present, as it must be whenever activity must be restricted. That dependency must be allowed to exist as long as the need for energy conservation continues, and it must be replaced with independence at a rate governed by the physical, as well as the emotional, needs of the individual.

The restrictive low sodium diet also creates issues for the patient in congestive failure. The ordinary gratification of food is denied, and it is not always easy—in fact it is rarely easy—to help the individual understand why he is being offered a diet he cannot enjoy. The ramifications of emotional response to food are as complex and varied in individuals who require a salt-poor diet as they are in all people. Each must be dealt with but always within the framework established by the individual's specific needs. There is perhaps no area in which "cheating" is more common than in the salt-restricted diet. Substitutes for sodium chloride are generally unsatisfactory. It is no more helpful to censure the dietary failures in this kind of a diet than it is in the diabetic patient. Once more, if the individual is allowed to help in the planning of his diet, he is more apt to honor its restrictions.

The patient who has had an episode of congestive heart failure faces the prospect of a rather complete alteration in his previous life style. It is totally unrealistic to expect that he will be able to change his employment, even if the work he does is inappropriate and dangerous for his cardiac status. Sometimes, it is true, the possibility of returning to his job is rendered out of the question by his physical condition. The alternatives to this, however, must also be sensible. Professional vocational counseling is available in many communities under the auspices of the Heart Association. Before the individual makes a decision, or is simply challenged to do so by the physician or nurse, concerning his future employment, the facilities available to guide him should be offered. For the homemaker, there is equal counsel available that will help her to organize her duties so that she minimizes the stress on her heart. The resources are excellent, and they substitute definitive knowledge for the frustration of radical adjustments without help or understanding.

The Conservation of Social Integrity

The anxiety created by cardiac disability in one member of a family is readily stimulated in the others. The activities within a household are related to the respective roles of the family members. Sleeping arrangements, bathroom facilities, dining habits, and the use of space within the home for all the activities that are localized there involve the interactions of all family members. Disabling illness in any member will have its effect on all the others, but in relation to the role that individual plays within the family. Cardiac disability influences so much of the daily pattern of activity that it may require major adjustments in the home to accommodate the sick member. The cardiac-disabled individual must have ready access to bathroom facilities, and his sleeping quarters should not require that he go up and down stairs. When he is seated in a chair, he should have his legs elevated for at least part of that time. If the disabled individual is the homemaker, the arrangement of kitchen shelves and accessibility of kitchen appliances may have to be modified to permit her to function in that role. Restructuring the physical facilities alone may be a task that considerably alters the entire family interaction. This is quite above and beyond the emotional involvement of the family members. Any prescription to restrict activity may be misinterpreted to mean over-solicitiude, on the one hand, or create hostility and resentment that leads to ignoring the restrictions, on the other. Only the afflicted individual can accurately judge the limits of his participation in daily affairs, but still he may need the watchful attention of a family member in order to protect him from excessive activity.

If his role in the family centers on its financial well-being, his ability to continue in this role will affect the family's welfare. In may mean that another member of the family, or even a public agency, will have to assume responsibility for maintaining the family unit instead. The continuing economic burden of illness, including the purchase of medications and the necessary expense of a special diet as well as medical and hospital costs, may well prove excessive, even in families where there has been relative socioeconomic independence. All of these alterations in its basic structure have a decided influence on the interpersonal relationships within the family unit, and the members should have professional guidance in making the adjustments required.

What the patient knows about his condition and its continuing treatment must be shared with the family as well. The salt-restricted diet bears little resemblance to most of the cultural and ethnic diet patterns in America, and if the usual diet in the home must be altered for one member, it may well influence the others as well. The food habits of a household are as emotionally determined as those of the individual; furthermore, in the home there is the pattern of mealtimes, which in themselves are essential aspects of the social life of a family. A special dietary pattern cannot fail to influence all the dietary habits in a family.

The threat of recurrent episodes requiring hospitalization and the question of the survival of the individual establish an emotional tone within the family that may be reflected in their behavior in the hospital setting. The individual who is being treated for congestive failure may be surrounded by strange equipment, not the least frightening of which is for oxygen therapy. Many people interpret such treatment as a genuine life and death measure, and, although it may be, it just as often is not. The nurse may be quite casual about the accumulation of equipment in the hospital room of a cardiac patient, but families are apt to be terribly upset by such surroundings. The modern electronic monitoring equipment is welcome as an adjunct to treatment by the nurse, but the wires leading to the monitors, usually misunderstood by family members, represent danger to the uninitiated. Most such wires are designed to pick up tiny electrical potentials produced by living tissues, and to carry them to amplifiers which allow them to be measured. It is difficult to convince some patients and their families that no electric current is being run towards the patient by the complex machinery to which the wires are attached.

Convalescence from any serious illness must include the re-establishment of the individual in the family and social milieu from which he came. A continuing need for restriction, and with it the possibility of recurrent problems, makes that return difficult for all patients. And yet, unless there is a niche into which the patient, and only the patient, can be fitted, he cannot be considered to have recovered at all. The best hope lies in understanding, and the family members must be taught, just as the patient is taught, to achieve an adaptation to the new reality they must face together.

Model IV: Pressure Gradient Systems in Nursing Intervention (Fluids)

OBJECTIVES

1. To understand the dynamics of adaptation of the human organism to the physical environment where all physiological parameters are influenced by gravity and atmospheric pressure.
2. To understand responses to alteration in body function created by pathophysiology affecting closed and semiclosed pressure gradient systems, and to recognize the signs and symptoms thus created in the individual patient.
3. To understand the criteria for interposing therapeutic pressure gradient systems into existing physiological systems as detemined by physical laws and biophysical response.
4. To understand the results of manipulation of pressure gradients when therapeutic pressure systems are imposed upon existing body systems.
5. To insure the safety of the individual patient by control of imposed pressure systems, prevention of trauma, and aseptic prevention of infection, when visualization of nursing process is limited to external orifices of the body.
6. To understand the emotional and psychological response of the individual patient to the symptoms of alterations of pressure gradients and the effects of therapeutic intervention.

ESSENTIAL SCIENCE CONCEPTS

1. The human organism is adapted to function in its physical environment so that gravitational force and atmospheric pressure are determinants of physiological response.
   - 1.1 The physical characteristics of the environment participate in essential physiological feedbacks.
     - 1.11 The effects of gravitational force have exercised continuing influence on the evolution of the organism itself.
       - 1.111 The body size is related to the effects of the forces operative on it.
       - 1.112 The cardiac pump must move the circulatory fluid volume against gravity.
       - 1.113 The skeletal-muscle systems are designed to work against gravity.
       - 1.114 The nervous control and sensory feedbacks identify the organism in relation to its gravitational postures.
     - 1.12 Gravitational force may influence the organism by contact or by interactions in a field of force.
       - 1.121 Mobilization against the field of force of gravity requires more energy than when the movement is parallel to the force.

1.122 Contact between two surfaces results in friction in proportion to the interaction of interlocking imperfections in each surface.

1.13 Gravitational force holds the atmospheric gases to the earth's surface.

1.131 Atmospheric pressure varies with altitude (i.e., distance from sea level).

1.132 Atmospheric pressure at sea level exerts a force of 15 lbs. per square inch and will raise a column of mercury 760 mm.

1.133 All objects on the earth's surface are continuously subjected to the effects of atmospheric pressure.

1.2 Structural components of living systems reflect the influence of the physical environment.

1.21 Living tissues are distensible (elastic).

1.211 Distortion in shape does not result in structural change within a normal range of distensibility.

1.212 Excessive distortion of size or shape results in physiological response to distention.

1.2121 Localized or referred pain.

1.2122 Sensation of "fullness."

1.2123 Discomfort from pressure on adjacent organs.

1.2124 Interference with physiological function of organ or system.

1.22 Fluid systems which establish pressure gradients are essential functional components of organs and systems in the body.

1.221 Fluid systems which are required to maintain structural integrity of organ.

1.2211 Aqueous and vitreous humor of eyes.

1.2212 Cerebrospinal fluid.

1.2213 Cardiovascular system.

1.2214 Interstitial fluid compartment.

1.2215 Intracellular fluid compartment.

1.222 Fluid systems which are essential to the physiological function of an organ or system (fluid used as transport medium).

1.2221 Gastrointestinal fluids.

1.2222 Kidney and excretory system.

1.2223 Extracellular fluid compartment, including intravascular fluid and lymphatic system.

1.2224 Respiratory exchange.

1.2225 All mucosal surfaces of the body.

1.223 Fluid systems which are communicating media.

1.2231 Endocrine glands and hormones.

1.2232 Synaptic junctions.

1.2233 Exocrine glands and secretions.

2. The performance of physiological pressure gradient systems is dependent upon the physics of fluids.
   2.1 Resting fluids—the physics of hydrostatics.
      2.11 Fluids conform to the shape of their container.
      2.12 The fluid exerts an equal force per unit area on the walls of its container in a closed system (Pascal's principle).
      2.13 In a fluid of uniform density acted upon by gravity, the pressure increases with the depth of the liquid: pressure is therefore determined by the height of the fluid column and is modified as the height is varied.
      2.14 Regardless of the shape of the container, fluids of equal height exert the same pressure on the base of the container (Pascal's vases).
   2.2 Fluids in motion—the physics of hydrodynamics.
      2.21 Frictional forces created by movement of liquids against the walls of the container influence the rate of flow.
         2.211 Laminar flow takes place in a straight tube when layering of liquid occurs, because liquid in the center is less affected by friction than are layers in contact with walls of the system.
         2.212 Turbulence in flow is created when there is alteration in direction or size of container causing liquid to flow back into the stream of flow.
      2.22 The rate of flow of a liquid varies in direct proportion to the diameter of the tube to the fourth power (thus 1 ml./min. from 1 cm. diameter, 16 ml./min. from 2 cm. diameter, 256 ml./min. from 4 cm. diameter) (Poiseuille's law).
      2.23 The energy of a moving liquid is conserved when the tube is constricted, so that the fluid moves more rapidly through a constriction than on either side of it (Bernoulli's principle).
      2.24 The viscosity of a liquid influences the rate of flow because of frictional forces between the molecules.
      2.25 In elastic containers, the rate of flow is influenced by the distensibility of the walls.
      2.26 A gradient is established when there is a pressure differential in a closed or semiclosed system, with movement from higher to lower pressure area.
         2.261 Siphon is established by a continuous fluid (liquid) connection from a volume of fluid at higher level to a lower level.
            2.2611 Liquid in connecting tube must be uninterrupted (no gas bubbles).
            2.2612 Flow continues until water levels are equalized.
         2.262 Suction is established by decreasing pressure in a system below atmospheric pressure, so that atmospheric

pressure pushes on fluid surface and forces liquid into subatmospheric regions of the systems.

2.263 Osmotic pressure is established between solutions, dependent upon concentration of nondiffusible solute in solutions separated by a semipermeable membrane.

2.264 "Gravity" drainage occurs when there is a difference in fluid heights, from the higher to the lower level.

3. The structure of pressure gradient systems in the human body influences response to physiological and pathophysiological demands.

3.1 Closed systems maintain integrity of function by homeostatic control of pressure gradients within them.

3.11 Volume of circulating blood is maintained at 5% of total body weight by colloid osmotic pressure and nervous and hormonal control of vascular size.

3.111 Effective pumping action of heart results in periodic maintenance of pressure within system by control of volume of blood forced into the circulation.

3.112 Viscosity of blood creates frictional force and resistance to flow.

3.113 Distensibility of large vessels and patency of peripheral circulation influence total pressure by regulation of volume of closed system.

3.114 Posture of body regulates height of "fluid column" and the consequent influence of gravity on hydrostatic pressure within the circulatory system.

3.12 The tension within the eye is maintained by controlled and constant pressure of fluid to allow maximum refraction and vision.

3.121 Drainage system in eye regulates pressure of contained fluid volume.

3.122 Increased pressure compromises circulation of retinal vessels and thus interferes with reception of stimuli.

3.123 Loss of fluid volume in eye results in loss of distending pressure and permanent loss of structure.

3.13 Cerebrospinal fluid system cushions vital tissues against positional change resulting from movement of the organism.

3.131 Bony cage of cerebrospinal system has no elasticity (distensibility), so that increase in pressure within it results in embarrassment of contained tissues.

3.132 Relief of increased pressure in the system must be imposed by therapeutic means.

3.1321 Alteration of osmotic pressure of fluids to remove fluid volume.

3.1322 Mechanical opening of bony cage by surgical intervention or aspiration of excess fluid.

3.2 Semiclosed systems develop alterations of pressure gradients as necessary feedbacks to control function.

3.21 Contained fluids of semiclosed systems are not isotonic with other body fluids, so that movement of fluids rests with a pressure gradient.

3.211 Fluids of gastrointestinal tract are prepared for absorption or excretion.

3.212 Fluids of urinary tract are prepared for conservation or excretion.

3.22 Semiclosed systems have "storage" areas capable of distention within broad limits of physiological function.

3.23 Semiclosed systems have "sphincter" guarding of entrances and exits.

3.231 Sphincters establish closed system when physiologically closed, with physical characteristics of enclosed pressure.

3.232 Opening of sphincters is mediated by nervous control with large element of voluntary and learned participation.

3.233 Sphincters protect system from bacteriological contamination from external environment.

3.24 Size of opening of semiclosed systems varies with physiological function.

3.241 Sphincters and tubes leading to sphincters are lined with mucosal tissue.

3.242 Patency of openings threatened by inflammatory reactions including edema, and subsequent fibrous tissue substitution (scarring).

3.25 Capacity of storage organs reflects dynamic relationship with the entire system of which they are a part.

3.251 Fluids in storage organs remain in functional relationship to body; i.e., they may be reabsorbed if storage is prolonged.

3.252 Excess filling of storage organs results in organismic response.

4. Therapeutic intervention in pressure gradient systems always involves pressure systems superimposed on physiological ones.

4.1 Pressure measurement in closed systems requires a secondary closed system which reflects parameters of physiological system.

4.11 Sphygmomanometer develops air pressure in a closed system measured in millimeters of mercury.

4.111 Wrapped cuff occludes blood flow in arterial system of limb.

4.112 As pressure is lowered in sphygmomanometer, blood flow is allowed to resume in vessels.

4.1121 Turbulence in partially occluded vessel may be heard with stethoscope (Korotkoff's sounds).

4.1122 Changing sounds reflect decreasing turbulence as occlusion of vessel is terminated, and they equal the high and low values of the blood pressure.

4.113 Inertia of mercury creates a lag so that results are correct within 10% (±8 mm. Hg).

4.114 Non-mercury manometers are similar to "aneroid" barometers.

4.12 Measurement of closed system pressures may be attained by introducing closed system with attached manometer directly into fluid of system.

4.121 Venous pressure is directly measured when exact volume, returning to heart must be known (as after cardiac surgery).

4.122 Measurement of spinal fluid or cerebral fluid pressure utilizes water manometer and direct penetration of fluid space by closed needle (needle with trochar).

4.2 Pressure reduction in closed systems introduces an alteration in pressure within by control of instrumentation of procedure.

4.21 Alteration of osmotic pressures results from introduction of hypertonic or hypotonic fluids into dynamics of a closed system.

4.22 Alteration in total fluid volume results in change in pressure gradient in a closed system.

4.221 Phlebotomy removes blood therapeutically to reduce circulating volume.

4.222 "Dry phlebotomy" or rotating tourniquet reduces total circulating blood volume.

4.223 Reduction of intracranial pressure by surgery or removal of fluid.

4.23 Gravity results in alterations in closed system by postural differences in the individual.

4.24 Introduction of fluids into closed system, when pressure change is not desired, requires constant attention to the rate of flow (introduction of additional volume of fluids into system).

4.241 Administration of intravenous fluids is controlled by height of column, rate of flow, and size of opening to prevent rapid increase in blood volume.

4.242 Installation of solutions into cerebrospinal system requires removal of equivalent volume of fluid before administration.

4.3 Introduction of fluid into, or removal of fluid from, semiclosed system depends on pressure relationships.

4.31 Fluids in storage organs may be removed when distention threatens function of system.

4.311 Tubes used to drain accumulated fluids in storage organs must be introduced through openings and past sphincters.

4.312 Drainage via inserted tube is passive (gravity flow) or active (physiological response of the body) or induced (suction).

4.313 Occlusion of openings of tube results from improper placement against tissues or from closing by fragments of organic material contained in fluids.

4.32 Installation of fluids into storage organs imposes a pressure change in them.

4.321 Fluids may be introduced to increase pressure and stimulate physiological activity as a result (enemata).

4.322 Fluids may be introduced to bring medication to lining of storage organ or to cleanse it (bladder irrigation).

4.323 Rate of flow of introduction of fluids determines pressure gradient during process.

4.324 Diameter of tube used to instill fluids affects rate of flow.

4.325 Elasticity of tissues of storage organs and presence of pathophysiology determine safe level of pressure.

4.326 Volume of fluid introduced must be within safe limits of the capacity of the organ to handle pressure.

5. Introduction of instruments to alter pressure gradient systems requires aseptic precautions because body defense against infection is being bypassed.

5.1 Cautious introduction of instruments prevents trauma to tissues through which they pass.

5.11 Frictional resistance minimized by lubrication of tubes that enter mucosal tissues.

5.12 Resistance to passage cannot be overcome by mere force without resultant tissue damage.

5.13 Absolute visualization of body opening essential for safe passage of tubes past sphincters.

5.2 Surgical asepsis required when instrument enters a normally "sterile" body region.

5.3 Clean equipment required when instrument enters a normally contaminated body region to prevent cross-contamination.

5.4 Microorganisms utilize fluid as transport medium, so that ascending infection accompanies failure to keep tubes and system scrupulously free of microorganisms.

6. Therapeutic processes that alter pressure gradients create discomfort and threat to the individual patient.

6.1 Increased pressure relationships are frequently accompanied by some degree of pain and discomfort.

6.2 Use of parenteral needles of all kinds is threatening to many individuals, regardless of age.

6.3 Introduction of tubes into body orifices may be accompanied by embarrassment as well as discomfort.

6.31 Enemata create physiological discomfort.

6.32 Catheterization of urinary bladder requires visualization of meatus and produces embarrassment.

6.33 Passage of tubes into upper gastrointestinal tract is attended by choking and discomfort of stimulus to back of throat.

6.4 Individual may be fearful of consequences of therapeutic process.

6.41 Frequent blood pressure measurement creates anxiety in the individual and desire to know results.

6.42 Surgical asepsis required for spinal tap may be threatening to individual.

6.43 Individual may be apprehensive about whether system is functioning properly because of importance placed upon its function by personnel or because of his own evaluation of comfort.

NURSING PROCESS

1. Manipulation of pressure gradients by therapeutic means requires control of environmental variables by the nurse.

1.1 Proper selection of necessary equipment and instruments to achieve desired therapeutic result.

1.11 Measuring devices accurately calibrated.

1.12 Tubing, connectors, and appliances "air-tight" when pressure in system is vital to process.

1.13 Surgically sterile equipment where required and provision for necessary sterile fields to perform process (including sterile solutions as needed).

1.14 Functional stopcocks and other devices to regulate rate of flow.

1.15 Necessary equipment to stabilize height of fluid column.

1.16 Selection of tubes and catheters of proper size for process, and lubrication if required.

1.2 Effect of patient's position on pressure alteration.

1.21 Blood pressure measured with cuff at heart level, unless otherwise directed by physician.

1.211 Gravity effects may be measured if individual is standing erect.

1.212 Site selected varies with purpose of measurement.

1.213 Measurement at more than one site may be required for full information on heart action.

1.22 Positioning for enemata usually with sigmoid in dependent position (patient on left side).

1.23 Catheterization of urinary bladder requires lithotomy position.

1.24 Patient supported in sitting position for passing of gastrointestinal tubes.

1.25 Gravity drainage bottle always kept lower than body level.

1.3 Knowledge of the expected physiological response when pressure gradient system is altered.

1.31 Strict adherence to physical determinants when process precludes direct observation of effect on body tissues.

1.311 Absolute visualization of body orifices before insertion of tubes.

1.3111 Enema tube inserted only 2 inches to by-pass sphincter and control flow of fluid into rectal area only.

1.3112 Urinary catheter inserted past sphincter until flow of urine begins.

1.3113 Resistance to passage of tube reported to physician, and tube never forced past obstruction.

1.312 Predetermined height of fluid column in accordance with nature of procedure performed.

1.3121 Tubing on system restricted so that safe height is not exceeded during process.

1.3122 Regulation of rate of flow by lowering height if necessary.

1.3123 Gravity drainage always to lower site than body level.

1.313 Direction of flow clearly understood so that fluid enters or leaves body in accordance with the therapeutic process.

1.32 Increasing discomfort or pain expressed by patient evaluated in light of specific process.

1.321 Discomfort of enemata should be minimized by slow administration of fluid.

1.322 Distinction between anticipated discomfort and indication that procedure should be stopped.

1.323 Recognition of untoward response and prompt intervention to eliminate it.

2. Nursing intervention varies with purpose of therapeutic process.

2.1 Insertion of tubes through body orifices to drain storage organs of accumulated fluids.

2.11 All tubes passed through meatus and sphincters are lubricated with water-soluble gels to preclude trauma to mucosa.

2.111 Entrance to gastrointestinal tract, either upper or lower, must be clean but not sterile.

2.112 Entrance to urinary bladder must be sterile.

2.12 Size of appliance used determined by the size of the natural orifice.

2.121 Tubes to be left in situ are not inflated until position is absolutely determined to be in proper alignment.

2.122 Stress on tubes left in situ is always prevented by visualization and placing of drainage tubes during moving of patient.

2.123 Drainage tubes and bottles are cleansed or replaced every 8 hours, or more often if drainage requires it.

2.13 Results of irrigation, catheterization, or enemata described as to quantity and quality in recording treatment.

2.2 Instillation of medicated solutions through tubes placed in storage organs.

2.21 All solutions instilled in urinary bladder must be absolutely sterile.

2.22 Solutions instilled via gastrointestinal tubes must meet requirements of tonicity when electrolytes are being protected (frequent washing removes electrolytes).

2.23 Therapeutic enemata must follow prescribed recipe.

3. The safety and comfort of the individual patient includes consideration of his anxiety and embarrassment in performance of pressure gradient processes.

3.1 Participation by individual patient depends on his understanding of the process.

3.11 Relaxation of sphincters to allow passage of tube is voluntary and requires a relaxed and confident patient.

3.12 Draping and screening designed to minimize embarrassment and assure privacy.

3.13 Nurse and patient agree on "cue" words that indicate flow is stopped until he is able to tolerate the discomfort again (especially in enemata).

3.14 Time selected to perform procedure does not interfere with rest, meals, or other nursing plans.

3.2 Patient's condition and ability to withstand process evaluated before it is begun.

3.21 Sedative or analgesic drugs given if necessary to alleviate discomfort before process is begun.

3.22 Realistic assurance is offered, which does not exclude possibility of pain or discomfort.

3.23 Individual is not allowed to become overfatigued, especially when procedure must be repeated, as in enemata, until clear.

3.24 Explanation of procedure in language the individual patient understands.

3.25 Individual properly positioned and supported in proper position for duration of procedure.

3.26 Individual not left alone until procedure is completed.

3.261 Following enemata, individual is not left on bedpan longer than necessary.

3.262 If expulsion of enema is in toilet, nurse arranges for signal when patient is ready to return to bed.

3.3 Success of process evaluated by observation of individual's response following it.

3.31 Evidence of relief of pain or discomfort as distention of storage organs is relieved.

3.32 Examination of specimens removed includes quantity as well as specific details of its nature.

3.321 Presence of untoward substances (such as blood) reported to physician.

3.322 Description of stool following enemata.

3.323 Color, consistency, odor of drained fluids indicate pathophysiology and response to treatment.

Vocabulary

active transport
anion
catalyst
cation
colloid osmotic pressure
concentration gradient
congestive failure
dehydration
diffusion
dissociation
diuresis
edema
electrolyte balance
enzyme
equivalent
etiology
extracellular fluid
fluid compartments
gradient
hydronium ion
insensible fluid loss
intake and output
intracellular
interstitial
matrix
milliequivalent
millimicroequivalent
millimol
mol
oncotic pressure
osmosis
osmotic pressure
proton-acceptor
proton-donor
semipermeable membrane
specific heat
surface tension
univalent

General Bibliography

BLACK, D. A. K.: Essentials of Fluid Balance, ed. 4. F. A. Davis Co. (Blackwell Scientific Publications), Philadelphia, 1967.

BORDICKS, KATHERINE J.: Patterns of Shock. Macmillan Co., New York, 1965.

DAVIS, KENNETH, AND DAY, J. A.: Water: The Mirror of Science. Doubleday & Co., Inc., Garden City, N.Y., 1961.

MODELL, WALTER, ET AL.: Handbook of Cardiology for Nurses, ed. 5. Springer Publishing Co., New York, 1966.

SMITH, HOMER W.: From Fish to Philosopher. Doubleday & Co., Inc., Garden City, N.Y., 1961.

TAYLOR, W. H.: Fluid Therapy and Disorders of Electrolyte Balance. F. A. Davis Co. (Blackwell Scientific Publications), Philadelphia, 1965.

Articles

Correcting common errors in blood pressure measurement (progammed instruction). Amer. J. Nurs. 65:133-164, 1965.

ESTES, J. W., AND WHITE, PAUL DUDLEY: William Withering and the purple foxglove. Sci. Amer. 212:110-119, June 1965.

HOKIN, LOWELL, AND HOKIN, MABEL: The chemistry of cell membranes. Sci. Amer. 213:78-86, Oct. 1965.

KORN, EDWARD D.: Structure of biological membranes. Science 153:1491-1498, Sept. 1966.

Of water, salt and life. Lakeside Laboratories, Milwaukee, 1956.

Potassium imbalance (programmed instruction). Amer. J. Nurs. 67:343-366, Feb. 1967.

RAWLINGS, MAURICE S.: Heart disease today. Amer. J. Nurs. 66:303-307, Feb. 1966.

SIMEONE, F. A.: Shock: 1. The nature of shock. Amer. J. Nurs. 66:1286-1289, June 1966.

SIMEONE, F. A.: Shock: 2. The treatment of shock. Amer. J. Nurs. 66:1290-1294, June 1966.

SNIVELY, W. D., JR.: Toward a better understanding of body fluid disturbances. Nurs. Forum III: 60-77, 1964.

SPAIN, DAVID M.: Atherosclerosis. Sci. Amer. 215:49-55, Aug. 1966.

STAMLER, JEREMIAH, ET AL.: Coronary proneness and approaches to preventing heart attacks. Amer. J. Nurs. 66:1788-1793, Aug. 1966.

TURELL, DAVID J.: The cardiac patient returns to work. Amer. J. Nurs. 65:115-117, Aug. 1965.

5 Nursing the Patient with a Disturbance of Homeostasis: Nutritional Needs

Bodily Processes Depend on Adequate Nutrition

The process of living is one of constant activity at the cellular level. The multitude of biochemical reactions which constitute metabolism can continue to take place for as long as the materials required by the cells—the fluids, electrolytes, oxygen, and nutrients—are provided in sufficient quantity. The provision of these substances must, furthermore, be in a form that can be utilized at the cellular level—the simple amino acids rather than the complex protein of a T-bone steak. Thus, the introduction of nutrients into the body is designed so that the foods can be converted into nutrients the cell can use to perform.

Cellular well-being is quickly challenged by a lack of oxygen, the limit of nervous tissue to hypoxia providing the maximal degree of toler-

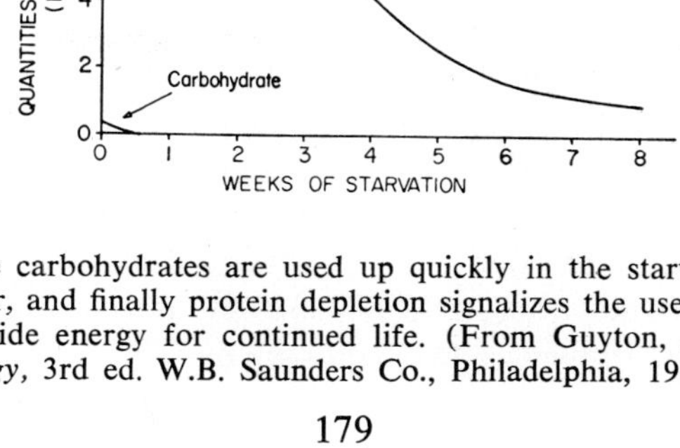

FIGURE 44. The carbohydrates are used up quickly in the starving individual, fat depletion is slower, and finally protein depletion signalizes the use of the body's own substance to provide energy for continued life. (From Guyton, A.C.: *Textbook of Medical Physiology,* 3rd ed. W.B. Saunders Co., Philadelphia, 1966.)

ance to such a lack. Within 72 hours, a failure of fluid supply produces the irreversible symptoms of dehydration. Because the tissues are capable of using their own substance when the ingestion of food is stopped for some reason, a lack of nutrients is tolerated for much longer periods of time. But even when the fluid balance is maintained to some degree, the inability to ingest food ultimately results in the death of tissue. In the utilization of its own substance to maintain energy requirements, the body uses carbohydrates first, but the stores of carbohydrates are entirely used up within 24 to 48 hours. Fats are used next, and in an individual with 15% of the body weight as fat, such stores are completely used in 5 or 6 weeks. Finally, the protein of the body is used to provide the energy for life, but once the fat is gone, the ability of the organism to sustain itself on protein stores alone is very shortlived.

These figures are based on the expectation in an otherwise healthy adult. During disease processes, the movement towards cellular starvation may be considerably increased, because an increased rate of metabolism often accompanies illness, and the total rate of usage is therefore hastened. In the course of these events, the organism displays gradually increasing signs of distress. Cellular embarrassment because of a nutritional failure is thus often a matter of degree. The specter of starvation is a widespread, world-wide problem of great political and social significance. It is also an extremely urgent reality in the wards of every hospital, since the ability of the organism to receive and properly utilize food is threatened in almost all disease processes and may be the central issue in many.

The supply of nutrients to the tissues provides them with their substance for the growth of the organism and for the replacement of tissues to maintain structure and function. But even this vital activity is dependent upon the *energy* available that allows these life processes to go forward. *Metabolism* is the total of *all* body activities—the sum of all the chemical reactions that characterize the life process. With only small exceptions, the energy produced in the process of metabolism is available in the form of *heat*. For this reason, the measurement of metabolic activity—the *metabolic rate*—is in terms of the rate of heat production during metabolism. And thus also, the measurement of the requirements of the body in the form of nutrients is in a unit of heat, the calorie: the amount of heat necessary to raise the temperature of 1 gram of water 1 degree centigrade. Food intake, described as calories, is a dynamic estimate of the energy source available to the body. Such a requirement varies remarkably with such parameters as age, sex, activity, and the presence of disease processes. The further division of foodstuffs by their chemical composition, and, therefore, their rate of utilization in the body, is also based on a variety of conditions which influence the requirement. The recent publicity given to dietary restriction of carbohydrate foods in reducing diets indicates that the entire story of individual utilization of specific nutrients is still a matter of considerable research, and conjecture. The very recent improvement of research methods that illuminate cellular biochemical function will doubtless clarify much of the controversy in the near future.

The purely physiological needs of the individual for food can be ascertained with some exactness in the laboratory, or in the laboratory analysis available in the hospital. But there are few areas of human need that are more involved in other determinants than food intake. Whatever the basic nature of the "drive" towards satisfying the organism's need for food, it must be sorted out of a welter of other influential behaviors, some of which are readily identifiable, whereas others are extremely difficult to pinpoint.

There are, for example, remarkable variations in how different cultures define "food." The most exquisite delicacy for inhabitants in one part of the world may be utterly revolting to others. The social and economic influences of availability of food often assist in this definition, but there are irrational factors as well that are equally, if not more, important. In the midst of plenty, the widespread occurrence of "food faddism" in the United States defies rational explanation on the basis of the organism's need alone. Philosophical and religious systems underlie the attitudes towards food intake, and these constitute a powerful rationale, capable of stirring great outbursts of emotion.

Food habits, fostered within the family group from infancy, are associated with feelings that are quite beyond the physiological requirements of the individual. Such habits involve not only food choice but also quantity and the frequency with which meals are taken. The family pattern established in childhood at mealtime may well influence this social ritual throughout the individual's life. Such patterns, deep-set in the relationships between family members, are not automatically turned off when the individual is hospitalized.

Food choice is, therefore, intimately associated with cultural value systems. But every individual also has entirely personal associations with foods, which influence his choice above and beyond those factors shared with his cultural, social, or family group. The folklore associated with food intake is correspondingly complicated by the individual's experience with specific food substances. Many of our feelings are expressed in the language of food. We "hunger" for material things that are inedible. We are "nauseated" by events that disgust us, even though food itself is not involved. Food is used as a "reward," and withholding it as punishment: the prisoner is reduced to bread and water. Food intake varies with the emotional predicament of the moment; in some individuals, the desire for food is so intimately related to the emotional state that the physiological need is utterly unimportant.

If such variables exist during health, it is no wonder that the problems of adequate nutrition and food intake in illness become rather critical. The lack of desire for food, anorexia, that accompanies many illnesses may substantially influence the course of the disease process. The factors that influence anorexia are multiple, but they include, for example, the defensive mechanisms of the body itself (the nauseated individual knows better than to ingest food), the withdrawal of the sick person into his own inner circle of introspection, the guilt feelings associated with illness that make it necessary for the person to punish himself by refusing food, the changes in the metabolism that alter the way foods taste and smell, and the differences in the diet offered the patient from what he is accustomed to eating. This last factor is always part of the problem in a sick individual whose condition requires a diet radically different from his usual food intake. The low-salt diet, the high-protein diet, the diabetic diet, and the low-calorie diet all represent a kind of deprivation from the usual, and the patient's acceptance of his diet is closely related to his feelings about food, his disease, and his sense of worth as an individual.

The nurse shares the responsibility for the nutritional management of the patient with the physician and the nutritionist. Prescribing the diet is the doctor's responsibility; planning it in consultation with the patient and his specific desires is the responsibility of the nutritionist. But the actual ingestion of the diet, the patient's response to it, the environment in which it is offered, and assistance with the mechanics of consuming it become the responsibility of the nurse. Close communication and frequent consultation with the doctor and the nutritionist are essential, and the evaluation of the success of the diet is shared by the nurse with the doctor and the dietitian *and the patient.*

Consideration of the physiological needs of the individual in health and illness continues to be the underlying rationale for dietary management. Many illnesses are susceptible to treatment by diet alone, and even when there are other medical therapies available, the emphasis on dietary management becomes a matter of education for the individual patient. The nutritionist makes great contributions in this area, but the nurse also shares this task. As in all teaching of patients, the approach must be realistic, sensible, and individualized.

The Provision for Cellular Nutrition Depends on the Integrity of the Gastrointestinal Tract

The problem of nutrition is the problem of maintaining the lifework of the cells by conveying to them the substances they need, when they need them, in the form for utilization, and in the quantity required. All the food taken into the body must be processed, therefore, to this degree, and all the food ingested is thus dependent upon the adequate functioning of the organs designed for food processing.

The structure of the gastrointestinal tract influences the way in which it carries out these functions. Food is composed of carbohydrates, fats, and proteins, which enter the gastrointestinal tract, usually in a rather complex form. Digestion consists of a series of chemical changes—all hydrolysis reactions—whereby the complex molecules can be absorbed and thus transported to the cells. But the chemical changes that degrade these substances take place within tissues that are themselves composed of carbohydrates, fats, and proteins. The food must be chemically acted upon. However, the tissues in which this takes place must *not* be. In other words, the digestive enzymes that mediate these changes must not digest the tract in which they occur. Structurally and functionally, then, there must be protective devices built into this system to protect it from its own activity.

Furthermore, chemical changes take *time*. Even those that are supported by enzymes are rarely instantaneous, and the complexity of the chemical task of breaking down foods into absorbable substances indicates that there is a progression of change—a series of chemical reactions, each dependent upon the previous reaction—so that there are a number of intermediate steps leading to the final product. Time is therefore an essential determinant in the successful change of food into usable substances, and the tract in which this takes place must be designed for the appropriate time expsoure so that the chemical changes can take place properly.

Once the final product is reached, it must somehow be transported to the bloodstream, because only the circulation of blood can bring the vital nutrients to all of the body cells. The gastrointestinal tract, therefore, performs two major functions: (1) the chemical change of digested food into transportable final products, and (2) the absorption of final products into the circulating blood.

In a sense, the gastrointestinal tract is really *outside* the body. The cells lining the tract are, indeed, mostly a type of epithelial cells which have a very high rate of regeneration. The passage of food through the tract constitutes a rather constant mechanical trauma to the lining of the tract; this is particularly evident in the upper tract where the ingested food, although chewed or masticated in the mouth, is still recognizable as food. The ingested food acts mechanically to rub and press and scrape against the lining of the tract, which, therefore, must be continuously replaced in order not to be utterly worn away from usage, as a stone is eroded by weathering.

Not all of the ingested food can be reduced to usable final products; there are, therefore, some waste materials that must be regularly removed from the tract, which is constructed with an "opening" at its beginning and another at its end. The tract itself is a patent tube protected at both ends and at crucial points in its course by muscular sphincters which can regulate the entrance or exit of materials. The materials in the gastrointestinal tract remain essentially outside the body then, except for those substances which can be absorbed through the walls and into the circulation.

The tube is rather long, as it must be in order to allow the materials in it the necessary time for the multiplicity of changes they undergo, as well as the time required for their absorption through the walls of the tract. The materials must move unhindered throughout its course for normal functioning. Any situation tending to block the tube immediately compromises its function and makes the digestion and subsequent absorption of nutrients impossible.

Some idea of the integrity of this system may be gained from a realization that the tube itself, from the oral entrance to the terminating anal sphincter is, in the normal adult, from 25 to 30 feet long. If it were a straight tube (and thereby largely dependent upon gravity), we would of necessity have to be considerably taller than we are. The small intestine alone is about 22 feet long, and since the tallest man is only slightly over 6 feet, it follows that the tube must be folded back and forth upon itself many times. The folding of the tube, thereby minimizing the effects of gravity, also makes it necessary that the propulsion of materials through the tract be accomplished by the ability of the tract itself to force the

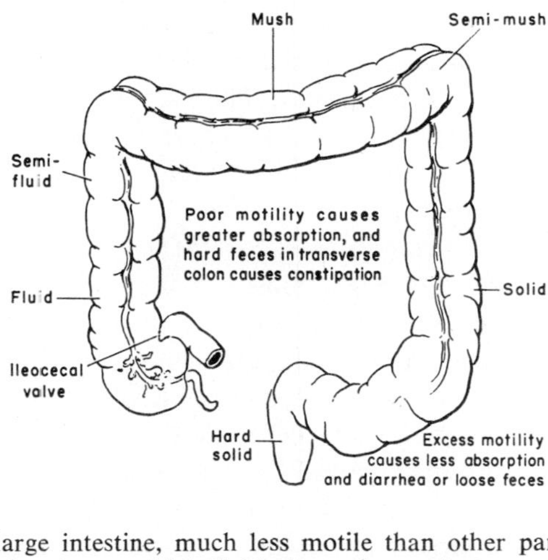

FIGURE 45. The large intestine, much less motile than other parts of the gastrointestinal system, is the site at which fluid absorption and storage of waste materials take place. (From Guyton, A.C.: *Textbook of Medical Physiology,* 3rd ed. W.B. Saunders Co., Philadelphia, 1966.)

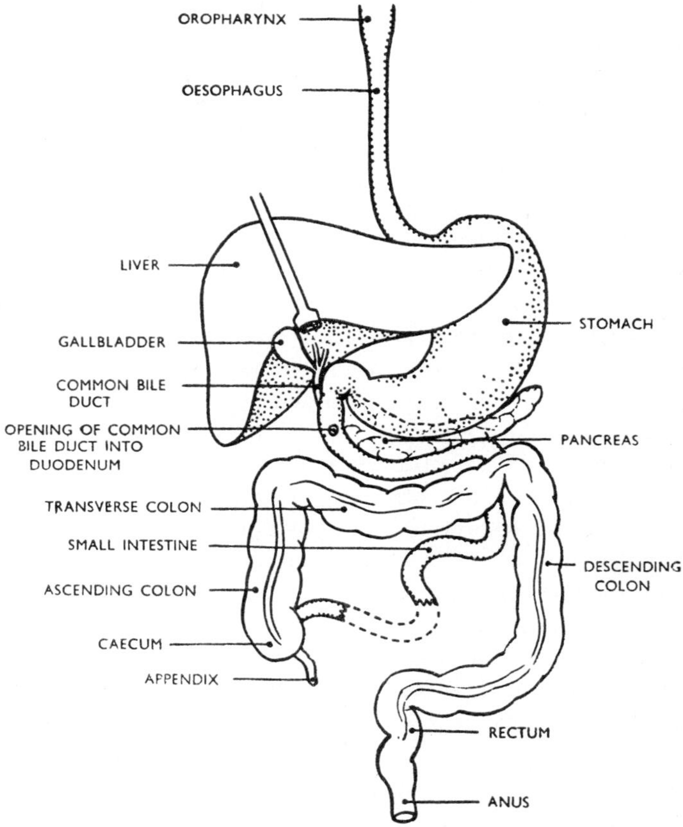

FIGURE 46. Schematic representation of the gastrointestinal tract. The systemic function is a factor of the individual function of the parts of the tract, anatomically and physiologically distinct. (From Sinclair, D.: *An Introduction to Functional Anatomy*, 3rd ed. F.A. Davis Co. [Blackwell Scientific Publications], Philadelphia, 1966.)

materials through. In other words, the tube must possess motility. Any factor influencing the motility will also influence the efficiency with which the tube performs its functions. A rapid movement of materials through the tract will not allow sufficient time for the digestive process or the proper absorption of nutrients prepared in the process. A slowed movement, on the other hand, may produce symptoms of more or less severity, depending on the degree of change in movement; frequently this is manifested early by an increase in the absorption of fluid normally found in the tract.

It is apparent, then, that all of these factors influence the total functioning of the gastrointestinal tract—a long, patent, motile tube, folded upon itself many times, and possessing muscular sphincters that separate some of its functional units. Interference with patency, motility, the condition of the lining, or the ability to absorb nutrients through the wall creates symptoms of disease.

The control of the motility of the gastrointestinal tract, as in any muscle system in the body, is nervous in origin. There is extensive parasympathetic and sympathetic nervous control, and, as is characteristic of the autonomic innervation, events elsewhere in the body that cause the discharge of stimuli in this system are reflected in changes in the gastrointestinal tract.

The motility of the tract also has a dual purpose. Not only must the contents be propelled towards the anal end, but, during the course of movement, the materials must be churned and mixed so as to afford the largest possible surface area for chemical reaction to take place. The chemical changes and the absorption that occur in the tract make the total surface area a crucial issue in the proper functioning of the digestive system. Most of the absorption takes place in the small intestine, and the walls of this section of the tract are therefore highly specialized, with an anatomical arrangement that vastly increases the total surface through which absorption can take place.

Protection of the lining of the tract is considerably enhanced by the presence of billions of single-cell mucous glands which secrete the material that acts as a protective coat for the surface of the tract. The mucus not only protects the walls, but also acts as a lubricant so that the materials can pass through the tract; the mucus itself is strongly resistant to the digestive enzymes normally found in the tract. This substance, therefore, lubricates the passage of food through the tract and also prevents excoriative or chemical damage to the epithelium. Its protective role becomes somewhat exaggerated when an irritation of the gastrointestinal tract occurs. As is true of mucous cells anywhere in the body, irritation stimulates an increased flow, presumably to wash away and dilute the irritant materials. When this occurs in the gastrointestinal tract, the excess fluid may increase the motility rate, and diarrhea, or the loss of liquid waste materials from the tract, may occur.

The gastrointestinal tract plays an important role in the regulation of body fluids too. After all, under normal circumstances, all fluids, as well as foods, are ingested in this way. But the secretion in the tract itself of the juices which contribute to the chemical processes of digestion reach a quantity ranging from 8 to 10 liters in a 24-hour period. For example, in 24 hours, the normal tract produces:

1200 ml. of saliva
2000 ml. of gastric juice

1200 ml. of pancreatic juice
700 ml. of bile
3000 ml. of succus entericus

Normally, 95% of this fluid is reabsorbed from the gastrointestinal tract, so that only 200 to 300 ml. of fluid is actually lost in the feces. The tract, therefore, becomes a major user of body fluids, and the normal conservation of this volume of fluid is essential to continued well-being. If the motility of the tract is increased so that the time for reabsorption is cut short, the fluid losses from this route become very important. This is a frequent problem in patients with diarrhea. The various medical therapies that remove fluid from the tract, such as the suctioning of the stomach or small intestine that frequently accompanies surgery on the tract, also create problems of fluid and electrolyte replacement which are a major medical and nursing problem.

Obviously, too, the supply of blood vessels to the walls of the tract must be great in order to accommodate the absorption of materials from it. The very active rate of regeneration of cells of the lining also requires a rich blood supply. Any erosion of the lining potentially exposes the individual to severe blood loss—such bleeding points are inaccessible without surgical intervention, and the bleeding into the tract may be large and acute, or slow but persistent over a period of time, with the same ultimate results. Any interference with the blood supply to the tract, by occlusion of the arterial supply, will create an immediate interference with its total function. Such failure of blood supply creates death of tissue in the walls of the tract, as it will anywhere in the body, but destruction of even a small part of the tract results in a failure of the entire system and constitutes a surgical emergency. In addition, the fact that the tract is really

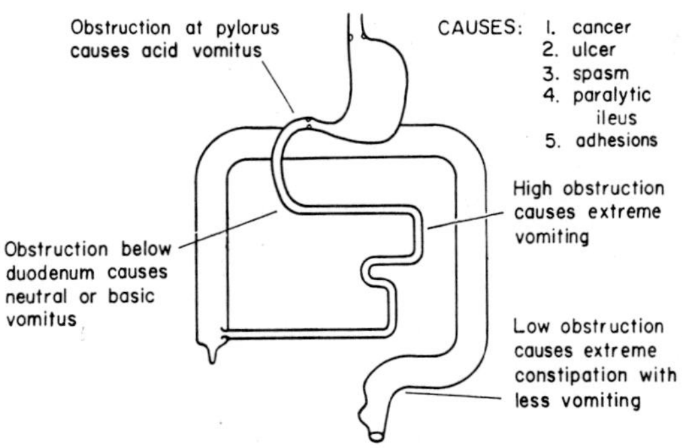

FIGURE 47. Obstruction in any part of the gastrointestinal tract alters the total function of the system, and this has inevitable and often serious implications in the well-being of the individual. (From Guyton, A.C.: *Textbook of Medical Physiology*, 3rd ed. W.B. Saunders Co., Philadelphia, 1966.)

outside the body is further emphasized by the presence of microorganisms, many of which are normally found there and actually contribute to the digestive processes, whereas others are pathogens and enter the body via the tract. Any interference with the integrity of the tract—an opening in the walls that will allow the digestive materials to escape into body cavities—also constitutes an urgent surgical emergency because of the danger of infection, as well as chemical assault on tissues that are not protected from the chemical activity of the digestive juices.

Although the gastrointestinal tract is a complex of several tissues performing separate functions, its response to assault is singularly unified. Since all materials brought into the body must enter via the tract, it is not strange that the mechanism for eliminating noxious materials involves the entire gastrointestinal tract, and, further, that the response is elicited by a wide variety of stimuli. Nausea and vomiting are frequent symptoms of disease, including many disorders in which the pathophysiology is not primarily in the gastrointestinal tract. The stimulus which sets off the vomiting reflex may arise anywhere in the gastrointestinal tract, and includes such factors as overdistention, irritant substance, or even over-excitation related to emotional factors. The mechanism of vomiting involves powerful muscular assistance from the abdominal muscles and the diaphragm, so that in repeated vomiting the element of muscle fatigue and pain may be evidenced. Nausea is a frequent precursor of vomiting itself and is often attended by excessive salivation, as if the extra liquid were intended to act as a diluent for the irritant elsewhere in the tract. Vomiting, however, may occur without nausea and is seen in diseases in which the vomiting center in the medulla is stimulated even though there is no such stimulus in the gastrointestinal tract itself.

The patient who feels nauseated, or who has actually vomited, will also be anorexic. The problem of the desire to ingest food, however, is usually much more complicated. While the physiological mechanisms of hunger per se are fairly well understood, the additional factors usually described as "appetite" are somewhat less so, because so many emotional and intellectual factors influence them. There is no doubt that the hunger mechanism itself is part of the basic and ever-present physiological need of the organism, which cannot survive too long without food. But the factors that make food desirable, and a specific food desirable at a given time, are much more difficult to determine.

Nursing Intervention in the Provision for Nutritional Needs

It is apparent that cellular nutrition will suffer from any interference with the integrity of the gastrointestinal tract. The cluster of nursing problems related to adequate nutrition thus includes the maintenance of proper function when the disease process is primarily in the tract, as well as when the tract is only secondarily affected by the disease process.

One of the most common nursing problems is concerned with the mechanism of swallowing food. Some of the preparation of food does take place in the mouth, where it is masticated and mixed with saliva, and a bolus of lubricated food is prepared for swallowing. The voluntary aspects of this process include the proper mastication and preparation for swallowing, factors that will be influenced by the condition of the oral cavity, the presence of teeth, and whether or not the individual has the sheer strength to perform this function without assistance. The diet can be adjusted to accommodate the lack of teeth or dentures which are ill-fitting (weight loss associated with illness often changes the shape of the mouth so that dentures that once fit no longer perform adequately). The diet can also be adjusted to conserve the strength of the very ill and weak patient. Assisting such patients during mealtime is a major nursing responsibility, and the ingenious nurse can assist such patients in many ways—by the size of portions offered, the way in which the portions are prepared, and by carefully pacing the activity to the patient's tolerance.

There is, however, a most serious consideration in assisting patients to eat: the passage for the swallowing of food is shared with the respiratory system. When food is swallowed, the glottis closes off the respiratory tree so that no food can enter the trachea or lungs. Ordinarily this mechanism works well, although even perfectly healthy and normal people occasionally get food "in the wrong throat." When the individual is very weak, or suffers some paralysis of the involved muscles, or even just because of the position in which his head is held when he attempts to swallow, the danger of aspiration of food into the respiratory tree is a very real threat. Foreign material of this kind in the lungs creates an inflammatory process that is always dangerous but is particularly disastrous for the individual already very ill. Liquids are even more difficult for the weakened individual to handle than are semisoft food masses. Positioning the patient to gain maximum advantage from gravity is often helpful, but even then, feeding such a patient requires constant watchfulness on the part of the nurse.

Consideration of measures to prevent aspiration is also vital in the patient who is vomiting, since vomitus may also be aspirated if the position of the head is not arranged to prevent it. Any patient with a nasogastric tube is susceptible to this kind of accident, particularly if nutrient liquids are being introduced into the gastrointestinal tract by this method.

Observation of the patient to determine the status of his nutritional needs is a nursing responsibility. Any symptoms referable to the gastrointestinal tract, such as pain, distention, epigastric distress, heartburn, or complaints of nausea with or without actual vomiting, should be promptly reported so that the physician can prescribe for the nutritional needs with these factors in mind. The nurse should evaluate the actual nutritional intake on the basis of the foods actually eaten by the patient, and record the amounts of specific foods he has taken. When the intake is less than is consonant with his needs, this fact, too, should be promptly reported.

The very real physiological and emotional components that influence dietary intake should always be considered in the nurse's evaluation of the patient's progress. The surgical patient who is restricted in his food intake must be carefully guided back to an adequate diet over a period of time, and frequently the return of the appetite, or the interest in food, is an indication of recovery from the entire episode of illness. Recognizing that even the food habits of the nurse may influence how she evaluates the patient's desires for food, attention to the personal desires and idiosyncrasies of diet in the individual will hasten the time when he is able to take an adequate nutritional diet. The social nature of a good meal thoroughly enjoyed has as much significance in the hospital ward as anywhere else. This is an invitation to well-being and satisfaction, contributing in a real sense to the recovery of the sick individual.

The Pathophysiology of Peptic Ulcer

For many modern men, theological considerations notwithstanding, the soul rests in the stomach. The immediacy with which food provides gratification and well-being is matched only by the equally prompt response of the stomach to unpleasant experience. In very unusual human beings, food is not a daily symbol of satisfaction, but for most individuals, the waking hours are punctuated by periodic opportunities to satisfy the "inner man," and homemade apple pie represents all of the gustatory and emotional gratifications that spell security and well-being. The emphasis on food in the mass media of twentieth century America is compounded of a strange mixture of science and soul-saving. Nutritional principles are widely advertised and widely acknowledged by homemakers who suffer anxiety if they fail to provide their families with the "basic four" every day. But at the same time, the feature articles on the women's pages emphasize that the average American consumes far too much carbohydrate, more salt than the body needs or can safely use, too much fat for healthy blood vessels, and (with obvious sorrow) not enough protein because it is too expensive. By definition, the successful housewife and mother is that remarkable woman who provides a balanced diet, superbly cooked and economically purchased, with a positive talent for serving it in a restful atmosphere replete with good taste, good conversation, and merry family relationships. If some time in every day an adult confronts a meal that is less than satisfying to him, he may fantasize about the way "Mother" used to cook and thus engineer a disappointment somewhat more intense than that stimulated by the food he is eating. The moral tone of the question: "Does one live to eat or eat to live?" stirs only a little guilt in the hungry consumer. The focus on food is a sociological phenomenon. It is small wonder that it also creates a medical problem of considerable proportions.

The measure of the incidence of stomach disorders is evident, in a peripheral sense, in the annual expenditure for drugs that are capable, according to the advertisements, of soothing, coating, protecting, and otherwise restoring the recalcitrant organ to a state of well-being. The television viewer cannot spend an evening free of pseudoscientific "experiments" that show the "stomach acids" eating away at a cloth and the sponsor's product gallantly protecting another piece from disaster. Of course, the viewer himself, long before the evening is ended, has managed enough potato chips and appropriate beverages to make even this explanation of the sensation in his epigastrium a welcome bit of information. Ordinary abuse of the stomach is compounded by ready availability of food everywhere an individual may be—the movies, the ball games, even the outdoor band concerts—so that constant consuming of unnecessary foods is a way of life, and it is not at all surprising that the manufacturers of antacids have flourished in the face of it.

The fact is that the lining of the stomach is capable of producing a juice with a pH of 1.0—or less—representing a proton concentration 4,000,000 times that of the arterial blood. The "acid" condition that is the target of the television advertisement is a normal and necessary attribute of every healthy stomach. Utilizing tremendous amounts of cellular energy, the stomach lining manufactures from 1200 to 1500 ml. of this caustic juice every day. The gastric secretions are not pure hydrochloric acid, of course. The stomach lining also secretes pepsin, an extremely active proteolytic enzyme, which is effective as a digestant of proteins, but only in a pH of 5.0 or less. The importance of this acidic fluid in digestion becomes clinically apparent when the secretion of hydrochloric acid is restricted. In such clinical entities, it is not unusual that the patient be given hydrochloric acid as part of his therapy. It was clearly nature's intention that the defensive means of the stomach be sufficient to prevent the gastric juice from digesting the lining of the stomach itself. The problem of peptic ulcer arises when that defense breaks down and the wall of the organ is attacked by its own physiological secretions.

Many questions related to hunger and its characteristics have yet to be answered, but the distinct influences on gastric secretion are fairly well understood. The first phase is called "cephalic" (head) because it is a response to stimuli which suggest food, although it occurs well before any

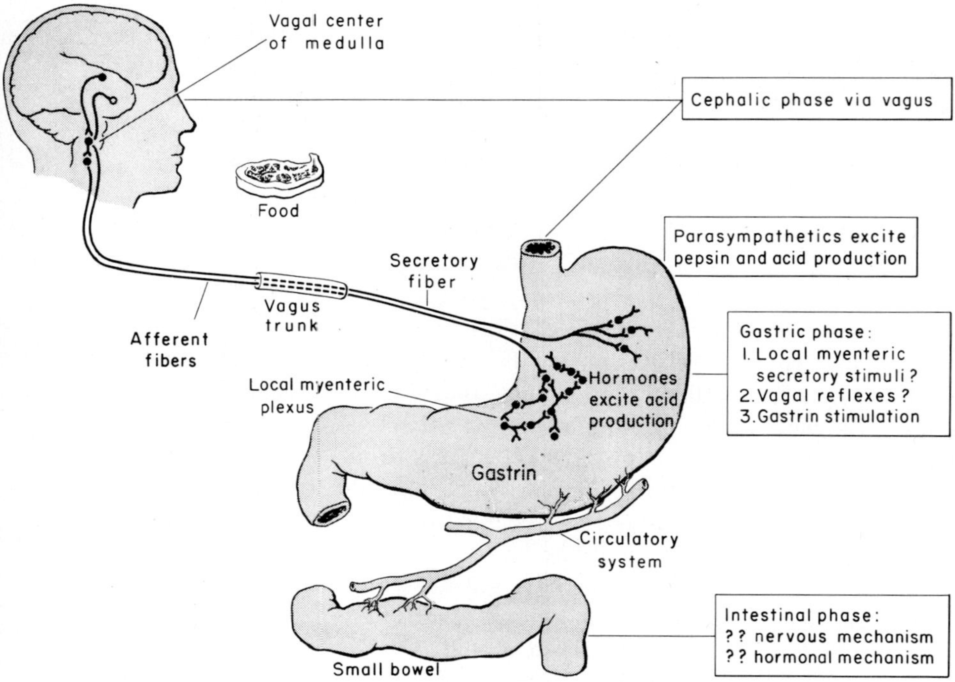

FIGURE 48. Gastric secretion is a complex process, mediated by both nervous and hormonal control, and occurring in identifiable steps. (From Guyton, A.C.: *Textbook of Medical Physiology,* 3rd ed. W.B. Saunders Co., Philadelphia, 1966.)

food is actually ingested. It is a preparatory phase, necessary to establish the conditions for the ingesting of food. The sight, smell, or even thought of food can stimulate a production of gastric juice of as much as 500 ml. per hour, and even if food is not readily available, the secretion will continue for 10 to 20 minutes after the stimulus is received. This preparation of the stomach exactly duplicates that which occurs when the individual is about to sit down and consume a meal. It is elicited by the fight-flight mechanism as well, because this response includes the engorgement of the stomach lining and the increased secretion of gastric juice. The readiness to consume a meal associated with the fight-flight mechanism reflects the more primitive behavior when the confrontation with a food source meant that the victor consumed his victim. The human stomach is prepared to "consume a victim," even though such a response to the environment is useless and even dangerous in modern man. Since anxiety is a stimulus for the fight-or-flight response, the incidence of the production of excess gastric secretion must be remarkably high.

The second phase of gastric secretion arises in direct response to the presence of food in the stomach. Although the mechanism is not understood, the stomach lining produces hormones which prompt the secretory cells to manufacture gastric juice. The tactile presence of food, moreover, stimulates the flow of mucus in the stomach. During this phase of actual contact, then, the digestive juice and the protective juice are simultaneously provided. The third, or intestinal, phase is characterized by a continuing flow of gastric juice so long as there is chyme in the small intestine. Although the major function of digestion in the stomach has been completed, as much as 10% of the gastric juice produced may arise during the intestinal phase. This, too, is probably mediated by hormones, although the mechanism has not been described. The three phases of gastric juice secretion emphasize the interaction which makes this highly localized physiological response a systemic type of process. The relationship between gastric function and that of the rest of the gastrointestinal system includes many refinements of interaction which serve to coordinate the diverse activities of the entire system. Distention of the small bowel or the presence of acid in the upper regions of the intestinal tract stimulates the enterogastric reflex, which slows down the emptying of the stomach, and thus integrates this process into the total activities of the entire system. Stomach-emptying time is also delayed by high fat content, and when the pH of the empty stomach falls to 1.5 or less, the protective reflex prevents the spillage of the gastric juice into the small intestine.

The factors that permit the digestion of the stomach wall, and thus the presence of peptic ulcerations, are diverse. Any number of factors are capable of causing sufficient irritation of the gastric mucosa to produce symptoms of discomfort, clinically a gastritis, but more familiarly known as "heartburn" (especially to the snacking television viewer). Irritant

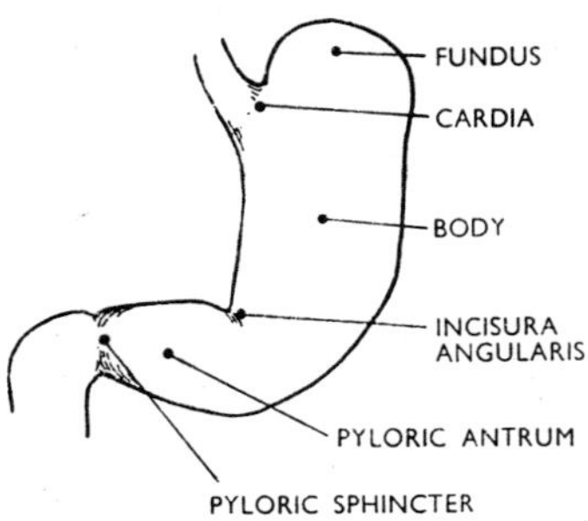

FIGURE 49. The stomach is anatomically described in several subdivisions. The site of ulceration influences the development and nature of the symptoms. (From Ellis, H.: *Clinical Anatomy*, 3rd ed. F.A. Davis Co. [Blackwell Scientific Publications], Philadelphia, 1966.)

foods or beverages are frequent culprits, and infections, both bacterial and viral, may also cause an acute inflammatory response in the stomach lining. Alcoholic beverages, of course, are notorious irritants. But gastritis in itself is not equivalent to peptic ulcer. An acute gastritis usually responds to abstention from food and fluids for a brief period, followed by a bland diet for a while longer. A peptic ulcer, however, arises when the relative pH and proteolytic action of the gastric juice overwhelm the normal defensive capacity of the gastric mucosa. When this happens, an excoriation in the wall of the stomach is formed, and the usual response of the tissues to any insult occurs here too: an inflammatory reaction is established.

Destruction of the integrity of any organ interferes with its function, but damage to the hollow viscus presents additional threat to the individual. The excavation, first of all, may erode a blood vessel large enough to initiate a serious hemorrhage. Within the hollow tube, it is impossible to apply pressure to the bleeding site, and because, even in disease, the gastrointestinal tract is in motion, it may be very difficult to stop such bleeding before a great deal of blood has been lost. Bleeding from ulcerations is not always sudden, dramatic, and unmistakable, although it may well be. Often there is a small but consistent blood loss identifiable only because the stools of such individuals assume a characteristic tarry color caused by the digestion of their own blood. Since many individuals do not observe their own stools, this symptom may not be noticed until there has already been considerable blood loss. It is not usual that the individual will vomit blood unless there has been a rather large and sudden hemorrhage. When the vomitus is bright red and clearly identifiable as blood, the individual is undoubtedly having a *serious* hemorrhage. The "coffee-ground" color of stomach contents, however, arises when the blood remains in contact with the gastric juice for a brief time; usually this indicates that the bleeding has not been as massive. It is nevertheless dangerous, as indeed bleeding always is. Blood loss leads to shock, and treatment must be instantaneous and often heroic.

Any erosion of the hollow viscus also creates the danger of perforation of the wall, and with it a spilling of the contents into the abdominal cavity. This is a critical emergency requiring immediate surgical intervention, because other body tissues are not able to withstand the assault of the highly acidic stomach contents, and the additional danger of spreading infection into the peritoneal cavity is great. Sometimes perforation occurs but results in fistula formation between the site of erosion and another organ in the immediate vicinity. The acute symptoms of perforation may be absent, but, since the pancreas is often involved in this kind of accident, a severe pancreatitis may develop, which is in itself a threatening turn of events.

The subsidence of the inflammatory reaction is usually accompanied by a scar formation, typical of healing. When the healed region becomes grossly scarred, there may be a distinct tightening or stenosis (narrowing) of the lumen. This represents another serious interference with the normal function of a hollow viscus. Sufficient scarring, or, indeed, sufficient inflammation with accompanying edema, may create narrowing that is equivalent to obstruction. This, too, may require surgical intervention.

The symptoms of peptic ulcer may exist for a long time before a serious turn of events sends the patient to the hospital emergency room. The frequency of stomach "distress" in the general population suggests that many more individuals have peptic ulcers than present themselves for treatment thereof. Characteristically, the pain and discomfort of peptic

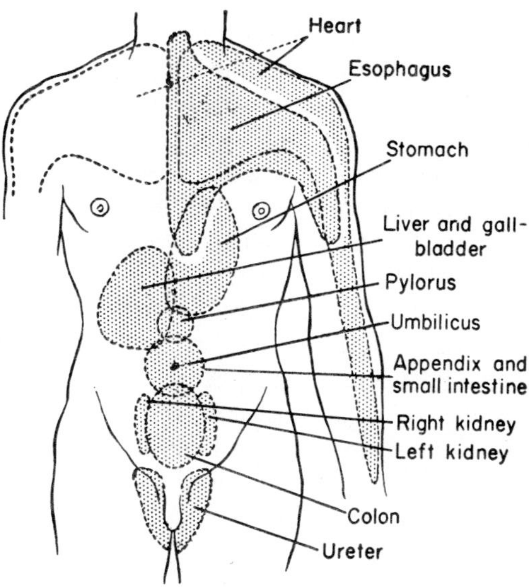

FIGURE 50. Pain in the viscera is referred to body regions on the surface, but often lacks the precision of pinpointing the exact cause without a careful medical work-up. (From Guyton, A.C.: *Textbook of Medical Physiology,* 3rd ed. W.B. Saunders Co., Philadelphia, 1966.)

ulcers, though relieved by food and antacids, are a persistent and periodic manifestation. The pain is highly localized over the site of the ulcer, and while identified as being in the epigastrium, it often radiates to the back as well. The occurrence of the pain accompanies the cyclic changes in the digestive function through the course of a day. Although it is generally absent before breakfast, it appears regularly within one to four hours following each meal that is taken. Another characteristic is the incidence of pain during the early hours of night. Between midnight and 3 a.m. the individual is often awakened from sleep with pain and must seek antacid or food relief. The etiology of peptic ulcer remains a mystery, but its association with emotional instability is rather well fixed, even in the lay mind, and recent research has indicated that the sufferer has a significantly higher secretion of gastric juice during the dream portion of his sleep than does the non-ulcer individual. While the significance of this fact is impossible to pinpoint on the basis of present knowledge, it seems well established that the physiological change that accompanies sleep contributes to the progress of the erosion in the stomach wall in susceptible individuals. Many persons resort to self-medication with soda bicarbonate to relieve the symptoms of ulcer pain; actually, several of the commercial antacids are essentially sodium bicarbonate. This is so characteristic that the use of this substance is called "soda-relief." The difficulty is that the relief is very limited, because soda bicarbonate is not a true buffer, and the temporary relief following the combination with hydrochloric acid in the stomach is accompanied by an "acid rebound," which soon results in more discomfort than before. Some individuals have used soda bicarbonate in such quantities in their search for relief that they have actually created an alkalosis (i.e., a raised blood pH) and may have distinct symptoms of electrolyte imbalance as a result.

The emotional component in the pathogenesis of peptic ulcers is widely recognized but poorly understood. In the high-powered, fast-moving, and tension-provoking atmosphere of the modern world, the sufferer from peptic ulcers enjoys a certain "status" in having a disease that characterizes him as an aggressive and ambitious member of society. It is not unusual that some diseases have more social acceptance than others. This has been true throughout history, and many diagnoses have enjoyed the distinction of social approval through the years. The pallid and waxen Victorian lady was distinguished by her tuberculosis. There is a social struggle now as to whether high blood pressure is more indicative of the young man "on the way up" than peptic ulcers, but an inordinate satisfaction accompanies the diagnosis in the individual whose digestive juices are consuming the lining of his stomach. The discomfort is real, and the threats posed by the ulcer even more compelling. It seems entirely possible, however, that the organismic nature of disease is nowhere more evident than here. There is a decided pathophysiological change, mediated at least in part by emotional instability and the gentle approval of society. The treatment of the patient with a peptic ulcer must therefore concern every aspect of the individual's life-style. The little package of antacid with the candy flavor available at every drug counter and in every supermarket has hardly solved the problem of peptic ulcer.

Care of the Patient with Peptic Ulcer

The Conservation of Energy

Ulceration of the stomach lining, with its threat of sequential complications, fundamentally represents a nutritional impasse for the individual. The treatment of peptic ulcers always involves dietary management, but in the highly specific manipulation of the pathophysiological response of the organ itself. The food is the therapy, and the diet is planned to alleviate symptoms, as well as to provide adequate nourishment. In its simplest form, the threat to energy sources is always present in the peptic ulcer patient. The focus of therapy in these patients is to bind the hydrochloric acid in the stomach so that the irritant effect is removed, thus allowing the ulcer to heal. This is a localized emphasis, but it cannot be achieved without consideration of the total effect of treatment on the entire body. Weight loss is not uncommon in older individuals who develop gastric ulcers, but a paradoxical weight gain is more apparent in young individuals. The weight gain is often due to the ingestion of high-calorie foods taken to relieve the discomfort. The ulcer victim quickly learns that milk —and even cream—will alleviate his discomfort promptly, and, in fact, that food in the stomach has the same effect, no matter what that food may be. The weight gain is due entirely to overeating in the sense of calorie intake, but it usually conceals some degree of nutritional or electrolyte dysfunction. This, of course, is a threat to the energy utilization in that individual.

The development of the serious complications of insult to a hollow viscus may bring about a very rapid threat to the energy balance in the individual. The loss of blood obviously upsets the entire functioning of the body, and its replacement, along with restoration of the integrity of the circulatory system, is extremely urgent. Bleeding in the gastrointestinal tract is an immediate indication to withhold oral food and fluids. The presence of ingested food in the tract stimulates motility, and withholding food permits the resting of the gastrointestinal organs. This often must be assisted with drugs, but, even with medication, complete cessation of gastrointestinal activity is neither desirable nor possible. With the loss of blood and the attendant degree of shock, conservation measures directed at the energy balance of the individual are identical to all nursing intervention required by survival needs in the patient. Bedrest and the provision for basic hygienic needs are required in order to make the least demand possible on the individual's available energy potential. The total abstention from food intake over a period of time—and in these circumstances such a restriction may be necessary for days—further compromises the energy resource of the individual, because the nutrients are not being supplied in balance with his daily need.

The other acute-emergency event associated with progressive gastric ulceration is perforation of the hollow viscus. This, too, is often accompanied by shock and demands the immediate institution of survival nursing intervention. The additional and grave danger of widespread intra-abdominal infection represents another demand on the individual's energy resource which may be life-threatening. Once more, oral intake is stopped and energy production is dependent upon the individual's potential. The gradual closing of the tube that accompanies stenosis is less dramatic and sometimes not apparent to the individual until the obstruction is rather well established. But, during the period of time in which this is taking place, the effective transportation of nutrients to body tissues must be embarrassed.

Conservative therapy in the individual with gastric ulcers aims to promote healing of the defect without the development of these serious complications. In the early stages of such treatment, the diet is extremely limited in content. The aim is to keep the stomach sufficiently supplied with substances that will bind the gastric juice but to do so in as quiet and as limited a way as possible. Neutralization of gastric juice is often accomplished by use of buffer drugs, so that the proton concentration is regulated over a period of time. The ingestion of such buffering compounds is frequently repeated throughout the day and night. An hourly dosage of such medication is not unusual, and there have been numerous efforts to make the medication continuous by administration through a nasogastric tube directly into the stomach. The use of a milk and cream mixture may be alternated in the hourly schedule with a buffering drug. Such a routine, lasting often as long as a week or more, very clearly does not provide an adequate diet. When foods are reintroduced into the diet, they are often given in small meals over the course of the day. The foods selected are "bland" and there is a restriction of all foods that tend to stimulate excess volumes of gastric juice. Such foods are called "secretagogues"; they include alcohol, coffee, tea, spices, and roughage in general. A fairly wide variety of selection may remain, but the food is given in a puréed form to eliminate as much of the roughage and bulk as possible.

Even in the most carefully planned "ulcer" diet, food restriction is apparent. The individual who must satisfy his nutritional needs with this diet is often one with long-time habits of poor food selection, and the restrictions may create a great deal of emotional disaffection. This, too, exacts a cost in energy utilization. The stereotype of the ulcer sufferer as a hyperactive and tense individual is far from the reality of clinical experience. But the evidence of an emotional component in this disease entity is overwhelming, and it may well be that the observable behavior of the individual patient, while disagreeing with the familiar stereotype, nevertheless indicates a degree of difficulty in his adjustments to the demands of life that will require sensitive nursing assessment. The frequent injunction to provide a restful environment, free of emotional stress, for the individual with a gastric ulcer is a generalization that frustrates the nurse and excludes the patient. No brief period of hospitalization can permanently or completely alter a life-pattern of behavior which in itself has precipitated the disease. The time of hospitalization, although theoretically capable of providing a restful atmosphere, must by its very nature also pose a threat to the ulcer patient. While his reaction to the anxiety of hospitalization, and the experiences that frustrate or upset him, cannot be eliminated, those aspects of care that are controlled by the nurse can be made as satisfying as possible. This requires, however, a nurse-patient interaction based on the individual's behavioral response to his care. He soon learns that the hourly administration of his antacid drug is an essential aspect of his treatment. Often the drugs are left at the bedside and the patient is responsible for taking them himself. It should be obvious—but unfortunately sometimes is not—that, if the patient is to take an hourly dose, he should have some bedside means of telling the time. Hospital admission policies encourage patients to leave valuable jewelry at home—including wristwatches. And very few hospital rooms are equipped with clocks. This simple environmental factor may be very distressing if it is ignored. Furthermore, the patient must have a constant supply of such medication. It must be replaced as it is consumed, and delay in doing so may be very upsetting to the patient. If his therapy also includes hourly intake of milk or cream, such foods must be kept at the bedside and must be refrigerated if they remain there. The problem of keeping an ice bucket filled with ice cubes sometimes becomes an administrative problem entirely out of proportion to the task. Such minor details of care can create major frustration and hostility in an individual who has already proved that he handles such stress in a very unsatisfactory way. The subtleties of his energy expense that are related to the emotional disturbances underlying his problem can rarely be handled by the nurse. The physician may offer the patient essential support and reassurance which is psychotherapeutic in its intent and may back it up with sedative drugs during the hospitalization. He may forbid activities that seem to upset the individual. Often this includes a ban on his usual business activities, and if the physician knows of family turmoil, he may enjoin against certain visitors. The nurse, on the other hand, must depend upon a relationship with the patient which spells security to the patient. Perhaps the most significant contribution to sparing the individual the cost of emotional energy fruitlessly wasted lies in the demonstration to him that the nurse is knowledgeable and competent to care for him. His security rests in his safety.

The development of progressive change in the ulcer patient that ultimately leads to serious sequelae is the usual factor that sends him to the operating room. The emergency situations, such as uncontrolled bleeding and perforation, require surgery very promptly upon diagnosis. Preparation of such individuals for this experience must focus on the urgency of the survival needs created by it. While every nurse strives to provide the patient with the comfort and security of proper emotional care, a hemorrhaging individual cannot be "reassured" out of his difficulties. He faces a seeping loss of his life itself and, when that threat exists, the nurse contributes to his emotional well-being by a quick and responsive attention to the danger he is in. Every surgical procedure is fraught with danger—some of it real but a tremendous proportion of it imagined. When the procedure is anticipated and planned for, the energy requirements that are apparent in nutritional and fluid needs, the hemoglobin and hematocrit, and the general state of the individual's health can be balanced and supported by preoperative preparation. However, an emergency surgical procedure does not allow time for this kind of preparation. The surgeon tries to compensate for the risks that he must take with the patient when the emergency arises. He may delay as long as it is safe to do so, in order to eliminate the shock by previous treatment, but he cannot always delay as long as he would like. If the situation is serious enough, he must compromise with complete preparation and compensate as best he can during the procedure and postoperative treatment. In effect, this represents conservation of the patient's energy in order to focus as much of it as possible on the defense he can muster to withstand the stress of the experience. But even surgical preparation that is not restrained by urgent questions of survival is essentially a planned program for conserving energy, so that the individual will have all he needs to withstand the procedure and convalesce without incident. Thus, preoperative nursing care includes an evaluation of the patient's energy exchange, and postoperative care measures the return of his energy capability. Nutritional intake is always restricted in any surgical procedure involving an anesthetic, but it is most severely restricted when the surgical procedure itself involves the gastrointestinal tract. Restoring nutritional balance to such patients is gradual but essential to ultimate recovery. It is often striking that the recovery of the surgical patient is directly proportional to his food intake and particularly to his ability to handle proteins. The increasing strength and freedom to move about are behavioral measurements of his increasing energy resource.

The Conservation of Structural Integrity

The presence of a peptic ulcer is a patent infringement on the structural integrity of the gastrointestinal tract, and the therapeutic process is designed to restore it as promptly as possible. The specific sequelae that arise when a hollow viscus is injured outline the dimensions of the clinical problem, but restoration of function of the entire system is essential to the total well-being of the individual. The ideal healing process, of course, is to foster repair of the defect so that no sequelae will follow. This can never be predicted in any patient because of the individual ways in which the human body responds to injury. Unlike the case of ulcerations on the surface of the body, visualization of the injury inside the gastrointestinal tract is not possible without employing specific technical means. Most often this involves x-rays of the tract, utilizing radio-opaque liquids which the patient drinks immediately before the x-rays are taken. While this is a valuable diagnostic tool, it is not always possible to definitively demonstrate a lesion in the wall of the stomach by this method. During the procedure, the radiologist observes the passage of the radio-opaque dye through the stomach by means of direct fluoroscopy. The motility patterns of the gastrointestinal tract, the emptying time of the stomach, and the behavior of the stomach sphincters may also indicate the presence of an ulceration, even if the direct visualization is not possible. The ingestion of this substance and the x-rays which follow are not possible if there is already evidence of bleeding in measurable amounts or perforation of the stomach. In such instances, identification of the source of the difficulty rests with the surgeon in the operating room.

It is characteristic of all inflammations in the body that they respond best and heal most satisfactorily if they are treated very early in their course. Although this does not always assure the individual that he will be free of later episodes of the disease, the earlier treatment is instituted, the better are the chances for lasting relief. As the ulceration and its attendant inflammation become prolonged, the increase in probability of bleeding, perforation, or obstruction is marked. Because there is so decided an advantage to early treatment, the widespread "self-diagnosis" and "self-medication" with antacids are particularly disastrous to the individual. Delay in seeking treatment for persistent symptoms of peptic ulcer means increasing structural change which not only may expose the individual to great hazard but may render future therapy less satisfactory.

Successful medical management of peptic ulcers is possible as long as the ulceration has not proceeded to severe symptoms requiring immediate surgical intervention. Dietary control and the use of drugs may, however, be required as a continuing way of life so long as the individual continues to confront the stress in his environment in unsatisfactory ways. It is frequent that, when the symptoms are alleviated, the individual does not respect the dietary restrictions, and the causes that created the original episode may remain operative and produce subsequent ones.

Surgical intervention of all kinds is essentially designed to restore the structural integrity of the gastrointestinal tract. There are numerous surgical procedures used to accomplish this in patients with peptic ulcers. The effect of the surgical procedure is to re-establish the patency of the tract by excising the diseased portion of the stomach and anastomosing (opening) the residual portion to the small bowel. If it is possible to leave a portion of the stomach, this is done, because the physiological function of the stomach is essential to the total digestive process. An individual without a stomach is able to eat and even gradually consume fairly normal meals, but the hormonal interaction involving the stomach is essential and is therefore conserved if possible. The procedure of removing the diseased portion of the stomach and establishing a new opening into the small intestine is often accompanied by a concurrent procedure that interrupts the vagus nerve fibers that normally influence stomach motility. This is done to decrease motility and the excessive secretion of gastric juice following the surgery.

The re-establishment of a patent structure to the gastrointestinal tract, especially if a portion of it is surgically removed, represents a new pattern of function as well. The initial postoperative period is devoted to the proper healing of the incisions so that, with resumption of digestive processes, the restored tube will remain intact. Food is reintroduced very slowly and in small amounts, because the revised structure of the gastrointestinal tract must become established over a period of time. Ultimately, the individual may resume a more normal diet, but for many weeks his food intake is restricted in both content and quantity. The individual himself prefers small meals, served at frequent intervals during the day, because he quickly feels "full." Re-establishing bowel function is essential after such surgical intervention. All kinds of anesthetics tend to depress gastrointestinal motility, and narcotic drugs, administered to relieve postoperative pain, have a similar effect. Distention of the gastrointestinal tract following surgery is prevented by continuous suction, which removes the accumulation of liquid secretions and gas (often swallowed air). Suction of secretions from the gastrointestinal tract, however, is always accompanied by electrolyte, as well as fluid, loss; obviously, both of these factors must be compensated for in the treatment. During the time the individual is not allowed oral ingestion of food, all fluid, electrolytes, and some nutrients must be given parenterally by intravenous fluids. The amount of drainage by suction, and the nature of the drainage, must be recorded by the nurse. She is also responsible for maintaining the fluid intake, and when intravenous fluids must be given over a period of days, this requires constant attention to make certain that the fluid is, indeed, entering the vein (and not the tissues around it), and that it is being administered at the proper rate. The re-establishment of bowel function and the passing of a stool usually occurs within three to five days of the surgery. A mildly stimulating suppository or a low enema may be used to assist the individual in having a bowel movement. Once this has been established, the ingestion of a more liberal diet is allowed.

Some of the most important issues of structural integrity arise in the care of the surgical patient. Proper positioning on the operating room table is based on careful physiological and anatomical considerations by the skilled personnel in the operating room. Postoperative positioning first emphasizes maintenance of the patent airway and a maximum of respiratory excursion following the anesthetic. Subsequent mobilization is extremely important and includes turning the patient every hour, as well as encouraging him to cough and deep-breathe in order to fully re-expand the lungs and prevent complications related to inhalation of anesthetics. Postoperatively, the individual is ambulated—in spite of the attached tubes and equipment, he must be gotten out of bed and actually walked. This procedure, which seems so cruel to the surgical patient and so difficult to the nurse, is the best insurance against the development of circulatory emergencies in the postoperative patient. It stimulates the flow of blood in the periphery and prevents the formation of clots in the legs which might break loose and travel to a vital organ such as the lungs or heart. In addition, the mobilization improves muscle tone and actually enhances the return to vigor that must come following surgery. Early ambulation is an essential factor in maintaining structural integrity, and although it is often very difficult, after the first time most individuals recognize that it is helping them and look forward to it. It is, of course, important that the patient be given sufficient assistance to prevent falling or injury, until the nurse is absolutely certain that he can mobilize himself without danger.

The onus of emotional components in peptic ulcer patients must never obscure the fact that structural changes have taken place, regardless of the etiology. The structural change threatens well-being in several ways, and, therefore, it must be dealt with, even if the emotional instability of the individual is not understood. Psychotherapeutic assistance may be offered the patient by his physician, and such help may be essential in some individuals following treatment in order to preclude the development of another structural insult.

The Conservation of Personal Integrity

The patient with a peptic ulcer comes to treatment already seriously in contention with his own personal integrity. While the emotional concomitants of his life-pattern may not be clearly apparent either to him or to his physician, the likelihood that such determinants have influenced his pathology is great. It is extremely probable that the social definition of the "ulcer" type is familiar to the individual, and even though there is the quietest approval associated with the diagnosis, the tensions and difficulties that create the stereotype are never socially satisfactory ones. The psychosomatic label accompanies the patient to his physician. Providing for the patient the kind of treatment that will definitively deal with the emotional problems rests with the physician, either through his own efforts at psychotherapy or by referral to psychiatric care. Once the symptoms are well-established, however, the treatment must emphasize the disease process itself and continue to do so until all physical threat has been eliminated. In the presence of active disease, no substitute can be offered for treatment of the altered physiological pattern and its attendant structural change. It is extremely unwise to approach the care of the peptic ulcer patient from a predominantly psychosocial bias. He is physically ill, and until physical well-being is restored, emotional well-being is impossible.

The factors that influence hospitalization, the presence of pain and discomfort, the anticipation of uncomfortable therapeutic procedures, restriction of dietary intake, and perhaps even a life-threatening episode of bleeding or perforation add to the already disturbed emotional tone in the patient. They are stimuli for dismay in any patient, but in the care of the peptic ulcer patient, they are additional tensions which he must be helped to face. Every individual must be assessed on his own terms, and the influence of his emotional difficulties specifically identified in his own behavior.

It is impossible for the peptic ulcer patient to escape even briefly from the therapy he must follow during hospitalization. Some form of medication or food will be administered *every hour on the hour*. It is soon apparent to the patient and the nurse that the time for another dose comes quickly, and the focus on the hourly administration concentrates much of his waking attention on his illness. The restriction of food also emphasizes his problem. It is rarely an emotionally satisfying diet, excluding specifically those foods that have a high taste index, and the use of puréed foods may create some problems in itself. By definition, puréed foods are "baby foods" and, for the aggressive, anxious individual, such a diet may be even more intolerable. The monotonous texture of a puréed diet eliminates the satisfactions of chewing and perceiving the nature of the food taken into the mouth, and this contributes in some degree to its lack of interest. Each meal, because it is so different from the usual food offered an adult, reinforces the emphasis on the stomach problems of the patient, and he cannot find satisfaction on an adult level because he is often also forbidden to smoke and is not allowed coffee or tea—the "adult" beverages. The variety of foods available in a hospital menu may increase the problem; it is not uncommon that, when the gelatin is always "red," the patient reacts to it in the manner of the Spanish bull. There is, of course, little that the nurse can do to make an unpalatable and deliberately bland diet truly satisfying for the patient. The manner of serving it, the environment in which it is eaten, and the sympathetic recognition of the patient's feelings about it can lower the emotional tone somewhat. If, in addition, he can be helped to understand that, during treatment, the food is designed to provide therapy, then the purpose may relieve some of the reaction to the diet. Often this routine eliminates symptoms, and the reduction of pain and discomfort in response to the diet may also convince the individual that it can be tolerated. It is equally true that the relief of symptoms will stimulate a desire for a broader diet, but the individual must understand why this cannot be immediately provided for him.

When he must confront a surgical procedure, the peptic ulcer patient —like all patients—must experience some fear and apprehension. It is essential that he understand, within his own capacity for doing so, exactly what is going to happen to him. The nasogastric tube is a source of constant difficulty for many people, and passing it is never entirely free of discomfort for the patient. When procedures are uncomfortable, the patient should not be regaled with assurances that they are not. Recognizing that he is uncomfortable—and that some degree of discomfort must persist—is kinder than ignoring or underestimating it. Whatever measures can be used to insure his comfort in other respects can be tried, and sympathetic attention to his complaints will assure him that the nurse cares about his discomfort, even if it cannot be entirely removed.

The most skillful technical care is required by the postoperative patient, and during the first few days after surgery, attention to his physical and therapeutic needs is the best assurance that he is safe. There is always a medication ordered for pain, and it should never be withheld during the immediate postoperative period. Attention to fluid and electrolyte intake and provision for hygiene and elimination needs are important aspects of postoperative care. Ambulation, breathing exercises, and position change should be provided with sufficient assistance so that he can perform these activities without danger of injury. The restoration of bowel function within five days of surgery may be physically difficult and emotionally trying for the individual; this, too, must be approached by the nurse with his individual needs clearly in mind. Gaseous distention after surgery may be extremely uncomfortable, although the nasogastric suction usually eliminates most of the likelihood that this will occur. The placing of a rectal tube in the anus may relieve gassy discomfort in the lower gastrointestinal tract, and this can be ordered by the physician if necessary. Sometimes drugs are given to help the patient expel flatus (a blowing).

The social niceties, of course, forbid this kind of behavior under ordinary circumstances, and many patients are terribly embarrassed when it is necessary to freely expel gas in the presence of a nurse. Since it is important that the bowel function be restored, the nurse's business-like approach to this event will spare the individual embarrassment as well as encourage him to do so, rather than suffer the pain of holding back.

The individual may also have rather strong feelings about the surgical incision. It is a source of pain in the first place and a permanent reminder to him of the hospitalization and its discomforts. He knows that he faces a time, within the week, when the sutures will be removed, and most individuals await this event with apprehension. He may have some fears that the sutures will not hold and will want to guard his activities to protect himself. The nurse can offer support when he is moved and demonstrate to him how he can support himself to eliminate some of the discomfort. The factors that influence his emotional response to the wound are as diverse as are the people who have operations, but the disfiguring aspects may be very real to him. Men react with as much concern as women to disfiguring scars on their bodies, even though they may not express their feelings about it as directly. In addition, there may well be some questions and apprehensions in their minds concerning the alteration that has been created inside of their bodies. While there is considerable humor regarding the social value of an operation for subsequent bridge-table conversation, few individuals are ever truly sanguine about the experience, and many disguise their apprehension by joking about it. The few who relive it in every possible social situation are probably displaying an inordinate degree of concern, which, unfortunately, is rarely pacified by their relatives and friends. The weakness and helplessness that inevitably attend a surgical procedure are frightening in themselves; in young men and women, the questions asked about future sexual capability are a direct reflection of that fear. Such questions deserve an honest and attentive response; if the nurse is unable to answer, the physician should be informed so that he can discuss it with the individual. Most such fears are completely unfounded, but they should be dealt with promptly when they are expressed.

The Conservation of Social Integrity

Every human being confronts situations in his life which he cannot "stomach." But for some individuals, that muffled rage allows the gastric juice to digest the walls of the organ that manufactures it. While every individual experiences with confining intimacy the physiological effects of the fight-or-flight syndrome, the stimulus that arouses this organismic response arises from his relationships with other persons. It is a most "social" kind of body defense, establishing an organic bridge between human beings. The original purpose of defense in a realistically hostile environment has left the physiological intensity of the response inappropriate to an environment where it is rarely necessary to fight for existence. But the sympathoadrenal discharge of chemicals that stir the entire organism to a plane of combative readiness still fortifies a man to defend his social role in the competitions and challenges of an environment where the struggle to survive is measured by dollars, social privilege, and group recognition. Despite personal goals as diverse as becoming the president of the company or just getting a job in the stock room, the physiological assault in the susceptible individual produces precisely the same structural change in the lining of the stomach. No one knows why this kind of change takes place in some individuals and not in others. There is probably some genetic predisposition, because it is not uncommon that the disease recurs in succeeding generations of one family. There is also some environmental predisposition, inasmuch as gastric ulcers occur frequently in high-altitude areas where adaptation to low oxygen concentrations has taken place; interestingly enough, the incidence is statistically higher in individuals with certain lung diseases in whom oxygen utilization is impaired. The environmental factors may also relate to the dietary patterns of a group, and the disease may occur more frequently in certain areas, even though no definitive evidence exists as to the food habits that are predisposing. Some drugs are known to be ulcerogenic, but one of the accused drugs is aspirin, and though it is consumed by the ton, only certain individuals develop an ulcer therefrom. The most specific and identifiable characteristic, however, is the physiological response of the stomach to the fight-or-flight stimulus: it becomes engorged with blood, and gastric juice is copiously excreted.

The nurse confronts, in the peptic ulcer patient, an individual who has had chronic difficulty in assessing his own social integrity. Conserving it during an acute episode of his illness may be difficult, because the added stress of the illness itself represents still another frustration in the pattern of striving that characterizes his life. That pattern involves the family group to which he belongs and must continue to involve them during a hospitalization. The importance of a tension-free environment for the peptic ulcer patient is often stressed; perhaps for some individuals the period of hospitalization itself represents a removal from the scenes of combat, which is perfectly justifiable and therefore protective during that period of time. The same aura of surcease, however, is not permitted the family members, especially if the patient is the young, male breadwinner in the family group, as is so often the case. For them, the fact of his illness is exaggerated by the need for hospitalization and the threat that the condition often leads to a surgical procedure. In many subtle ways, the family group contributes to the interactions that establish the necessary conditions for a peptic ulcer. They belong in the social milieu of striving and seeking, which is the background against which the pathophysiology develops. What those dynamics are cannot often be known to the physician or to the nurse who cares for the patient. It is, however, necessary to evaluate the family relationships as they are displayed in the patient's hospital room and to deal with the family members when their presence and concern demand it. Like the patient, they must understand the need for the therapy instituted. The dietary restrictions that may continue after hospitalization can be observed best when the homemaker understands what they are and how to prepare the individual's diet accordingly. A diet as specialized as the ulcer diet, furthermore, cannot avoid making some radical change in the dietary pattern in the home. When a diet must be observed following hospitalization, instruction should be as thorough for all the parties concerned as it is when a diabetic is taught how to control his food intake.

The success of conservative management of a peptic ulcer patient rests very clearly with his ability to participate in his own care. That always involves an extended period after hospitalization, because, while healing may proceed satisfactorily during hospital care, the conditions that precipitate symptoms cannot be entirely excluded in a brief time. Thus, most of the success of this kind of treatment depends on the posthospitalization activities of the patient *and* his family. Without professional help, realignment of life patterns rarely occurs, and the incidence of recurrent episodes is very high.

A quarter of the patients diagnosed with peptic ulcer suffer a hemorrhage at some time during their life span. Such episodes, occurring in the home, are terrifying to the patient and his family, and, of course, they require very urgent treatment. In addition, if an individual has had one hemorrhage, the chances are that he will have others, so that, even after the emergency has dissolved, the ever-present threat may well remain in the family psyche. Extensive bleeding requiring many transfusions of whole blood during the treatment places another burden of participation on the family that nurses sometimes do not properly assess. Family members are often asked to donate their own blood or to locate donors to replace the blood used for the patient. Such a contribution to his welfare emphasizes the deep involvement of a family in the welfare of the patient, and it is not an experience that they can ignore.

If symptoms persist so that complications develop, the peptic ulcer patient ultimately faces the necessity of surgical intervention. It is always best if there is sufficient time before surgery to properly prepare the patient. The emergency surgical procedure is a dramatic and demanding experience for the patient and his family—as well as for the hospital staff. Under circumstances in which the individual's life is at stake, it is not unusual that family members are shunted aside in the interests of the patient. But under these circumstances, as well as when there *is* time for adequate preparation, the traditional folkways of the hospital often compound the difficulty that the family members of a surgical patient must face during this critical period. The rationalization that focuses all of the energy and interest of the professional staff on the patient is sound enough. He must come first because he is the human being whose life is threatened. The ritual of exclusion from the operating room of all those who are not actual participants in the operation itself is indispensable. To maintain the aseptic environment where the natural defenses of the individual are being encroached upon by the surgical procedure is absolutely essential to the *patient's* well-being. The individual who goes to the operating room must go alone, but at the same time he is never alone. He must place himself utterly in the hands of the surgeon and his team of physicians, nurses, and technicians, completely dependent upon their skill, wisdom, and concern for him. There is no personal experience more frightening, more lonely, and more personal for the patient. Some of that isolation is borne by those who love him, and as they watch the stretcher leave the ward, they turn over their emotional involvement to the efficiency and devotion of other persons.

Often, for hours, there is nothing to do but wait. It is not uncommon now that the modern hospital has set aside a place where the family may wait during the operation of a family member. The facilities vary considerably, but in some, at least, the environment is comfortable, and there is a telephone communication with the operating room which permits the notification of the family when the surgery is completed. Most surgeons try to see the family as soon as possible after the procedure is completed, to inform them of the patient's condition, and to explain what has been done. This is not always a satisfactory or even feasible interview. If the surgeon has scheduled several patients, he may be unable to come to the family for several hours after the operation is over, or he may not have the time to satisfy all of the doubts and apprehensions they may be experiencing. Nurses have not often interpreted their responsibilities in the reassurance of family members as part of their concern for the patient, and removing the family to a designated waiting area serves to isolate the nurse from the family even more. Only rarely will the nurse have more information than the family does about the patient's condition, but the family frequently assumes that the nurse does know. The use of postoperative recovery rooms, where all of the technical equipment will assist in the individual's recovery from the anesthetic, prevents any family visit—often for hours—after the surgery is completed. The isolated placement of the operating rooms can be defended on sound scientific ground: they must be kept as free of contaminants as possible. But the isolation of the recovery room and the restriction placed on family members from seeing the patient after surgery are much more difficult to justify. The increasing trend towards intensive care units of all kinds, with the isolation of the patient from the family members, has begun to create questions as to whether this is a wise procedure. All of the technology of modern medicine may be gathered in a single place, and expert nurses may focus all of their attention on the very sick patient. In such units, the issue of sufficient care and observation by nursing personnel is eliminated, and it is just plain fact that the patient's physical well-being is thereby protected. However, the definitive effects of even this kind of social isolation for the patient very much need to be explored. It has become increasingly clear that the very rigid visiting restrictions in hospitals create more problems than they solve. The members of a family *do* get in the nurse's way. They *do* demand the attention of the nurse, and they *do* increase the complexity of caring for the patient. But they do something else too. They offer the support and concern and interest in the individual that are important to him during his illness, and they establish the sharing of the experience with him that will be meaningful after it is over. The shielding of the patient from his family members during hospitalization produces more unpleasant memories of his care than any other factor. He may soon forget how much pain he had after the operation, but he will remember for years that he did not see his wife until nightfall. Nurses expect families to understand their brusque efficiency in caring for the patient's needs, but families want to know that the concern is real; unless there is a warm and sympathetic expression of interest, all of the nurse's skill fails to provide nursing *care*. The judgement that must respond sensitively to the physical needs of the patient is not enough to insure adequate care unless it derives from the humanity of the nurse. And the patient is not only the still figure in the bed: he is the emotional center of the frightened wife who sits silently in the room. When she is ignored or pushed aside, something of the patient is too.

Model V: Nursing Determinants in Provision for Nutritional Needs

OBJECTIVES

1. To provide nourishment and fluids to the individual patient in accordance with his specific needs.
2. To learn nursing skills designed to assist the individual patient to derive the optimum benefit from his diet.
3. To identify and take appropriate measures for food preferences or dyscrasias for the individual patient as determined by:
   - 3.1 His individual psychological approach to food habits.
   - 3.2 His cultural and religious antecedents which influence his food habits.
   - 3.3 His socioeconomic background as it affects his food habits.
   - 3.4 His therapeutic needs for specific dietary and fluid control.
4. To insure the safety and comfort of the patient during the ingestion of food or fluids.
5. To teach sound food habits to the individual patient in accordance with his ability to tolerate and understand such instruction.

ESSENTIAL SCIENCE CONCEPTS

1. Individual nutritional requirements are created by metabolic processes at the cellular level.
   - 1.1 The energy production essential to well-being is dependent upon food intake.
     - 1.11 Even at complete rest, energy is required to support living processes.
     - 1.12 Energy utilization is a variable related to age, sex, activity, body size, environmental conditions.
     - 1.13 In the absence of food intake, the body substance itself is utilized for energy production.
       - 1.131 Carbohydrate stores will be exhausted within 24 to 48 hours without daily supply.
       - 1.132 Fat stores are depleted in 5 to 6 weeks.
       - 1.133 Use of body protein for energy quickly results in inanition and eventual death.
   - 1.2 Balanced food intake is necessary to insure all necessary elements for cellular activity.
     - 1.21 Proteins are absolutely indispensable for the processes of life.
       - 1.211 Proteins contribute the essential "building blocks" of cellular structure.
       - 1.212 Proteins are essential in production of constituents of physiological processes.
         - 1.2121 Genes.

1.2122 Enzymes.
1.2123 Hormones.
1.2124 Antibodies.
1.213 Proteins regulate oncotic pressure and thus maintain fluid balance.
1.214 Proteins are essential in acid-base balance as buffer systems.
1.215 Normal "attrition" of proteins amounts to 30 gm. per day in average adult, so that replacement must exceed this amount.
1.216 Daily protein intake is recommended as 1 gm. per kg. of body weight in adult.
1.217 Proteins provide 4 cal. per gram when utilized as energy resource.
1.22 Fats provide a ready and high-energy source, as well as contributing to cellular structure.
1.221 1 gram of fat provides 9 cal.
1.222 The body stores excess food as fat for subsequent energy use.
1.223 Fats are constituents of essential compound substances, such as lipoproteins and phospholipids used in cell structure.
1.224 Dietary fat requirement is not established, but ranges around 40% of intake in U.S.
1.23 Carbohydrates are the foods that provide the immediate energy resource for the body.
1.231 Carbohydrates provide 4 cal. per gram.
1.232 Excessive carbohydrate intake results in deposition of fat in the body.
1.233 Daily requirements are not established, but they should be sufficient to prevent use of body protein for energy.
1.24 Vitamins are essential because they act as coenzymes which mediate important body processes.
1.25 Minerals fulfill numerous vital roles in the physiological processes of the body.
1.251 Minerals are important regulators of the pH of body tissues.
1.252 Minerals as electrolytes influence the osmotic pressure relationships.
1.253 Minerals are constituents of essential substances, such as hemoglobin.
1.254 Minerals are incorporated into the cellular structure of many tissues.
1.3 Food is ingested by the individual in response to physiological sitmuli.
1.31 Central nervous system control is demonstrable for the devel-

opment of hunger (physiological craving for food).

1.311 Hunger is accompanied by painful sensations related to contractions of the stomach.

1.312 Hunger is the stimulus (drive) that sends the organism in search of food.

1.32 Appetite is not accompanied by sensations of the gastrointestinal tract, but reflects a desire for specific kinds of food.

1.33 Satiety is mediated by the central nervous system and reflects satisfaction, which causes the seeking for food to cease altogether.

2. Pathophysiological conditions result in an alteration of nutritional requirement and balance.

2.1 Protein use becomes a critical factor in the body's defense against disease processes.

2.11 Nitrogen balance reflects the relationship between protein intake and attrition in the body.

2.111 Positive balance is assurance of protein required for healing.

2.112 Negative balance threatens the use of the body's substance for necessary defense.

2.12 Excessive loss through disease increases demand above that required by normal attrition.

2.121 Failure of gastrointestinal absorption accompanies many disease entities, including those that result in diarrhea.

2.122 Excessive amounts may be lost in purulent drainage from wounds (including decubiti) and massive burns.

2.123 Severe kidney disease is characterized by protein loss.

2.13 Protein is indispensable for the mobilization of the body's defense against disease.

2.131 Blood clotting mechanisms depend on protein supply.

2.132 Antibodies are made of proteins.

2.133 Repair of tissues requires proteins for healing.

2.2 Deficient intake of essential vitamins results in development of disease syndromes.

2.21 Subclinical signs may exist, even when individual is able to eat, because of poor food choices.

2.22 Except in specific instances, vitamin failure usually involves more than one vitamin.

2.221 Vitamin K, essential for blood-clotting, is manufactured by intestinal bacteria.

2.222 Vitamin B_{12}, essential for maturation of red cells, cannot be absorbed in the absence of *intrinsic factor,* a component of gastric juice.

2.23 Therapeutic diet requires supplement of vitamins unless calculated into daily food intake.

2.24 Absorption of fat-soluble vitamins is deficient when there is failure of fat-absorption (Vitamins A, D, E, K).

2.241 Biliary disease (jaundice) prevents proper fat absorption and is thus accompanied by delayed clotting time (Vitamin K).

2.242 Rapid movement of food through gastrointestinal tract results in inadequate fat absorption (severe diarrheas).

2.3 Deficient intake of mineral substances may result in evidence of disease processes.

2.31 Though iron is conserved by the body, some is lost daily and must be replaced to prevent development of iron-deficiency anemia.

2.32 Thyroid function depends on adequate iodine supply, with enlargement of thyroid (goiter) if deficient.

2.33 Calcium is essential for continued strength of skeletal system.

2.34 Phosphates are indispensable in tissue structure.

2.35 Trace elements must be supplied to avoid deficiency disease (copper, zinc, cobalt, manganese).

2.4 Alteration in metabolism requires control of carbohydrate and fat intake (as in diabetes mellitus).

3. Individual food choices are determined by psychosocial factors more than by physiological needs of the body.

3.1 There is wide variation in the substances defined as "food" by various social groups.

3.2 Cultural, ethnic, and religious influences are potent factors in the individual selection of foods.

3.21 Food habits of the family or group have deep roots related to value systems and moral codes.

3.211 Individual foods may be classified as sinful to consume.

3.212 Food preparation may have to follow a ritual prescribed by group (as kosher foods).

3.22 Meal patterns are important aspects of the environment for ingesting foods.

3.3 Socioeconomic status influences food selection.

3.31 Foods available in the region are generally the basic foods of a social group.

3.32 Ability to purchase foods, and their costs, vary with socioeconomic status.

3.33 Food usage is widely disseminated in public media with both good and bad trends developing.

3.34 Deprived groups select less expensive carbohydrates in exchange for expensive proteins and fats.

3.4 Emotional and psychological factors influence individual food choices.

3.41 Previous experience with food predetermines acceptance.

3.42 Common food "folkways" ascribe medicinal or curative powers to some foods.

3.43 Foods are used as rewards for good behavior and may be denied in expiation of "sins."

3.44 Foods are used as symbols of love and approval and may be interpreted as such by the individual.

3.45 Craving for specific foods is rarely related to biological need, but often a response to emotional needs.

3.46 Quantity of food consumed at a meal becomes habitual, and may persist even when need is less.

3.47 Food intake is often influenced by bowel habits of the individual.

3.48 Food ingestion is often blamed as cause of disease when relationship is not cause-effect.

4. Adequate ingestion of foods is influenced by the individual's ability to accept it orally.

4.1 Anorexia is a frequent symptom of many disease entities.

4.2 Ability to swallow influences ability to ingest foods.

4.21 Shared airway threatens respiratory effectiveness unless individual can control swallowing.

4.22 Individual must be conscious and aware in order to swallow without endangering respiration.

4.23 Pain, obstruction, or weakness may limit ability to swallow foods.

4.3 Oral ingestion of foods must be withheld whenever there is interference with normal function of gastrointestinal tract.

4.31 Food is withheld following surgery until gastrointestinal tract recovers from effects of anesthetic and/or narcotics.

4.32 Disease of gastrointestinal tract requires limitation of oral intake until control is established.

4.4 Condition of teeth influences the type of foods offered to individual patient.

4.5 Environment in which meals are taken influences willingness to eat.

5. Therapeutic dietary restrictions always represent deprivation to the individual patient.

5.1 Altered diets may appear less palatable to individual.

5.2 Restrictions may be interpreted as punishment.

5.3 Restrictions may cause changes in family food patterns and meal habits with consequent friction.

NURSING PROCESS

1. Knowledge of therapeutic nutrient effects is the basis for nursing intervention in the provision of nutritional needs for the individual.

1.1 Food intake should assure the proper maintenance of the individual patient's energy requirements.

1.11 Observation and assessment of the individual's condition and behavior determine his energy resource.

1.12 Evaluation of food intake at each meal to indicate ingestion of necessary energy foods.

1.13 Evaluation of the 24-hour food intake to determine care plan in reference to ingestion of necessary energy foods.

1.2 Food intake should assure the proper maintenance of positive nitrogen balance.

1.21 Adequate protein support for healing assessed by observation of healing or convalescent process in the individual patient.

1.22 Evaluation of protein loss by observation of potential sources of loss, including drainage from wounds.

1.23 Recognition of the importance of protein in preventing localized nutritional failure of pressure areas and development of decubiti.

1.24 Continuing assessment of individual's returning strength and ability to function independently.

1.3 Food intake should assure adequate supply of vitamins and minerals to maintain essential balance.

1.31 Knowledge of foods rich in necessary vitamins and minerals so that individual can be encouraged to eat them.

1.32 Knowledge of exchange lists with comparable vitamin or mineral resources when individual refuses essential food items in his diet.

1.33 Emphasis on food that supplies essential substances required for a specific therapeutic effect, as iron in deficiency anemias.

1.34 Recognition of early and subtle kinds of deficiency, especially when dietary intake is restricted.

2. Pathophysiological requirements determine nursing methods for providing for nutritional needs of the individual patient.

2.1 Provision essential to insure safety of the individual during ingestion of oral food and fluids.

2.11 Prevention of choking or aspiration during eating.

2.111 Assessment of individual's ability to handle the type of food offered him.

2.112 Feeding of patient by the nurse with constant observation during the meal.

2.113 Proper positioning to allow maximum physiological function.

2.114 Alteration of the diet, or preparation of foods to permit maximum safety for the patient.

2.115 Individual allowed unhurried meal at his own pace, whether fed by nurse or self.

2.12 Knowledge of individual's ability to masticate food in preparation for swallowing.

2.121 Proper dietary preparation for edentulous individual.

2.122 Preparation for meals includes placement of dentures, if available and individual can tolerate.

2.123 Preparation of food at bedside to facilitate swallowing (as moistening bread).

2.124 Evaluation of individual's ability to chew foods if very weak or partially paralyzed.

2.1241 Small amounts of food offered and completely swallowed before given more.

2.1242 Soft masses of food more easily handled than liquids.

2.1243 Food placed on side of mouth where there is muscle strength in hemiplegic individual.

2.2 Knowledge of the therapeutic intent of the diet assists in promoting its therapeutic value to the individual.

2.21 Assessment of the individual's response and desire for food.

2.211 Determination of causes of anorexia.

2.2111 Refusal of food related to the disease itself.

2.2112 Presence of nausea or vomiting related to drugs, emotional upset, food dyscrasia.

2.212 Individual's knowledge of need for dietary restriction which intereferes with his desire to eat food offered.

2.213 Alteration in bowel function which may influence desire to eat diet.

2.22 Continuing teaching effort to help patient understand therapeutic diet and its intent.

2.221 Severe restrictions (as of salt) explained, and individual's response accepted without scolding or censure.

2.222 Interpretation of dietary needs to family.

2.223 Well-established communication with dietitian to assist in interpretation, teaching, and selection of allowed foods for patient.

3. Psychosocial requirements determine nursing methods for providing optimal nutritional value to the individual patient.

3.1 Preparation of the environment in which meals are taken.

3.11 Preparation before the meal to allow use of bedpan and handwashing.

3.12 Tidy bedside unit, with space provided to place tray when it arrives.

3.13 Elimination of unnecessary and unpleasant noise, odors, and equipment before mealtime.

3.14 Proper positioning of the patient to permit consumption of meal with minimum muscle stress.

3.141 Tray and necessary utensils in easy reach.

3.142 Recognition of social aspects by placing tray so that

meal is shared with wardmates.

3.15 Tray attractively set with hot foods kept hot and cold foods kept cold.

3.151 Necessary utensils and foods provided, including cream for coffee.

3.152 Napkin, condiments, utensils placed on tray as table would be set.

3.16 If patient is fed by the nurse, individual is allowed independence and decision for himself.

3.161 Finger foods offered to patient so that he can control some of the process.

3.162 Food offered in the sequence and at the rate patient desires it.

3.163 Protection of bed linens and napkin use to prevent soiling, dribbling, and other embarrassing accidents.

3.164 Knowledge of temperature of foods offered, using precautions with very hot foods.

3.2 Recognition of the individual's preference within the limits of the therapeutic diet and hospital policy.

3.21 Religious requirements on food intake scrupulously observed under all circumstances.

3.211 Consideration and respect for individual's needs communicated to him.

3.212 Even kosher meals available in frozen form, or family may bring food.

3.22 Substitutions made whenever possible in consultation with the dietitian.

3.23 Planning for therapeutic diet by consultation with dietitian and patient.

3.24 When individual is allowed choice and participates in planning, therapeutic restriction is better accepted.

3.3 Acceptance of the diet is influenced by patient's condition, and should be evaluated by the nurse.

3.31 Quantities of food actually taken recorded by nurse.

3.32 Complaints relative to food have social acceptance, and may substitute for hostility and fear related to other aspects of hospitalization.

3.33 Refusal of foods evaluated in terms of individual's previous food habits, ethnic and cultural considerations, and the quality of food preparation offered him in the hospital.

3.4 Nutritional value is enhanced if the patient is taught the implications.

3.41 Basic nutritional principles may be taught by using opportunities during all meals.

3.411 Recognition of areas of knowledge which individual requires.

3.412 Respect for deep-seated attitudes which cannot be altered.

3.413 Recognition of economic limitations which may influence individual's food choice.

3.42 Therapeutic dietary knowledge offered in formal and informal teaching situations.

3.421 Emphasis on the therapeutic value of dietary restrictions.

3.422 Explanations in terms individual can understand.

3.423 Air of censure and scolding absolutely avoided, so that guilt and anger are not superimposed on situation.

3.424 Use of community resources to aid in planning and preparation of diet in the home, as well as social worker aid in securing funds adequate to purchase diet.

Vocabulary

absorption
anastomosis
antacid
appetite
calorie
cephalic phase
contractility
diarrhea
digestion
distention
edentulous
epigastric distress
erosion
flatus
gastric phase
heartburn
hunger
idiosyncrasy
mastication
motility
mucus
nasogastric tube
nausea
nutrition
parenteral
peptic ulcer
peristalsis
peritoneal
saliva
secretagogue
soda-relief
sphincter
stenosis
ulceration
viscus
vomiting

General Bibliography

CANNON, WALTER B.: Bodily Changes in Pain, Fear, Hunger and Rage. Harper and Row, Publishers, Inc., New York, 1963.

MOORE, FRANCIS: Metabolic Care of the Surgical Patient. W. B. Saunders Co., Philadelphia, 1959.

MOYER, CARL A., ET AL.: Surgery—Principles and Practice. J. B. Lippincott Co., Philadelphia, 1965.

NECHELES, HEINRICH, AND KIRSCHEN, MARTIN: The Physiological Basis of Gastrointestinal Therapy. Grune and Stratton, Inc., New York, 1957.

PROUDFIT, FAIRFAX: Normal and Therapeutic Nutrition, ed. 12. Macmillan Co., Inc., New York, 1961.

Articles

Anxiety, recognition and intervention (programmed instruction). Amer. J. Nurs. 65:129-152, Sept. 1965

BIRD, BRIAN: Psychological aspects of pre- and post-operative care. Amer. J. Nurs. 65:685-687, June 1965.

BUCKLEY, BONITA R.: Feeding the aged person. Amer. J. Nurs. 59:1591-1593, Nov. 1959.

CARNEVALI, DORIS: Preoperative anxiety. Amer. J. Nurs. 66:1536-1538, July 1966.

DUMAS, R.: Psychological preparation for surgery. Amer. J. Nurs. 63:52-59, Aug. 1963.

Knicely, Kathryn H.: The world of distorted perception. Amer. J. Nurs. 67:999-1002, May 1967.

Leithauser, D. J., et al.: Immediate ambulation after extensive surgery. Amer. J. Nurs. 66:2207-2208, 1966.

Martin, Harry, and Prange, A. J., Jr.: Stages of illness–Psychosocial approach. Nurs. Outlook 10:168-171, March 1962.

McCarthy, Rosemary T.: Vomiting. Nurs. Forum III: 48-59, 1964.

Morris, Ena: How does a nurse teach nutrition to patients? Amer. J. Nurs. 60:67-70, Jan. 1967.

Newton, Marjorie E., and Folta, Jeanette: Hospital food can help or hinder care. Amer. J. Nurs. 67:112-113, Jan. 1967.

Sailor, Nelle M.: Nutrition knowledge applied to everyday living. Nurs. Outlook IX:756-758, 1961.

Tillery, Betty, and Bates, Barbara: Enemas. Amer. J. Nurs. 66:534-537, March 1966.

Von Mering, Otto, and Dorsey, Harry: The many faces of food. Part I. Hospitals 35:68-75, Aug. 1961.

Von Mering, Otto, and Dorsey, Harry: The many faces of food. Part II. Hospitals 35:109-113, Aug. 1961.

6 Nursing the Patient with a Disturbance of Homeostasis: Systemic Oxygen Needs

All Tissue Oxygen Must Be Provided via the Respiratory Tree

The work of living cells requires an unceasing supply of oxygen because this substance is the fuel of life. All earthly beings live in an environment surrounded by a blanket of gases that reach only a few miles into the atmosphere. A blanket of air weighs heavily on every individual, exerting a constant pressure on the surface of the earth and on all that stand or rest upon it. At sea level, the weight of the blanket of air exerts a pressure that is measured at 15 lb. per square inch, or 760 mm. Hg in a U-shaped manometer.

Human beings are oxygen-breathers, and thus possess a body structure adapted to survive within this blanket of air; the delicate but hardy relationship that we have with our gaseous environment is based on a subtle interaction with it. In some species, the intimacy of this relationship emphasizes the awesome reality of life in the environment of air. The tiny bird, for example, whose body size requires a rapid metabolism, is able to draw into his lungs with each breath several times more air than he requires, and then to use it gradually, while in the meantime the excess fills air sacs that give the bird buoyancy as he flies through the sea of air. Our respiratory tracts allow us to waste some air; it is this bonus that supports the human organism in disease—the extra endowment that permits adaptation. When even this bonus is used up in a disease process, the patient is often described as having a "pulmonary insufficiency."

Within definitive limits, the supply of oxygen to the cells is based on their requirement—the rate at which they utilize oxygen in the metabolic activities that provide energy for life processes. Not all cells require oxygen at the same rate of supply, but the vital tissues have a high rate of usage and are therefore protected by a variety of mechanisms so that they will receive the necessary oxygen, even at the expense of other body tissues.

This is particularly true of the nerve cells of the central nervous system—specifically those concerned with the so-called "higher" functions of living. The protective devices include a particularly ingenious blood supply and a means of shunting extra blood to the cerebral tissues when they are threatened with insufficient oxygen. Cerebral cells can survive a maximum of 3 to 5 minutes without an adequate supply of oxygen. This is, therefore, the outside limit of deprivation. A longer period without oxygen results in irreversible damage, and while an individual may survive the entire episode, he will no longer be a functioning person. Cerebral damage may leave him to vegetate, with basic functions continuing in an individual no longer able to participate in life.

Other tissues, deprived when the protective shunting of blood is operative, may also receive an insult from which they may never recover; the kidneys, for example, are often victimized when this otherwise protective mechanism is called into play. Thus, the maintenance of adequate oxygen to all cells is measured by its adequacy for cerebral cells. The term "anoxic" (without oxygen) is often mistakenly used in referring to tissue supply of oxygen. It is more correct to use the term "hypoxic" (minimal, or failing, oxygen supply) since many tissues can survive hypoxic conditions, whereas no living cell can survive a complete cessation of oxygen supply.

Functions of the Respiratory System

An examination of the structure of the respiratory system indicates how it functions. Fundamentally, it performs two major activities. The first is *ventilatory* and the second is *respiratory*. Respiratory functions, furthermore, may be divided into *internal* and *external* respiration.

The ventilatory functions are designed to deliver the vital gas to the place where it can be absorbed. The respiratory functions are concerned with the gaseous exchange that maintains the oxygen supply while regulating the elimination of the gas (CO_2) which is a waste end-product of the metabolic processes. Adequate ventilation depends on several factors. It has an obvious dependence on the supply of oxygen in the immediate environment. The human organism is capable of adaptation to a thin air such as occurs in high altitudes and in mountainous countries, but such an adaptation takes place rather slowly and involves structural changes in the thoracic cage itself to compensate for the decrease in the oxygen concentration. Usually, when the exposure to lower oxygen concentrations is brief, as, for example, in a high-flying airplane or in a spacecraft, oxygen must be supplied under pressure in order to prevent the effects of the lowered concentration on the total body economy.

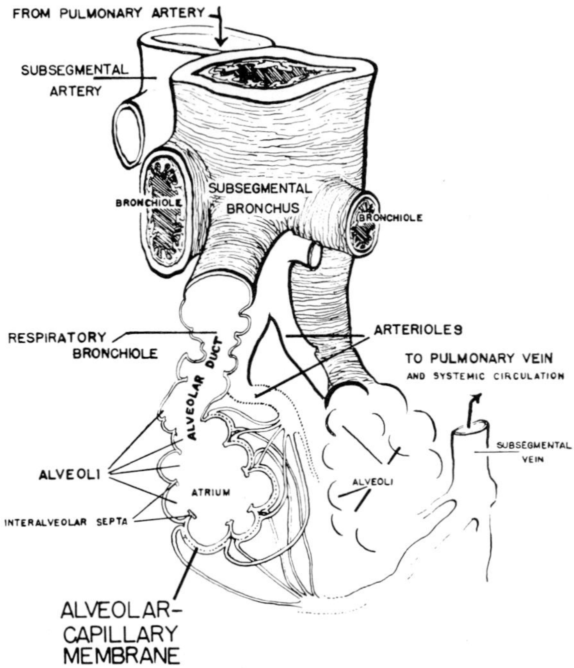

FIGURE 51. Schematic representation of the primary respiratory unit emphasizes that the gaseous exchange via the ventilatory pathways is intimately dependent upon the circulatory competency largely responsible for the respiratory functions. (From Pace, W.R.: *Pulmonary Physiology in Clinical Practice.* F.A. Davis Co., Philadelphia, 1965.)

The second factor vitally affecting the ventilatory function is the patent airway. The freedom of movement of air in and out of the lungs must be maintained at all costs, and this factor is zealously guarded by a number of built-in defense mechanisms that protect the patency of the respiratory tract in the healthy organism. During illness, interference with these mechanisms, either directly as a result of the disease process, or indirectly because of weakness, paralysis of muscles, or other factors, creates urgent problems demanding prompt nursing intervention. The ventilatory function of the respiratory system, therefore, depends upon the health and integrity of the passageway: the nasal passage, pharynx, larynx, trachea, bronchi, bronchioles. This part of the respiratory tract is often called the "dead space," because while no gaseous exchange can take place here a considerable volume of air can occupy these passages.

The mechanics of ventilation are dependent upon the fact that the lung tissue itself is an elastic tissue. Thus, it is distensible and, after being stretched, can return to its original shape. In other words, like any truly

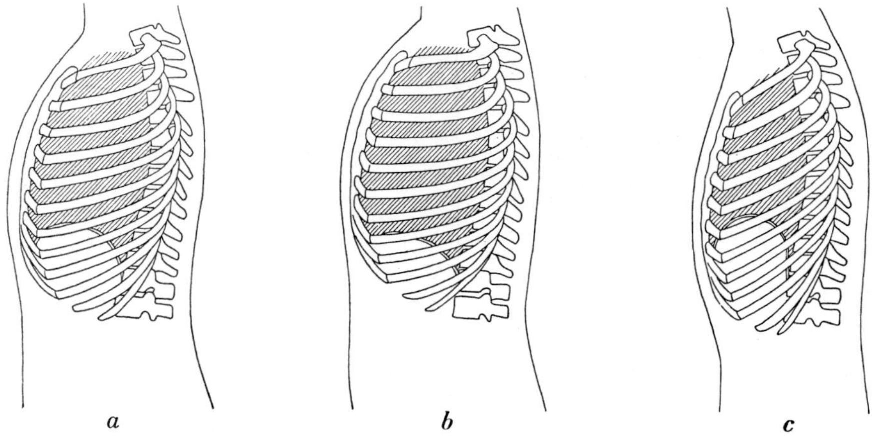

FIGURE 52. The changes in the shape of the thoracic cage are accomplished by muscular movement. In (A), at the end of a normal expiration, the respiratory muscles are relaxed. At maximum inspiration (B), the chest is enlarged by the flattening of the diaphragm and the raising of the rib cage. At the end of maximum expiration (C), the diaphragm is pushed upward by the abdominal muscles, while the ribs are forced down so that the chest cavity is made smaller. (From Fenn, W.O.: "The Mechanism of Breathing." Copyright ©1960 by *Scientific American, Inc.* All rights reserved.)

elastic substance, it *tends to return* to its resting position. Normally, the lungs are always distended with air, but this tendency for lung tissue to collapse is called *compliance*. Obviously, there must be forces in operation which successfully counteract the tendency of the *lungs to collapse*. These are the intrathoracic-environmental pressure relationships. The lungs completely fill the thoracic cage in the healthy individual, conforming to shape so closely that there is only a *potential* space at the pleural margins. When, during the respiratory excursion, the cage changes shape, the lungs must conform to this change too. As the cage enlarges during *inspiration,* the pull on the distensible lung tissue (working against the compliance of the lungs) tends to create a slightly sub-atmospheric (or negative) pressure in the thorax, i.e., a pressure that is 2 to 7 cm. H_2O less than the atmospheric pressure in the immediate environment (see Boyle's law below). As long as the lungs are intact, there is no communication between the inside of the lung and the thoracic cage, but the inner lung space is open to the atmosphere via the patent airway. When sub-atmospheric pressure develops within the thorax, air from the outside environment rushes into the lung space. The gas in the atmosphere, as anywhere else, moves from a higher pressure to a lower pressure, and thus is sucked into the lung space until the pressure within the lung is nearly atmospheric again. At this point, muscular activity of respiration forces air out of the lung space by making the thoracic cage temporarily smaller. This of course is *expiration*. This completed cycle emphasizes how important it is that the tissue integrity of all parts involved in respiration be maintained. Any communication between atmospheric pressure and the pleural space, as may occur in a penetrating wound to the chest wall, or in perforation of the lung parenchyma from injury of some kind, results in a situation in which these normal pressure relationships cannot be sustained. When this occurs, an urgent emergency situation exists. The aim of treatment must be to once more close the parts of the respiratory tree so that the usual pressure relationships can be re-established. It should be emphasized, too, that respiration involves muscular work. The weakened, debilitated, stuporous, or comatose patient requires cautious nursing care in order to maintain adequate ventilation in the face of inability to perform this muscular work.

Ventilatory function is also influenced by the behavior of the gases themselves. The gas laws, which describe the behavior of gases under varying physical conditions in the laboratory, also affect the way in which the gases are introduced into the body and utilized by the tissues.

The Gas Laws

Boyle's law states that, with the temperature remaining constant, an increase in the pressure on a gas in a closed space results in a decrease in its volume. Conversely, a decrease in the pressure results in an increased volume. This, of course, is related to the fact that in a gas the molecules are relatively far apart, and when pressure is put on the gas the molecules come relatively closer together and thus occupy a somewhat reduced space. Boyle's law states that this relationship is mathematically predictable, that is, the increase or decrease in pressure is inversely proportional to the increase or decrease in volume.

Dalton's law, also known as the Law of Partial Pressures, states that, in a mixture of gases, each gas exerts a pressure as if it were the only gas present. Therefore, the total pressure of a mixture of gases is the simple numerical sum of the individual pressures exerted by each gas in the mixture. Air is a mixture of gases, and thus it demonstrates Dalton's law.

Components of Air	%	Pressure, mm. Hg
Nitrogen	78.62	597.0
Oxygen	20.84	159.0
Carbon dioxide	0.04	0.3
H_2O (vapor)	0.50	3.7
Total	100.00	760.0

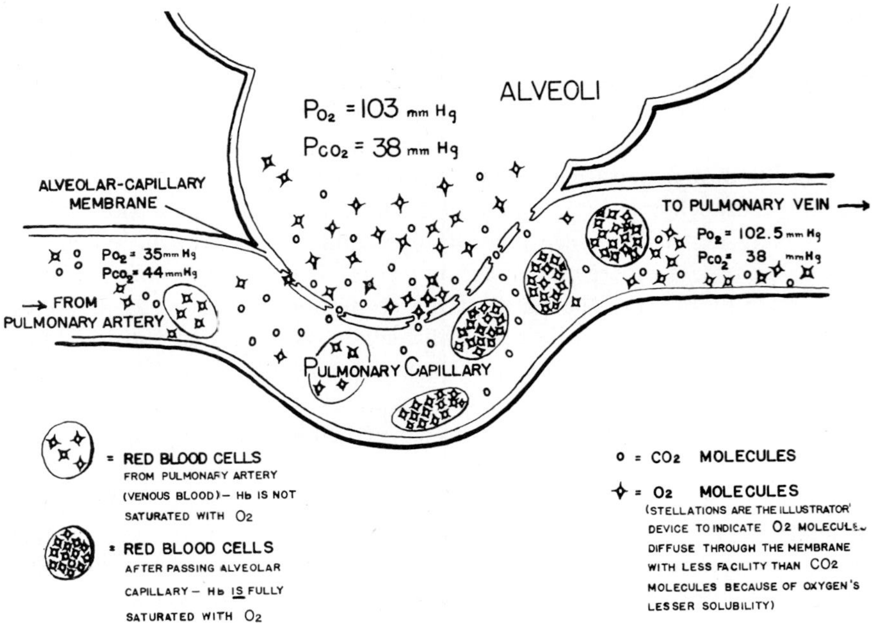

FIGURE 53. The partial pressures determine the direction of the movement of gases across the alveolar membrane and into the capillary, as well as in the corresponding transfer of gases from the circulation to the alveoli. (From Pace, W.R.: *Pulmonary Physiology in Clinical Practice.* F.A. Davis Co., Philadelphia, 1965.)

The partial pressure of a gas in a mixture exerts its own pressure as related to its concentration in the mixture. Nitrogen is the chief gas found in air and is therefore responsible for the major share of the pressure exerted by the atmosphere. The partial pressure of nitrogen in the air becomes a major issue whenever the pressure relationships change radically. It is the high concentration of nitrogen, for example, which causes nitrogen to dissolve in the bloodstream of the deep-sea diver and cause "bends," unless the diver is decompressed slowly over a period of time, i.e., unless the nitrogen is allowed to diffuse gradually back into the respiratory tree and be exhaled. The astronauts are maintained in space suits that simulate atmospheric pressure in order to prevent this occurrence. In recent years, the development of hyperbaric treatment centers has re-emphasized the effect of increased atmospheric pressure on the normal gaseous exchange from the respiratory tract.

Henry's law states that, at a constant temperature, the quantity of gas that will go into solution is directly proportional to the partial pressure of the gas. Anyone who has opened a warm bottle of soda pop will testify that the gas escapes so rapidly that the fluid boils over. The gas in the soda pop has been dissolved under pressure and at a lower temperature, and then the system is sealed. When the cap is removed, the gas bubbles off rapidly. Henry's law indicates the amount of gas that can be *dissolved* directly in body fluid—specifically in blood plasma.

The respiratory phase of breathing takes place only in the alveoli, or air sacs. This complex anatomical structure of the lungs provides, in a relatively small area, an almost unbelievable surface of semipermeable

Table 9: Partial Pressures of Respiratory Gases—in Air, at Sea Level (as mm. Hg)

	P_{O_2}	P_{CO_2}	P_{N_2}	P_{H_2O}	P_B
Atmosphere (dry)	159	0	601	0	760
Inspired gas (BTPS)	149	0	564	47	760
Expired gas (BTPS)	116	28	569	47	760
Alveolar gas (BTPS)	100	40	573	47	760

(From W. R. Pace: *Pulmonary Physiology in Clinical Practice*, F. A. Davis Co., Philadelphia, 1965.)

Table 10: Partial Pressures of Blood Gases (as mm. Hg)

	P_{O_2}	P_{CO_2}	P_{N_2}
Arterial	95	40	573
Venous	40	46	573
Tissues	<30	>50	573

(From W. R. Pace: *Pulmonary Physiology in Clinical Practice*, F. A. Davis Co., Philadelphia, 1965.)

Table 11: Arterial Blood Gases—Normal Values

O_2 content (breathing room air at sea level)	17.5 to 20.5 vol. %
O_2 per cent saturation (breathing room air at sea level—resting or exercise)	$> 94\%$
O_2 per cent saturation (breathing 100% O_2) (plus 1.9 ml. O_2 dissolved in plasma/100 ml. blood)	100%
O_2 capacity	$1.34 \times$ Hb. (in gm./100 ml.) $+ 0.3$
O_2 tension (breathing room air)	95 to 100 mm. Hg
O_2 tension (breathing 100% O_2)	600 to 640 mm. Hg
CO_2 content, whole blood	49 vol. % or 21.9 mM./L.
CO_2 content, plasma	59.6 vol. %
CO_2 tension	40 mm. Hg
pH	7.4

(From W. R. Pace: *Pulmonary Physiology in Clinical Practice*, F. A. Davis Co., Philadelphia, 1965.)

membrane, all richly supplied with blood vessels, where the exchange of gases actually takes place. The adult requirement of surface area for gaseous exchange is 1 square meter of such membrane per kilogram of body weight. In the average adult, the total membrane area thus available for respiratory exchange is the size of a tennis court. And, at that, not all alveoli are utilized all the time in health. But they must be maintained as open, gas-filled sacs where the free diffusion of gases across the membrane can occur without interference. Any situation that blocks off the supply of gas to the alveoli, substitutes fluid for gas within the alveoli, or interferes with the integrity of the semipermeable membrane will create respiratory embarrassment for the patient. Thus, the initial phase of respiration involves the delivery of a proper concentration of oxygen through the ventilatory passages of the respiratory system to the open and functional alveolar membrane for diffusion into the circulating blood. The removal of excess CO_2 from the pulmonary blood vessels and the diffusion of this gas into the alveoli for removal from the body with the expiratory stream of air are equally essential to the adequate functioning of this system. The exchange in the alveoli is called *external* respiration. Internal respiration is concerned with the gaseous exchange at the cellular level in all other body tissues and is discussed in Chapter 7.

Nursing Intervention to Enhance the Protective Mechanisms of the Respiratory System

The air brought into the lungs is the air in the environment; it is dirty, contains varying amounts of moisture, and may range in temperatures from very hot to subfreezing. Thus, before it actually reaches the alveoli, the air must be cleansed, properly humidified, and brought to body temperature.

A major part of the cleansing process takes place in the nasal passages, where the moist, warm turbinates, covered with ciliated epithelium, meet the incoming stream of air and thus filter contaminants out of it, moisten it, and, if it is cold, begin to warm it. Interference with the function of the nasal passages affects the respiratory cycle. Diseases of the upper respiratory tract are common and frequent. In addition, there are a number of medical treatments that cause nursing care problems because of their local effect on the nasal passages. A nasogastric tube, for example, may act as an irritant to the mucous membrane and create much discomfort for the patient. The mucous sheet in the nasal and pharyngeal areas sweeps the store of contaminants to a point in the back of the throat where it can be swallowed or removed by blowing the nose. The area of the mucous membrane in the upper respiratory tract is richly supplied with blood vessels. This aids in the warming of the incoming air, as well as in the defense of the area from invasion by microorganisms. As in the response of mucosal tissue anywhere in the body, irritants stimulate the formation of excess mucus; once more it seems likely that this is intended to dilute and to wash away the offending material. The "runny" nose of the bad cold is familiar to everyone, and, of course, the materials so discharged are grossly contaminated with the virus as well as with all other microorganisms residing in the passages. Handling such materials requires cautious asepsis. Frequent handwashing, the correct use of facial tissues, and disposal into bags, so that a clean area is left for later handling, become very important. The responsibility of the nurse to remain off duty when she has an upper respiratory infection is another real contribution to the patient's welfare. The control of the spread of microorganisms by droplets during conversation, as well as by sneezing or coughing, is particularly important when the field in which the nurse is working is sterile. This is why, for example, a face mask is worn when surgical dressings are changed.

The cough is a major defensive reflex of the respiratory tree; as with most such bodily mechanisms, its effectiveness may be great, or it may simply compound the misery already present. The purpose of the cough reflex is to forcibly remove accumulated foreign material, including excess mucous secretion, when the normal pattern of ciliary movement cannot handle it. It is therefore purposeful and useful if it is productive. The act of coughing involves the trapping of air behind the glottis by a deep inspiration of air. With the glottis closed, the contraction of the muscles of the chest wall and the abdominal wall develop a positive pressure, and with the sudden opening of the glottis, the air under pressure is forcibly expelled, carrying the excess mucus or foreign material with it. It is significant that the act of coughing also involves muscular work. This factor becomes very important when the cough begins to tire an already very sick patient. It is equally important in the postoperative care which requires that thickened secretions be mobilized by coughing to prevent the obstruction of alveoli and serious postoperative respiratory complications, including atelectasis and pulmonary infection. The postoperative patient is urged to cough in order to assure that pulmonary complications will not arise, and often this is a difficult task for the patient to perform. The increasing trend in surgical nursing to teach patients the importance, as well as the skill, of coughing *before* surgery is a positive approach to this important nursing problem. Frequently, after surgery, the presence of the incision and general discomfort make the patient unwilling to cough. But the coughing is so vital to the patient's recovery that it must be encouraged, even when it is a painful and difficult procedure. A variety of nursing measures are available to minimize the discomfort.

If a cough is not productive, as often happens when the disease process involves the tracheobronchial passages themselves, then careful observation by the nurse is essential to aid the doctor in his decision as to whether or not the cough reflex should be depressed. In the very weak, debilitated patient, a persistent, non-productive cough results only in increasing fatigue, and frequently this is compounded by interference with sleep. In some instances also it is severe enough to compromise the patient's ability to eat. If the cough is not useful, there are drugs available to depress it. Sometimes an effort must be made to make the cough useful by increasing its productivity; for this reason, the nurse must accurately describe what the cough is producing, including an estimate of the quantity, if possible.

If the cough mechanism fails, as it may following some surgical procedures in unconscious patients or in patients who are becoming overly fatigued or weakened, it is often necessary to actively intervene by suctioning out the materials from the airway. The technique must enhance the patient's own protective mechanisms, which means, specifically, protecting the integrity of the mucous membrane. The technique should be aseptic, and extreme caution should be taken to prevent traumatizing the mucous membrane. It should be done gently but effectively, and as often as necessary, although obviously the decision will rest on the nurse's observation of the patient's respiratory activity.

The movement of the mucus also takes place deep in the bronchi, but even this mechanism does not entirely protect the lung tissue. Particles of 10 microns or less in diameter may easily get past the body's defense against foreign contaminants. The final line of defense consists of phagocytes deep in the lung, which ingest the particles and carry the indigestible matter to the mucous sheet and the cilia for disposal. This mechanism works better with dry particles than with wet ones, so that liquid drainage from the upper respiratory tract, from chronic sinus drainage, bronchitis, or other disease processes, may get past all the barriers to the alveoli where it becomes a potential instigator of serious infection.

It is, of course, possible to manipulate the external environment to some degree in order to support the normal defense mechanisms of the respiratory system. An environment of filtered, humidified, and temperature-controlled air can be provided when necessary. It is remarkable that normally the alveoli are sterile and free of foreign matter. Dirty air is estimated to contain 100,000,000 particles per cubic foot, while so-called clean air may still have 3,000,000 particles per cubic foot. The effectiveness of the filtering and cleansing action of the respiratory tract, in the face of this, is truly amazing.

The nurse must be more than merely aware that the patient is having respiratory difficulty. There are many patterns of rate and quality of respiration that are significant in gauging the progress of the patient or his response to his therapy. Considerable hypoxia of tissues may be present with only minimal signs of respiratory trouble. The respiratory rate is intimately associated with activity, so that it may be used as a measure of the patient's tolerance to activity of various kinds. It is also highly influenced by the metabolic activity and reflects changes in the chemistry of the body that are not exclusively related to the oxygen requirements. The role of the respiratory system in the control of pH by the elimination of CO_2 is one example of this. Respiratory distress is most dramatically evident when it is obvious that, although the patient is working very hard to get oxygen, he is not succeeding in doing so. Such efforts require intervention in the form of increasing the oxygen in the local environment by the administration of oxygen, and often in the use of drugs to help support respiration. One frequent sign of futile muscular effort to improve respiration is the retraction of the sternum, not normally observed in the breathing pattern. Sternal retraction, especially in the young child, indicates serious respiratory distress.

Anatomically, the critical point in the respiratory tract is at the larynx, where there is a natural narrowing of the airway. Any factor that causes further narrowing of the airway usually affects this point. It is here that aspirated foreign bodies often become lodged so that the airway is completely cut off. The larynx is also a frequent site of infection, and since swelling, or edema, often accompanies infection, the possibility of laryngeal edema is a serious problem. In maintaining a patent airway, one of the really crucial issues is to keep the laryngeal area patent and to observe the patient carefully to detect the first signs of interference. Sometimes a sign is stridor, or a whistling of air, caused by the turbulence of the narrowed opening, often accompanied by sternal retraction.

Proper positioning for maximal respiratory benefit is another nursing responsibility. The consideration must be two-fold. The first concern is for the patency of the airway, i.e., maintenance of a straight airway with no interference in the flow of air. The second is to accommodate the muscular activity that controls the size and shape of the thorax. In each instance, proper positioning can make the difference between comfortable respiration and the possibility of real danger to the patient.

There is probably no cluster of symptoms commonly seen in the sick that are accompanied by more anxiety than interference with freedom in breathing. Respiratory distress is always accompanied by anxiety. Manipulating the environment and providing respiratory support in the form of oxygen or drugs will perform only part of the task of relaxing and reassuring the patient. Individuals who are having difficulty in breathing need the comfort of knowing someone will be near to help them, if needed. The patient should have the assurance that he is being watched, including the confidence that, when he sends for the nurse by signal, she will come promptly to his bedside. In the face of the agitation and fear often evidenced in the patient with difficult breathing, the nurse has a positive obligation to remain calm and certain. If the patient is very distressed, the nurse should remain with him, at least until her presence has aided him to realize that he is all right.

Close observation and the prompt reporting of changes in the rate or pattern of respiration should be emphasized again. The patient receiving oxygen may be extremely apprehensive because so often this is interpreted by the layman as a desperation measure. Members of the family may also require explanation and reassurance on this score. The protection of the environment, when oxygen is being used, is another nursing responsibility. This involves control of any appliances which may spark, since oxygen does support combustion, even though it is not in itself explosive. Thus, any factors that may create the potential of combustion must be excluded from the environment of a patient receiving oxygen therapy.

Finally, the presence of pulmonary disease places on the nurse the responsibility to assist the patient to utilize most effectively whatever pulmonary function he retains. This often involves instruction as to how he can best limit his activities, and may include teaching him a variety of breathing exercises designed to increase the effectiveness of his pulmonary function. Obviously, protection from the commonplace, acute upper respiratory diseases is extremely important when the pulmonary competence is already compromised by disease.

The Pathophysiology of Emphysema

Only a deep-sea diver, an astronaut, or jet pilot must prepare himself for daily experience with variations in atmospheric pressure. Alterations in external temperature are common, everyday experiences for all human beings, and such variations are readily adapted to by the human organism. But, in spite of the fact that the welfare of the individual literally hangs on every breath he draws, changes in barometric pressure at ordinary altitudes are so slight that there is as yet no scientific identification of their influence on the individual. Alterations do, however, exist in the pressure relationships between the individual and the environment, but such alterations always reflect a change in the respiratory system itself. In other words, in ordinary experience, changes in the pressure relationship between the external and the internal environment occur only when disease processes of the respiratory system have developed.

The lungs are like a bellows, encased in the thoracic cage, a rather

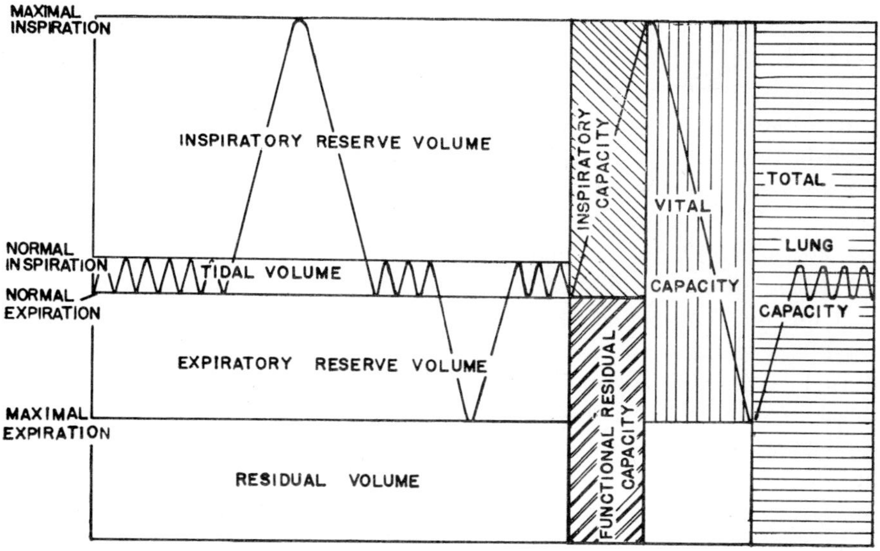

FIGURE 54. The relationship of lung volumes and capacities. Alterations in the relationships reflect the nature of the pathophysiology. (From Pace, W.R.: *Pulmonary Physiology in Clinical Practice.* F.A. Davis Co., Philadelphia, 1965.)

rigid structure which can modify its size only by a relatively fixed change in its shape, a change dependent upon the ability of the intercostal and diaphragmatic muscles to expand and contract, carrying with them the structures to which they are attached. The lung tissue is distensible within the limits of its rigid cage; in the adult male, if the thorax is expanded as far as it can be, the lungs may be filled with a total volume of about 5800 ml. of gas. This maximum to which the lungs can be forcibly expanded is the *total lung capacity.* Unless one makes a concerted effort to do this, however, the actual total of air in the lungs is always somewhat less than the total lung capacity.

The lungs can contain this volume of gas because they are capable of being stretched, but that capability is directly related to the atmospheric pressure in the environment in which the individual finds himself. The deep-sea diver must carry with him an artificial mixture of gases at atmospheric pressure in order to keep his lungs expanded. As he descends, the pressure around him increases so that, by the time he has reached a point 100 feet under water, the external pressure is four times that of the atmosphere. In accordance with Boyle's law, when this occurs, his lung volume shrinks to one-fourth its normal size. If he were not protected by his equipment, he would not have sufficient alveolar surface to allow an adequate gaseous exchange.

Even at atmospheric pressure, no individual can voluntarily expel all of the total lung capacity for air—5800 ml.—no matter how hard he tries. In relation to the atmospheric pressure, the lungs always remain inflated, so that the pressure outside of the body and that within the distensible lung tissue remain in dynamic balance. Thus, the most concerted effort to exhale air from the lungs will always leave some air in the alveolar space. The air left behind, called the *residual volume,* averages about 1200 ml. in the young adult male. The forcible exhalation of air requires tremendous muscular effort on the part of the individual; it can be successfully accomplished only if the airway is absolutely unobstructed and the individual capable of the expense of effort required. Since the total lung capacity is 5800 ml. and the most determined effort leaves 1200 ml. of air in the lungs, at best a forced exhalation of air can send only 4600 ml. out of the lungs. This amount represents, then, as much air as an individual can possibly draw into his lungs by the most concerted effort he can muster. For that reason, this volume of air is called the *vital capacity.* The measurement of vital capacity is made by having the individual inspire as deeply as he can and then measuring the volume of air he can expire, using all of his energy to do so. This is a measure of the individual's ability to expand his lungs to their fullest volume.

Any factors that limit the individual's ability to expand his lungs fully will necessarily limit his vital capacity. One of the most common elements restricting vital capacity is the individual's posture at bedrest; this is therefore an area in which nursing intervention is very important. The strength of the individual, and specifically his ability to perform the work of muscular contraction, is another determinant in establishing the vital capacity. The very weak individual, as well as the postanesthetized patient, may not utilize their potential vital capacity because they are not able to perform the work required to do so. Obviously, any partial paralysis of the muscles of respiration will also limit the individual's ability to increase his thoracic size and thereby limit his vital capacity. And, of course, any alteration in the integrity of the lung tissue itself compromises the vital capacity of the patient.

It is unusual for an individual to expand his lungs to their fullest volume, or, indeed, to expire air forcibly until all that can be pushed out of the lungs actually is. The ordinary respiratory rate involves a relaxed exchange of air volumes with each breath, most of the time without conscious effort on the part of the individual. The volume of air that is normally drawn in, without extra effort, in every inspiration is called the *tidal volume.* It is about 500 to 600 ml. of air, and, like the tides, it is brought in and out in the ordinary exchange of quiet and effortless breathing. The difference between the total lung capacity and the amount of air in the tidal volume indicates the difference between a conscious and maximal expansion of the lungs and the casual intake of gas that occurs with every breath.

Disease of the respiratory system is often accompanied by a loss of the individual's ability to breathe effortlessly in order to maintain an adequate gaseous exchange in his respiratory system. The ventilatory function of the respiratory system must, furthermore, always include the filling of the "dead space" with air, and there is no gaseous exchange in this region.

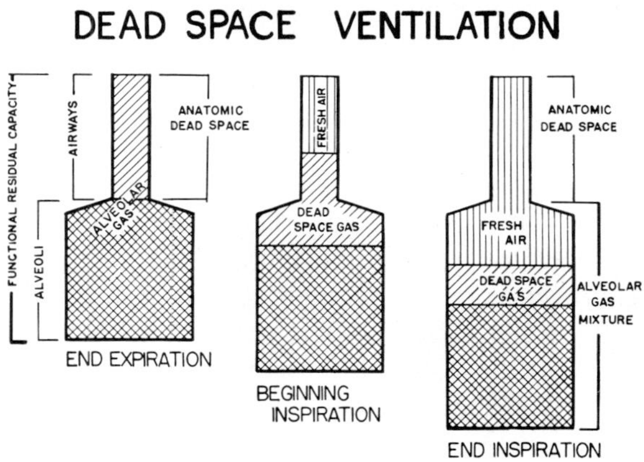

FIGURE 55. The "dead space" represents a volume of gas that cannot be utilized because it is not at a site where diffusion can take place. While the anatomical and physiological dead space always represents some portion of the total lung volume, in disease "dead space" is increased wherever the tissue is nonfunctional. (From Pace, W.R.: *Pulmonary Physiology in Clinical Practice.* F.A. Davis Co., Philadelphia, 1965.)

The tidal volume includes that amount of air that is left in the dead space of the respiratory tree. Even under normal circumstances, this space is difficult to measure. It is generally assumed to be approximately 1 ml. of gas for every pound of body weight. Thus, in the average young male adult who weighs 150 pounds, the dead space is about 150 ml. The tidal volume, therefore, can at best deliver 350 ml. of air to the alveoli, where there is an effective exchange of gas across the membranes. Any interference with the free movement of gas into the functional alveoli, or any interference with the permeability of the alveolar membrane, increases the "dead-space" volume proportionately. Adequate ventilation of the lungs actually means delivering enough oxygenated air to the membrane for transfer into the bloodstream, and it is interfered with and compromised by any factors limiting that function.

Changes in the respiratory function that limit the delivery of even this volume of air to the alveoli are often compensated for in the body by an increase in the rate of breathing. Instead of breathing 14 to 16 times per minute, the individual may take 20 to 40 breaths per minute in an effort to supply enough oxygen to the body tissues. The medullary center that controls respiration responds to the increasing concentration of carbon dioxide in the circulating blood—an increase that results when the usual exchange of oxygen and carbon dioxide does not occur at the alveolar membrane. Usually this is accompanied in the individual by a sensation of respiratory difficulty. Such a sensation of suffocating is called *dyspnea* (difficult respirations), but this is a subjective symptom, reflecting only the individual's awareness of difficulty, and therefore not a measure of his problem. The degree of awareness of difficulty varies tremendously from one individual to the next; there is often no clear correlation between the actual interference with gaseous exchange and the individual's assessment of his degree of breathlessness. In addition, increased respiratory rate, called tachypnea (rapid respirations), is often associated with very shallow breathing. Unless the thoracic cage, and thereby the lungs, are fully expanded during an inspiration, the air that remains in the dead space is proportionately increased. Greater conscious effort may expand the lungs further, and this is the basis for frequent deep-breathing exercises for the postoperative patient. During anesthesia, and for some time during recovery, the individual tends to breathe in a shallow, or "thoracic," manner. Encouraging him to breathe deeply at regular intervals during the day aids in the total re-expansion of lung space compromised during anesthesia and prevents the development of postoperative pulmonary problems, such as collapse of the lung (atelectasis) or fluid accumulations that lead to infection. This is particularly difficult when the surgical procedure has taken place in the abdomen, since full expansion of the lungs includes the use of abdominal muscles, and the patient may resist such activity because of incisional pain.

The free exchange of gas at the alveolar membrane presupposes that the exchange of air volumes with atmospheric air is unhindered. This is the basis for the urgent concern for a patent airway free of obstruction. The emphasis on nursing measures that protect the patent airway is directed at the free passage of air to the alveoli. The most frequent nursing problem associated with a patent airway is that of keeping the airway cleared of its own secretions. The defensive response of the mucosa is to produce increased secretions to wash away irritants. In many situations, the patient is unable to keep the excess mucus moving and cleared. The presence of any irritant capable of stimulating increased mucous secretion is always accompanied by an inflammatory reaction in the bronchial tissues where the mucus is produced. Respiratory infections are widespread and common, and each time such an infection occurs it is accompanied by inflammatory changes in the bronchial walls. Acute situations, such as those accompanying a severe cold, produce a bronchitis characterized by increased mucous production and a consequent increase in the stimulus to the cough reflex in order to keep the passages cleared of the extra secretions. In general, once the acute bronchitis has subsided, the tissues return to normal.

Not all irritants are infectious in nature. In the modern environment, many irritants exist which create an inflammatory reaction in the bronchi in the absence of infectious agents. Much of the concern centered on the cigarette smoker has grown out of research that clearly indicates the irritant effect of this habit on bronchial tissues. The cigarette "cough" (in spite of the ancient assurance that there is "not a cough in a carload") is a symptom of chronic bronchitis and reflects a definite insult to the integrity of the bronchial tissues. The irritants in the smoke itself, when it is inhaled, are probably no more culpable than the heat of the smoke, but, taken together, they represent a severe insult to the defensive capability of the bronchial lining. Other irritants are also common. The incidence of chronic bronchitis has always been highest in individuals working in an environment where there was much industrial dust in the air, especially in open mining operations and in many industrial plants. This danger is now minimized by public health control of the industrial processes and by the use of face masks where workers are exposed. There are notoriously more contaminants in the air of urban areas than in that of rural areas, and in recent years the problems of air pollution in cities have focused on automobile exhaust. Thus, the pollutants generally found in the air of cities, plus those to which the individual exposes himself, such as cigarette smoking, have created an alarming increase in the incidence of chronic bronchitis and its sequelae. There may also be a relationship between climate and bronchitis, since the incidence in Great Britain is higher than almost anywhere else in the world.

The public emphasis on air pollution and attendant lung disease has been in connection with the increased incidence of malignant tumors of the lung. Although the danger of malignant change hovers over the issue of air pollution, it is not the only serious problem that results. Pulmonary disease that severely endangers the individual has increased so remarkably that the true measure of the problem of chronic bronchial irritation must include not only the victims of lung cancer, but the army of victims of emphysema as well. This irreversible change in the lungs shortens life and creates helpless invalids in far greater number than does cancer of the lungs, and the likelihood is that the number of sufferers will continue to increase so long as air pollution control measures are not widely undertaken. While the organism is capable of adaptation to many variables in his environment, the impact of industrialized and mechanized society on the bronchial tissues is a sobering indication that there are decided limits to what man can perpetrate in the world he lives in.

It is characteristic of every chronic source of irritation in body tissues that the structural changes in the inflamed cells are progressive and that a positive feedback (vicious cycle) is often thereby created. As the scarred and altered tissue is produced, the symptoms that stimulated it in the first place become progressively worse. Chronic inflammation of the bronchial tree (including bronchi and bronchioles) leads to a permanently altered structure of the bronchial walls. They become thickened, scarred, and incapable of producing either the mucus with which to wash away the irritants or, indeed, the functional cilia to move the sheet of mucus out of the lungs. The bronchi and bronchioles are, in addition, tubes that can alter their diameter because of the smooth muscle that is normally part of their structure. As the thickening and scarring progress, the tubes become less and less capable of changing their diameter by muscle action. Their patency is thus compromised, and the space through which the air must pass both into and out of the lungs becomes more and more narrowed and less and less capable of responding to the demand. However, long before the opening in the bronchioles has been closed completely by inflammatory change, the physical changes in the gaseous exchange become manifest. The alteration of pressure gradients reflects structural changes in the lung tissue which make the minute-by-minute task of supplying oxygen to body cells virtually impossible.

Any irreversible narrowing of the bronchiolar lumen creates in those tubes a kind of check-valve that makes the free passage of the gases in and out of the alveoli impossible. As air is drawn into the lungs, there is a great deal of push behind it created by the atmospheric pressure forcing the air into a region of sub-atmospheric pressure and aided by the stronger inspiratory musculature. But when the air is expelled from the lungs, it must be forced out entirely by the muscular effort of the individual. As air enters the bronchiole under the push of atmospheric pressure, the lumen of the bronchiole is slightly widened, and the air is forced past the narrowed portion into the alveoli. But when the air is forced out by the individual, the same slight widening of the narrowed bronchiole does not take place, and, in fact, the bronchiole may collapse and shut altogether. As a consequence, some of the air is retained in the alveoli, beyond the narrowing, which would otherwise have been exhaled. Small amounts of gas are retained in the alveoli with each breath, and because the lung parenchyma is capable of being stretched, as the gas accumulates in the alveolar space, the alveoli begin to "blow up" almost like a balloon. As this process continues and the alveolar sacs are increasingly distended, the stretch may break down some of the walls between them so that larger areas of distended air sacs are created beyond the narrowed lumen of the bronchioles. It is not possible for the individual to bring sufficient fresh air into these distended sacs to permit an adequate supply of oxygen for diffusion across the membranes that are still intact; in any event, the distention of the air sac tends to eliminate the capillaries that supplied it, so that diffusion into the blood in these sites is impossible.

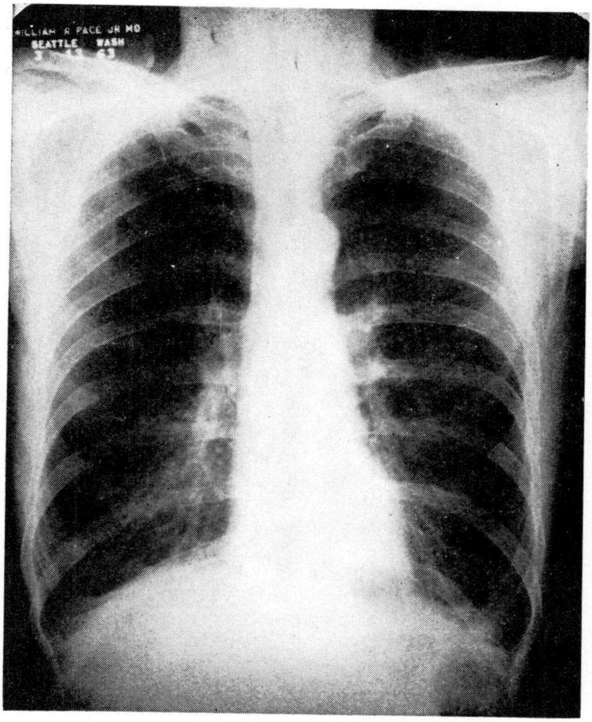

FIGURE 56. X-ray of the chest showing the typical signs of emphysema. The diaphragm is low and flat, and the lung fields are enlarged, reflecting the retention of air in the alveolar space. (From Pace, W.R.: *Pulmonary Physiology in Clinical Practice*. F.A. Davis Co., Philadelphia, 1965.)

With some air being trapped and retained with each breath, the individual with emphysema gradually builds up a relatively high residual volume—or retained air that he cannot succeed in moving out of his lungs, no matter how hard he tries. It should be apparent that his total lung capacity may be considerably increased, but, because so much of the volume is residual air that cannot be exchanged, the vital capacity is markedly decreased. The difficulty is further compounded as the alveoli become distended with air, because the pressure within the thorax gradually rises, and the necessary sub-atmospheric pressure that permits inhalation of air is almost erased. In extreme situations, it even becomes slightly positive (i.e., above atmospheric pressure). When all of the pressure gradients essential for respiration are altered in this way, the individual becomes a respiratory cripple, and there is no way in which the structural change can be reversed.

In addition, his own defenses have been seriously compromised. The production of mucus does not fulfill its defensive role in removing contaminants in the respiratory tree, and the thickened secretions are moved, if at all, only with tremendous effort by the patient. His cough reflex no longer protects him either, because the closure of the glottis and increased intrathoracic pressure necessary for coughing cause a collapse of the alveoli and bronchioles. The secretions are not effectively moved because the cilia are nonfunctional, or ciliated tissues are replaced by fibrous tissue.

Thus, the individual with emphysema must work hard to exhale every breath of air. After a while, a compensatory change seems to take place in the thoracic structure itself. The individual tends to become "barrel-chested," but whether this change is actually a compensatory one that aids in respiration is not certain. His respirations are characterized by a noisy inspiration as the air whistles past the narrowed bronchiolar walls and a wheezing expiration as he forces the air out of his lungs by the most determined muscular effort. The early signs of these pressure changes may develop as an "exertional" dyspnea. The individual discovers that otherwise usual activity is attended by increasing respiratory distress, from which recovery comes at first very slowly, and later not at all. His activity range is narrowed as his ability to breathe freely is restricted.

Moreover, the problems of the developing emphysema are not limited to these alterations. In the absence of effective defense, the incidence of respiratory infection, including pneumonia, is high, and following each acute episode the degree of disability is somewhat more advanced. Finally, as the altered pressure within the lungs closes off the capillary blood flow more and more, the increased vascular pressure in the pulmonary circulation creates increasing stress on the right heart until it, too, fails. Right heart failure, or "cor pulmonale," adds all of the dimensions of decompensation of the circulatory system to the already serious problems faced by the individual. His respiratory distress remains even when he is absolutely quiet. He is obviously hypoxic, and his skin color is characteristically a dark cyanotic hue.

However localized the structural changes may have been at first, the ultimate organismic reaction to the deprivation of oxygen involves every tissue of the body. The alteration in metabolism is marked by the chronic increase in carbon dioxide tension in the circulating blood. The increased CO_2 blood level (hypercapnia) poses difficult problems for both the patient and his therapy because of the importance of carbon dioxide as the stimulant maintaining the homeostasis of the respiratory rate. Under normal conditions, the CO_2 level in the blood is the regulator for the respiratory feedback, probably through its effect on the respiratory centers in the medulla. When the individual becomes hypercapnic, the increased CO_2 tends to depress the respiratory centers. Carbon dioxide in sufficiently high concentrations was, in fact, tried as a general anesthetic during the late nineteenth century. When the level is chronically increased, chemoreceptors in the carotid arch and the aorta, which respond to low oxygen tensions, take over the maintenance of the respiratory rate. These receptors respond only to hypoxia and represent a second line of defense in maintaining the respiratory function for the individual. The desperately hypoxic individual who must receive oxygen as a life-saving measure is in danger of losing the only stimulant he has left to maintain his respirations. As the oxygen tension is improved by administration of this gas, the hypoxic stimulant to the chemoreceptors is removed, and the ventilatory function of the individual is thereby inhibited. This creates the paradoxical situation in which administration of oxygen actually results in an *increased* retention of carbon dioxide because of the decrease in the ventilatory volume of gas. In an individual who already has a high carbon dioxide retention, the excess CO_2 produced is enough to cause serious symptoms of carbon dioxide narcosis. The inhalation of a 25% concentration of carbon dioxide is sufficient to produce surgical anesthesia in a normal individual. As the carbon dioxide blood level is increased in the emphysematous individual, he begins to develop the signs of central nervous system depression. The most obvious is a lethargy that rapidly proceeds to somnolence and finally to coma. For this reason, the administration of oxygen to the patient with emphysema is always a calculated risk, and the oxygen is given *very* slowly at no more than 1 to 2 liters per minute. Even at this rate, the individual must be constantly observed, and the earliest signs of narcosis are an indication to stop the oxygen at once and notify the physician.

The distention of the air sacs may create still another very serious problem for the emphysematous patient. If the ballooning sac is near the surface of the lung, a disruption of the wall may actually open the lung to the pleural space. Such an event is called a "pneumothorax," because air will promptly escape into the pleural space and, as it builds up in the chest, will exert more and more pressure on the vital organs in the chest. The lung itself may be forced to collapse, and the increased pressure inside the thorax encroaches on the heart and great vessels. Such an escape of air from the lung must be dealt with very promptly to avoid the sequelae of increased pressure on the cardia. Usually, this means emergency surgical insertion of an airtight drainage tube into the chest to prevent the build-up of gas inside the thorax.

The chronic cough associated with chronic bronchitis may be the first sign of severe and intractable changes in the respiratory tree. As a symptom of disease, it should never be ignored or rationalized by the individual. While the emphysematous patient can be helped to a degree, the full return of pulmonary function is rarely possible, and learning to live with what remains often requires drastic alteration in the individual's entire living pattern.

Care of the Emphysematous Patient

The Conservation of Energy

Oxygen is the fuel of life, and when it is restricted or denied to the cells, energy production immediately decreases. So fundamental is this relationship that the measure of metabolic activity is often made by determination of the rate of oxygen utilization by the individual in a specified period of time (the basal metabolic rate). Only a very limited amount of energy is available to the organism in nonaerobic chemical change, and even when this occurs, recovery depends upon subsequent oxygen utilization. The limitation of his energy resource is directly related in the emphysematous individual to the limitation of his oxygen ventilation.

The early signs of "exertional dyspnea" signal the necessity to limit activity and, thereby, energy utilization. The sensation of fatigue and oxygen hunger that accompanies vigorous exercise is familiar to every individual. Such unusual energy expense is attended by rapid respiration as the body demands extra oxygen to provide for the oxidative reactions created by the increased activity of the tissues. When the individual becomes fatigued and tachypneic, he stops and rests; the signal that he is ready to resume activity is a respiratory rate which is slowed and quiet once more. In other words, everyone has exertional dyspnea, but the issue arises in the kind of exertion which creates the altered respiratory rate and is compounded by the length of time it takes to recover from the episode. It is not alarming to become breathless following an unusual expense of energy, but when that same degree of breathlessness accompanies the most ordinary of daily activities, the concern must be very real. If, in addition, the individual withdraws to inactivity to await the return to effortless breathing—and it does not occur very soon or very completely—then the full impact of his difficulty is established. Whatever the emotional components of this situation may be, and they usually are considerable, the physiological implications are extremely important. Not only is there a default of oxygen delivery to the cells that makes it possible to move comfortably in the environment, but there is an additional demand placed upon the individual with every breath he draws. In order to breathe at all, he must breathe consciously, expend effort, and work hard at a task which he could ordinarily ignore. And this is the crucial issue in energy conservation in the care of the emphysema patient: he must have an energy resource available just to do the work of breathing itself.

Any therapeutic effort in the care of emphysema must first be designed to minimize the energy requirement of the individual during the act of respiration itself. The ideal, of course, would be some means of increasing the size of the bronchiolar lumina so that the obstruction woud be relieved. There are many drugs which dilate the bronchioles, but they depend upon their effect on the smooth muscle that lines these tubes; when there has been extensive scarring and fibrosis, the effect on the smooth muscle is limited. Some individuals may obtain a great deal of relief with the administration of bronchodilating drugs, and, of course, response to this kind of therapy establishes the simplest and most rapid assistance to the work of breathing. Unfortunately, such drugs do not always help the individual with emphysema, in which case other and less satisfactory therapeutic measures must be employed. If the therapy can be directed at the bronchitis and thus relieve the obstruction to free air movement in the lungs, the subjective distress of the individual may be rather promptly alleviated, even in the absence of any real alteration in the pathology. For this reason, acute episodes of bronchitis caused by infectious agents are treated vigorously with antibiotic drugs to combat the infection and minimize the constricting effects of the inflammatory process on the bronchiolar air space.

The logic of supplying oxygen to the individual who is deprived of it is so reasonable that it is difficult to realize that it is a treatment undertaken for emphysema with the utmost caution. The rationale is sound, and oxygen is widely used in the treatment of pulmonary and cardiac disease, but in every instance in which the disease has resulted in long-standing increased carbon dioxide blood levels accompanied by hypoxia, the ever-present danger of carbon dioxide narcosis demands the most outstanding kind of nursing care. Decisions which are vital to the individual's welfare in respect to oxygen administration are clear-cut evaluations of his energy utilization. If the oxygen treatment, even at slow administration, is accomplishing its purpose, the individual will respond with increased evidence of renewed energy resource. The failure of oxygen therapy is immediately apparent in a decreased energy utilization, characterized by the increasing depression of central nervous system activity. It cannot be emphasized enough that constant observation is the individual's only guarantee against a life-threatening insult.

When an individual is obviously having great difficulty in breathing, the most natural reaction of the observer is to, somehow, help him to breathe. Mouth-to-mouth resuscitation is the simplest and most ancient method for substituting pressure gradients when an individual is obviously unable to maintain them himself. Many devices have been developed which accomplish the same thing. The earliest mechanical devices were respirators, or "breathers," which stimulated an individual to breathe by creating a pressure environment that re-established the necessary gradients. The entire body was placed in an airtight tank which had cycles of alternating pressure inside that substituted for the individual's own chest movements. The increased pressure within the tank compressed the chest and forced air out of the lungs; then, as the pressure was decreased inside the tank, atmospheric air rushed into the lungs to fill the void of pressure thus created. Sophisticated modifications of the respirator included tanks which enclosed only the chest and thus made the individual more accessible for nursing care. Such respirators are still in use and are usually employed for individuals who have paralysis of the respiratory muscles, including the diaphragm. The use of respirators in the care of patients with bulbar poliomyelitis, for example, is widely known. During World War II, devices were developed which altered the pressure gradient by direct influence on the respiratory tree. Using a closed mask, the system created increased pressure at the mouth, which forced air into the alveoli during inspiration and then decreased the oral pressure so that the air would leave the lungs on expiration. Such devices, really mechanical substitutes for mouth-to-mouth breathing, are called Intermittent Positive Pressure Breathing apparatuses, or IPPB. The principles underlying IPPB therapy recognize that, in order for the gas to flow, it must move from a point of higher pressure to one of lower pressure, just as the gradients are established during ordinary breathing cycles. A number of different IPPB systems are available. Some of them essentially establish pressure gradients for the patient during both inspiration and expiration. Some, on the other hand, are essentially instruments for delivering specific volumes of air to the individual's respiratory system, also in a cycled pattern. The use of IPPB, however, must always take into consideration the individual's own structural requirement and physiological need. Whenever this kind of cyclic alteration in pressure gradients is mechanically established for the patient, the machine must exactly duplicate the individual's respiratory pattern. Unless it does, he is susceptible to injury and additional insult to his respiratory needs. All IPPB mechanisms function within a system of a gas under pressure, and most frequently that gas is oxygen. Air under pressure may also be used, and, indeed, mixtures of gases are available for a number of therapeutic purposes.

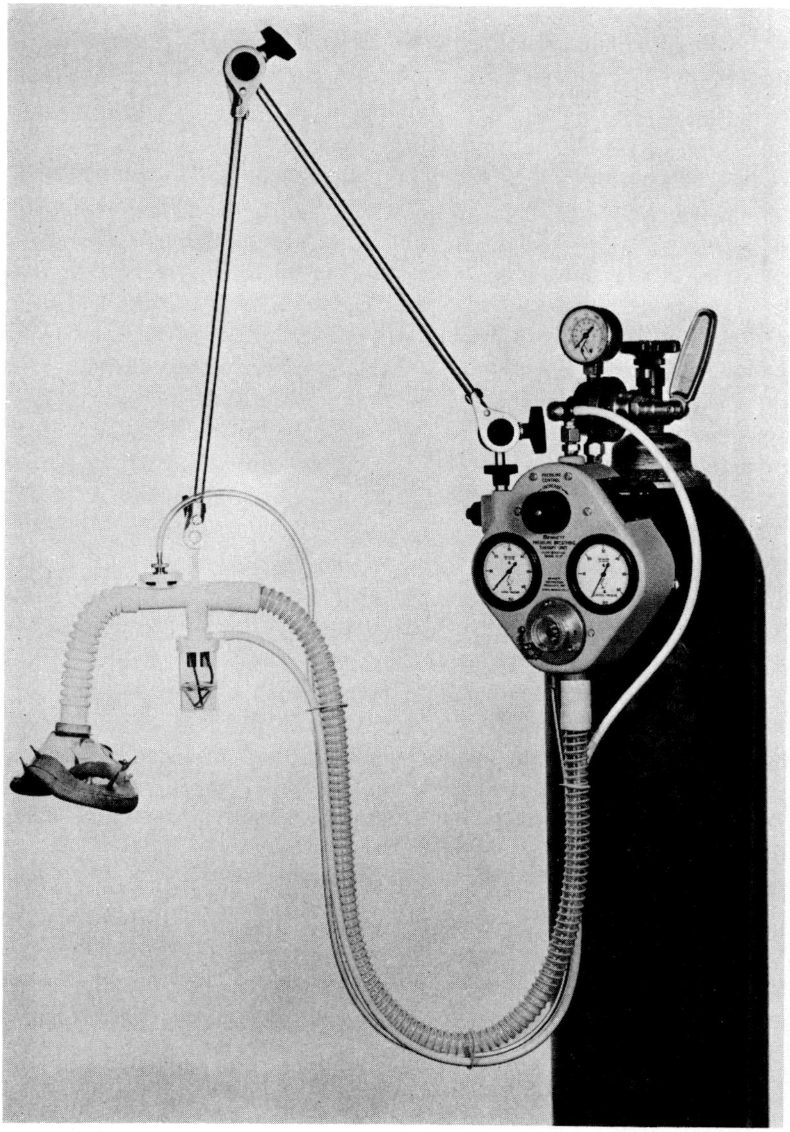

FIGURE 57. The Bennett pressure breathing unit is an example of assisted respiratory systems which impose another pressure gradient when the physiological relationships are not able to sustain adequate respiration. (From Pace, W.R.: *Pulmonary Physiology in Clinical Practice*. F.A. Davis Co., Philadelphia, 1965.)

Successful assistance with respiration, using IPPB machines, depends in large measure on the pathological condition that has interfered with the respiratory process. The patient with emphysema develops a serious failure of pressure gradients because of the retention of air and the increasing difficulty of forcing exhaled air past his narrowed and collapsing bronchioles. Such individuals often learn themselves that, if they purse their lips during expiration, thus slowing down the rate at which they push the air out of their lungs, they increase the effectiveness of their breathing pattern. In general, the problem in emphysema is not in inspiration, although dyspneic individuals tend to breathe in a shallow pattern that does not sufficiently inflate their lungs. The success of IPPB for such individuals depends on the benefit they may derive from having the inspiratory phase deepened, but obviously the expiratory phase, already hard work for them, must not be made more difficult by a pressure gradient that demands more energy in exhalation than they can possibly afford. IPPB may have the additional advantage of loosening mucous plugs as air is forced through the bronchioles, thus opening some areas for ventilation which the patient has been unable to open himself. The use of assistance in respiration is designed to minimize the individual's own energy expense during breathing, as well as to improve the ventilation of his lung space. In the earlier phases of emphysema, this treatment may be very helpful. It is often combined with the administration of drugs that loosen and liquefy the secretions, thus facilitating their removal by the patient with a minimum of energy expenditure. Because of the problems of carbon dioxide narcosis, IPPB treatments in emphysematous patients are often given using compressed air rather than oxygen. Any introduction of gases into the respiratory tree, whether under pressure or not, MUST, however, be accompanied by adequate HUMIDIFICATION. The gases used are dry, and, as they blow past the moist mucosa, they will dry it and damage the tissues. Some means of introducing water is, therefore, a part of every machine used to administer gases directly into the respiratory tree. It is a nursing responsibility to make certain that those water sources NEVER run dry.

The patient with emphysema may be taught to conserve his energy expense during respiration even without the use of mechanical breathing devices. The work of breathing involves muscular activity; if he can learn to modify and control his muscular movements, he can learn to breathe with less energy use. The muscles of the thoracic cage, the intercostals, are relatively small muscles, and there is considerable question as to whether exercising them will cause the compensatory hypertrophy that improves muscle function in other skeletal muscles. The diaphragm, however, is a large muscle, and, though it cannot be restored to a condition of optimal up-and-down movement, it is located so that its activity can be enhanced by other relatively large muscles. Those muscles, of course, are the abdominals, and exercises that help the patient to use his abdominal muscles during respiration may improve his ventilation considerably. The contraction of the abdominal muscles forces the contents of the abdomen against the diaphragm, thus helping to decrease thoracic size. One exercise commonly used is to have the patient breathe with a book on his abdomen so that he can see the book move up and down with each breath. The patient can also be taught to exhale slowly by pursing his lips, or by blowing up a child's balloon. He can also exercise a slowed expiration by using "blow" bottles. A volume of water can be forced through a glass tube from one bottle to another as the patient blows into the first bottle, increasing the pressure within it as he blows into it. Some authors emphasize the importance of teaching the individual a pattern of respiration that stresses a slowed and deep inspiration and a slowed expiration, thus conserving as much energy as possible. In some instances, the "learned" pattern of breathing becomes habitual and has been observed even when the patient is asleep. Every breathing exercise and the postural efforts that force the abdominal contents against the diaphragm are all designed to spare the patient as much effort as possible to thereby conserve for him the energy essential for other body functions.

Any unnecessary expense of energy must be avoided. This certainly includes a nonproductive cough, a problem that often accompanies emphysema. The cough is usually most pronounced in the morning upon awakening, and the mucus tends to be thick, viscous, and stringy so that the effort to raise and expel it may be considerable. Every effort must be made to make the secretions as liquid as possible, and therefore as easy to remove as possible. Certain drugs will aid in this goal, but it is extremely important that the patient have a liquid intake that also helps to liquefy the secretions. Sometimes IPPB administration of liquefactive agents is given at intervals during the day. Such therapy not only loosens the secretions but encourages the individual to cough them out, which may require a great deal of his energy. When treatment of this kind is anticipated, his day should be planned so that he is rested before the treatment begins and allowed sufficient time to recover afterwards before other activities are introduced.

The Conservation of Structural Integrity

The degree of disability that accompanies the structural changes of emphysema varies remarkably from one individual to the next. The process may be very rapid from onset to death, or it may proceed slowly over many years, usually attended by increasing disability. Emphysematous changes often occur in the aging individual, but this is rarely of clinical significance. There may, however, be a relationship between these changes that accompany age and the frequency with which immobilization in bed leads to pulmonary infection in older individuals. Whatever the degree of difficulty experienced by the patient, the threat of advancing pathological change always exists, and such individuals are constantly threatened by the occurrence of acute respiratory infection which can only compromise the bronchiolar space further. The prevention of respiratory infection in such individuals is of the utmost importance. Every recurrent bout of acute bronchitis leaves the patient somewhat less competent to ventilate his alveoli than before. With his own defense mechanisms ineffective, recovery from an acute respiratory infection may be very difficult. Nursing intervention is required to compensate as much as possible for the defense mechanisms that no longer provide the individual with enough protection.

The patency of his airway must be vigorously defended. Liquefacient drugs, sufficient oral fluids (or parenteral if necessary), and proper positioning to facilitate the removal of secretions are important aspects. It may be necessary to actively suction the airway if the individual is unable to remove the secretions by his own efforts. Both the quality and the quantity of secretions should be known and recorded by the nurse as a guide to further treatment. And, of course, in the presence of active infection, every aseptic precaution must be scrupulously observed. The individual must be taught to cough either into a container or into a tissue and to discard such tissues properly into a paper bag which can be removed and discarded regularly. Facilities and opportunities for frequent handwashing are necessary for both the patient and the nurse. Cross-contamination must always be prevented, but it is an urgent issue when the danger of superinfection threatens a patient who has already lost his ability to defend himself against infection. Every individual with emphysema must be taught the importance of avoiding upper respiratory infection if at all possible. This may curtail his presence in crowds and on public transportation and emphasizes the need for general hygienic practices that insure cleanliness. He must, of course, never be exposed to upper respiratory infection by hospital personnel or his own visitors.

In the severely emphysematous individual, the difficulty experienced in any activity that encroaches on his ability to breathe often leads to self-imposed immobilization. The sequelae of immobilization are as dangerous to his structural integrity as they are in any situation that limits skeletal muscle function. He may develop a rather marked atrophy of the skeletal muscles through disuse, and, of course, all of the nursing measures available to conserve his skeletal-muscle function must be employed. Frequent position change, particularly into positions that will support the maximum vital capacity available to him, will aid in his breathing problem, as well as prevent structural deformities related to lack of mobility itself.

The remarkable dyspnea that accompanies the late stages of emphysema may make it extremely difficult to adequately nourish the patient because of the great difficulty he experiences in swallowing oral foods and fluids. The airway must be closed during the swallowing phase, and when the respiratory difficulty is marked, this may create an exhausting experience with each meal. Every precaution must be taken to prevent the aspiration of food during meals; since the individual may need an extended time in which to eat, he must be allowed all the time he needs. Foods should be offered that can be handled with minimal chewing activity, thereby limiting retention in the mouth. In general, soft foods are easier to handle than liquids, but the individual's preference really determines the food selection and preparation. Complaints referable to the gastrointestinal tract must be carefully evaluated because of the high incidence of peptic ulcer in individuals with emphysema. With other symptoms creating the need for intervention, such distress may be overlooked or ignored by the patient.

When ventilatory function has been chronically impeded, the individual with emphysema develops a compensatory increase in the number of red blood cells in an adaptation analogous to that seen in populations that live at high altitudes. The increased number of red cells represents the body's effort to bring more oxygen to the cells, but when the percentage of formed elements in the circulating blood increases, the viscosity of the blood also increases, and with it the resistance to flow through the peripheral vessels. This factor, in combination with alteration of pulmonary blood flow and the subsequent development of right heart failure, creates a serious threat to the patient's cardiac status. Drugs to support cardiac action and treatment for decompensation must be given. In fact, the cause of death in emphysema is usually heart failure, particularly now that antibiotics have made it easier to combat acute infection.

Whatever structural competence is lost when the individual presents himself for treatment cannot be restored to him. The goal of therapy must be to prevent further structural loss, and that necessarily includes the elimination, insofar as possible, of all the irritants that could be responsible for perpetuating the cycle of damage. This, of course, must include smoking, but it must be remembered that the individual so enjoined has usually been a heavy smoker (more that a pack of cigarettes a day) for many years. Whatever the psychic or psychological dependence on cigarette smoking may be, relinquishing the habit, even in the face of respiratory difficulty, is frequently a terrible struggle for the individual. How he faces the problem depends a great deal on his own personality, but he must be helped to understand the logic of withdrawing from this practice, rather than be admonished against it without adequate explanation. Often the nurse casts herself in the role of a policeman, guarding zealously against infringements on the patient's part. As desirable as this may be in the treatment and prevention of further damage, the disciplinary role is rarely a satisfactory one for either the patient or the nurse, and just as often fails in its goal. The publicity afforded the dangers of smoking in recent years has made people who smoke defensive and guilty about the habit. When a serious alteration of body structure can be so definitely identified with this habit, then the individual must be helped past the point of abject guilt and offered understanding and knowledge instead. It is with disbelief that nurses have witnessed the efforts to smoke in emphysematous individuals who can barely breathe. The factors that drive them to persist are not known. But the physician and the nurse need better tools with which to help them than the dire threats and scolding now commonly employed. It is a matter of public record that even printing a gruesome warning on every package of cigarettes has not succeeded in eliminating the use of tobacco products. It is quite apparent that threat is not enough. It is equally apparent that the dangers are very real, and that thus far the awful reality has not been adequately communicated to the smoking public.

The utilization of breathing exercises and the use of abdominal muscles to aid in breathing are also designed to conserve the structural integrity still left to the individual. The importance of these activities requires that the nurse spend sufficient time with the patient to be certain that he is performing them correctly and frequently enough to make the effort worthwhile. Once more, he should understand the purpose in the activities prescribed, as well as the details of how they are done, so that he does perform them correctly. They must be repeated at intervals during the day but always terminated before the individual becomes overtired. The nurse bears a responsibility to help the individual use these exercises to help himself, recognizing that they conserve his remaining structural integrity.

The Conservation of Personal Integrity

The dramatic instant at which the infant gasps his first breath of air and cries his presence in the world marks the beginning of the unceasing pattern of respiratory action that ends only when his life is over. Every defensive resource of the organism—physical as well as psychological—is oriented to the repetition of the tidal flow of air in and out of his lungs. And no threat is more immediate and more fraught with panic than one which compromises the quiet and effortless respiratory function. Even the breathlessness that normally attends vigorous activity has its element of cautious anxiety, and the quiet that is sought in which to "catch one's breath" is a withdrawal involving the emotions as well as the physiology of the individual. When such a retreat, through long habit an effective means of restoring the placid interaction with the atmospheric sea, no longer provides such relief, then the emotional, as well as the physiological, dimensions become pathological.

In the first place, a man depends on the established pattern in order to survive at all, and, beyond that, the limit of his mobility through the demands of his daily life is measured by the availability of oxygen to his body cells. The initial aspects of panic associated with an intractable shortness of breath are disastrous in themselves. But the additional realization that the continuing struggle to draw each breath must alter every aspect of his life is even more significant. If there is a single characteristic shared by every air-breathing organism, it must surely be the morbid fear of suffocation. And the patient with emphysema is slowly suffocating.

As the severity of emphysema increases, the likelihood that therapeutic measures will relieve the difficulty in breathing decreases, and the nursing intervention, which can offer only minimal relief from dyspnea, must offer maximal relief from fear. Unquestionably, the first step is an awareness that, even when the dyspnea has been long-standing and the individual's adaptation to it, in the remarkable manner of mankind, seemingly substantial, the element of anxiety does not fade away. There is a certain comfort to be gained in the knowledge that the individual has survived months, and possibly years, of consciously difficult respirations. But the disease progresses and the difficulties mount; even though the expectations may be modified by experience, the individual faces, with every breath, the one that will fail him and call forth every panic signal he can muster. Those therapeutic measures that afford him relief—drugs, positive pressure treatments, exercises, or a controlled and properly humidified environment—must be given diligently, promptly, and with the same sense of urgency by the nurse as shown by the patient, in order to provide him with whatever support he can receive. For every individual, the nurse must assess the limits of the capacity to be active and help him to remain within them. The determination of the most fundamental aspects of nursing care must be individually scaled to the patient. The pace of his morning care is that which he tolerates best, and he should have a voice in deciding it. He must be spared the anguish that attends further demands and stress on his respiratory capacity than he can handle, even under the best of conditions. If he is struggling to breathe, he must be helped to contain his struggle.

Having lost the confidence of comfortable respirations, he must also depend on others to help him when physical or emotional demands encroach upon his breathing pattern even more. He must never feel that he is alone, or that, when he needs the active assistance of the nurse, it is not immediately available to him. He will soon identify for himself those aspects of his care that provide the most relief and comfort, and they will become the focus of his therapeutic goals. The use of positive pressure apparatus, for example, may initially frighten him, so that staying with him and teaching him the proper use of the instrument is extremely important. After he has learned that the therapy, however frightening, actually relieves some of his discomfort, then he will want the treatments performed promptly and as often as the physician has ordered them. It is the nurse's responsibility to do this in any event, but the special urgency of the emphysematous individual makes it even more essential that the responsibility be respected.

The patient must be observed and watched carefully. If he is receiving oxygen therapy, his personal integrity is directly related to absolute safety and confidence in the procedure. The prevention of accidental fires during oxygen therapy depends very simply on strict adherence to the rules that protect the individual, but the patient must depend on the nurse to see that this is done. If, in addition, the individual is in any danger of developing the signs of carbon dioxide narcosis, the nurse alone can save him from this serious event by adequate observation and sensitive awareness of his condition from one moment to the next. If such symptoms should develop, his life depends on the prompt action of the nurse. As he slips into lethargy and somnolence, he cannot signal his distress, and the nurse must see and recognize it in him.

He has probably been smoking heavily all his life, and by the time he has reached the hospital bed, he has been made well aware of the damage he has perpetrated upon himself. He has very likely been warned to cease and desist many times in the past. Yet here he is, the hapless victim of his own choosing. He ignored the injunction printed on every pack of cigarettes he smoked. He ignored the doctor's dire prediction of future troubles. Newspapers and magazines informed him of the disaster he was courting. And now he is, indeed, the victim who would not believe he could become one. This is punishment enough. It need not be extended by the nurse or the doctor through continuing exhortation or recrimination. The etiology of emphysema is not established, and, even though the cigarette is deeply implicated, there is no way to measure the actual factors in each individual instance against the wilful behavior of the patient. In fact, the wilful behavior of every human being is essential to his own sense of integrity, and it need not be challenged when he stands on the brink of disaster. That smoking is now forbidden must, of course, be made quite clear to the patient. It is often astonishing how an individual will attempt it anyway, even when he is unable to take a decent breath of air. The nurse must approach this problem with compassion, recognizing that years of scolding and warning have not worked before, and that the same approach has little chance of working now. Whatever he can be helped to understand, he should be taught as sympathetically and reasonably as possible. His psychic—or perhaps physiological—dependence on smoking as a means of relieving tension will not disappear with his first serious bout of respiratory distress. The difficulty is compounded by the fact that he cannot be given sedation freely, because most of the sedatives in common usage tend to depress respiration even more. There are no easy answers to the problems posed by the smoker who is not allowed to smoke. But certainly here, as indeed in every restrictive measure required for the treatment of disease, a sympathetic recognition of his difficulty will be more useful to him than the sharp and unyielding disapproval of those entrusted with his care.

The Conservation of Social Integrity

The word "cripple" is neither scientific nor sympathetic, but probably no term in common use more accurately reflects the social integrity of the afflicted individual. It is a word frequently used to describe the radical dependence of the emphysema victim when his disease has rendered him incapable of continued participation in life. The helplessness and hopelessness of utter dependency are summarized in the words "respiratory cripple." Unlike the unfortunate man whose limbs have betrayed him, the respiratory cripple is faced with complete devotion to every breath he takes, and there are neither crutches nor casts to support him.

Unless an individual can move freely and without restraint, he cannot pursue the ordinary activities of social life; when every energy he can muster is spent on managing the next breath of air, there is nothing left that allows him the freedom to live. The cost exacted in his relationship to his family, his job, and his aspirations for the future can hardly be measured in ordinary terms. It is often necessary for the individual with emphysema to give up his efforts to earn a living altogether. Although some individuals survive for many years with their disability, the limitation it places upon them tends to become increasingly more restrictive. The ordinary hazards in the environment become extraordinary, because even a common cold is too dangerous to be risked. Those aspects of his life which must obviously be limited are easier for him and his family to understand than, for example, the tremendous threat posed by exposure to upper respiratory infections. He can, furthermore, be certain that he will continue to require medical care and occasional hospitalization for the rest of his life. The expedient, which sometimes seems so simple, of moving to a more benign climate rarely proves satisfactory, and, in any event, few individuals can pull up all of their roots and seek new ones elsewhere.

The emphysema patient is, unquestionably, physically crippled. The structural distortion in his lungs cannot be reversed, and every new insult compounds and extends the damage. He is also physiologically crippled. Every cell in his body suffers for its lack of oxygen, and much of his voluntary activity must be restricted in order to provide the essential tissues with sufficient oxygen to function. He is, furthermore, emotionally crippled. He is beset by anxiety and the frustration that attends his inability to move freely and seek the satisfactions of everyday life. And he is socially crippled, because he is dependent upon others to provide for him the basic necessities of care. The noisy and labored respiratory sequence he endures must be borne also by others who witness it, and who can do so without a sense of dread? He is rarely silent; this in itself creates a social issue in many environments. If he shares sleeping quarters with another family member, that individual must learn not to listen to the respiratory wheeze, and yet, at the same time, to listen carefully in the event the individual should develop sudden difficulty. Conversation with other persons is a laborious task and is therefore also self-limiting. And the unpleasantness of coughing out his secretions may also add to the tension within the family group.

However, the interest in his welfare is rapidly growing in modern society. The tremendous increase in the incidence of emphysema has stimulated research foundations, as well as concerted public health efforts, to help him face the multitude of problems confronting him. Vocational guidance is available, and, as long as he is able to perform at all, he should be encouraged to attempt to do so. Knowledge of breathing exercises is becoming common nursing knowledge, and efforts to rehabilitate him and help him to manage his symptoms are far more concerted than was previously true. He cannot be expected to derive much comfort from the knowledge that others share his problems, and yet their experiences will help him to solve his own. The utter hopelessness that once accompanied his diagnosis need not be felt, because knowledge of the physical principles of his rehabilitation has led to a plan for his future care that aims to minimize the severity of his symptoms and slow down the progression of his disease.

Emphysema affects many more men than women, and frequently becomes clinically disabling in the middle years. The age of the usual patient with emphysema formerly contributed in large degree to the assumption that his was a lost cause. But it is increasingly apparent that a man's life should not be despaired of when he is in his 50's, and the new faith in rehabilitation skills devoted to older patients has stimulated much interest in aiding the emphysematous individual. The success of rehabilitation, however, is individualized by the ability of the patient to establish his own goals in cooperation with the physician and the nurse. The removal of the common sources of bronchial irritation can be accomplished only if the individual recognizes them and their implications for his future well-being. The goals he establishes for himself must, however, be realistic, and the measure of their validity often involves the way in which his family is able to assist him in attaining them. They must first have knowledge, because, without understanding, this difficult task becomes impossible. And the counseling offered them must recognize the existing limitations and problems realistically.

The individual with emphysema ultimately faces the need for radical revision of his entire life pattern. No aspect of his life can be left as it was, and the optimal use of his adaptation resources early in the course of his disease affords him the only hope of satisfaction in his lifetime.

Model VI: Pressure Gradient Systems in Nursing (Gases)

OBJECTIVES

1. To understand the pressure gradient systems that control the interaction between the atmospheric gases and the functions of the respiratory system in the indispensable provision of oxygen for body tissues.
2. To understand the anatomical, physiological, and physical determinants of effective pulmonary ventilation and the urgency of a patent airway.
3. To understand the anatomical, physiological, and physical determinants of effective gaseous exchange at the alveolar membrane.
4. To understand the effects of pathophysiology on the respiratory system and the systemic results of altered metabolic controls.
5. To recognize the emotional component as an influence in respiratory function, and the extreme anxiety that arises when respirations are threatened.
6. To understand the physical laws governing the use of apparatuses that substitute pressure gradient systems for oxygen delivery when the individual must be assisted in respirations.

ESSENTIAL SCIENCE CONCEPTS

1. The physical laws that govern the behavior of gases regulate the interaction between the external environment and the respiratory function.

1.1 Effective respiratory function is closely dependent upon atmospheric pressure at sea level (15 lbs. per square inch).

1.11 Pressure gradients in ventilatory function establish direction of flow of gases with the external environment.

1.111 During inspiration, intrapulmonary pressure is below atmospheric pressure (−3 mm. Hg) so air moves into lungs.

1.112 During expiration, intrapulmonary pressure is above atmospheric pressure (+3 mm. Hg), so air leaves the lungs.

1.12 Pressure gradient within the thorax establishes continuing mechanism for flow of gas into or out of the lungs.

1.121 The lungs normally occupy all of the intrathoracic space, attached only at the hila, so that they change shape as the thorax changes shape.

1.122 The intrathoracic pressure is normally −10 to −15 mm. Hg, thus holding lungs against the walls of the thorax.

1.123 Pleural space is only "potential" so long as lungs are fully expanded and no fluid or gas has accumulated in the region.

1.1231 Alteration of fluid or gas accumulation in pleural space results in changed pressure relationships.

1.1232 System must remain airtight to insure expansions of lungs.

1.13 Communication with atmospheric pressure is entirely within the lung space itself.

1.2 The physical gas laws determine pressure gradient relationships in the respiratory system.

1.21 Boyle's law: The pressure of a gas in a closed system is inversely proportional to its volume.

1.211 If atmospheric pressure is doubled, unprotected lung space would be one-half of normal.

1.212 If atmospheric pressure is halved, unprotected lung space would be doubled.

1.22 Dalton's law: In a mixture of gases, each gas exerts a pressure as if it were the only gas present.

1.221 The human organism is adapted to a mixture of gases (air) in which the oxygen concentration is 20% of the mixture.

1.222 Variations in the concentration of oxygen (and therefore its PO_2) occur whenever there is a change in atmospheric pressure.

1.2221 At high altitudes, the lowered oxygen concentration results in a lowered PO_2.

1.2222 When subjected to increased air pressure, alteration in PN_2 (nitrogen) may cause decompression sickness as pressure is restored.

1.223 At high altitudes, changed pressure of water vapor may result in "boiling" of body fluids (above 63,000 ft., with atmospheric pressure of less than 47 mm. Hg).

2. The anatomical and physiological determinants of the living organism establish the bases for respiratory exchange.

2.1 The ventilatory function brings air to the alveolar membrane.

2.11 The passage from the alveoli to the oral-nasal openings must remain patent and clear to permit free passage of gas in and out of the lungs.

2.111 The tracheobronchial tree is in direct communication with the external environment.

2.112 Turbulence is created by changing direction and diameter of tubes.

2.12 The lung parenchyma is capable of changing size.

2.121 The viscoelastic structure of the lungs makes it compliant: the measure of the distensibility, or ability of lungs to fill.

2.122 Increase of alveolar pressure by 1 cm. H_2O results in lung expansion of 130 ml.

2.13 Compliance of the lungs is restricted by the distensibility of the thoracic cage.

2.131 Stretching of the lungs requires alteration in the size and shape of the thorax.

2.132 Change in the size and shape of the thorax can only be accomplished by muscular work.

2.1321 Muscles of inspiration include diaphragm, intercostals, and sternocleidomastoids.

2.1322 Muscles of expiration are abdominals and intercostals.

2.1323 Two-thirds of the work of respiration is accomplished by muscle activity.

2.133 Compliance is reduced when there is any interference with alteration of the size of the thoracic cage.

2.14 Pathological change in lung parenchyma or bronchial tree reduces compliance.

2.15 Rate of ventilation is mediated by nervous and chemical control systems.

2.151 Nervous control is vested in the respiratory center in the medulla.

2.1511 CO_2 and H^+ are the principal stimuli of respiration.

2.15111 Increased CO_2 increases respiratory rate.

2.15112 Feedback is established when decreased CO_2 in blood decreases rate.

2.1512 Nervous circuits to respiratory muscles must be intact to permit thoracic cage expansion.

2.152 Chemoreceptors in aortic arch and carotids respond only to decreased oxygen tension when CO_2 stimulus fails in disease processes.

2.153 Hering-Breuer reflex regulates distensibility of lungs on inspiration and expiration.

2.154 Autonomic nervous system response to emotional stimuli affects respiratory rate.

2.155 Increased body temperature (rate of metabolism) increases respiratory rate.

2.156 Activity above basal demands increased oxygen and increases respiratory rate.

2.2 Respiratory function of the lungs takes place at the alveolar membrane.

2.21 External respiration involves the transfer of gases across the alveolar membrane.

2.211 Adequate exchange depends upon a normal alveolar membrane supplied by capillaries of the pulmonary circulation.

2.212 Alveolar ventilation is regulated by the P_{CO_2} (normally 40 mm. Hg).

2.2121 The higher tension of CO_2 in the capillaries (44 mm. Hg) causes diffusion of CO_2 into the alveoli.

2.2122 Oxygen tension in the alveoli (103 mm. Hg) is higher than in capillaries (35 mm. Hg), and so oxygen diffuses into the capillary.

2.22 Adequate hemoglobin in perfused capillary blood is essential to sufficient diffusion of oxygen through alveolar membrane.

2.221 Oxygen is less soluble than carbon dioxide, and thus diffuses more slowly through membrane.

2.222 Red blood cells are carriers of hemoglobin, which becomes saturated with oxygen after passage through alveolar capillary.

2.2221 Oxygen, 97%, is carried in combination with hemoglobin.

2.2222 Oxygen, 3%, is dissolved in blood plasma.

2.3 Respiration at cellular level takes place at membrane of every body cell.

2.31 Diffusion of oxygen and carbon dioxide takes place from region of high concentration to region of lower concentration.

2.32 Tissues are given preference of oxygen supply when there is threat to total supply, so that vital organs are sustained (e.g., nerve tissue).

2.4 Defense functions of respiratory tree support the integrity of the respiratory system.

2.41 Upper respiratory system prepares air for alveolar ventilation.

2.411 Air is warmed and humidified by passage over mucosa before reaching alveoli.

2.412 Ciliated mucosal surface removes microscopic contaminants from inspired air, thus cleansing air for passage to alveoli.

2.413 Reflexes defend tract from irritants.

2.4131 Sneezing forcibly removes irritants from upper tract.

2.4132 Coughing permits expulsion of contaminants trapped in mucus in bronchi.

2.41321 Closing of glottis builds pressure in lung, and opening forcibly expels mucus.

2.41322 Permits removal of foreign material

and contaminants after passage upward by cilia and mucosal sheet.

2.414 Constant exposure to environmental contaminants and irritants accounts for frequency of upper respiratory infection.

2.415 Mucosa produces increased secretions to wash and dilute irritants, which are moved out of tract by upward beat of cilia.

2.42 Lower respiratory tract maintains sterility by rich supply of phagocytes to remove irritants or organisms not removed by upper tract defenses.

3. Alterations in the structure of the respiratory system inevitably establish changes in pressure gradient systems operative with environment.

3.1 Obstruction anywhere in ventilatory passages results in interference with exchange of gas volumes.

3.11 Obstruction high in tracheobronchial tree may completely prevent movement of air to alveoli.

3.12 Obstruction of any portion of bronchi or bronchioles limits gaseous delivery to and from the alveoli they supply.

3.13 Progressive obstructive diseases of bronchi or bronchioles limits their patency and causes alteration of movement of gas volumes in or out of alveoli they supply.

3.2 Encroachment on lung parenchyma by space-occupying lesions, fluids, or inflammatory products results in limitation of alveoli available for gaseous exchange.

3.21 Interference with circulation to alveoli limits membrane available for gaseous exchange.

3.22 Stiffening or scarring in lung parenchyma reduces compliance and limits available alveolar membrane.

3.23 Trauma that reverses pressure gradients results in atelectasis, with resultant decrease in available alveolar membrane for gaseous exchange.

4. Mechanical devices substitute pressure gradient systems when the individual is unable to maintain adequate gaseous exchange.

4.1 Increased oxygen source may assist individual when he is unable to extract sufficient oxygen from inspired air.

4.11 Direct delivery of increased oxygen concentrations alters the pressure gradient for oxygen in the alveoli.

4.12 Delivery of oxygen to alveoli depends on a patent airway.

4.121 Dry gas must be humidified at all times to prevent irritant stimulus to increase secretions or traumatize mucosal surfaces.

4.122 Presence of nasal catheter itself stimulates mucous production in upper respiratory passages.

4.1221 Vasoconstricting nosedrops suppress nasal secretions.

4.1222 Nasal catheter changed from one nostril to the other minimizes continuing irritation to mucosa.

4.13 Oxygen supports combustion, although not itself explosive, so that sources of combustion are zealously prevented during oxygen therapy.

4.2 Assisted respiratory patterns depend upon instruments which control gaseous exchange.

4.21 Control of pressure gradients by administration of gases under pressures regulated for inspiratory and expiratory phases (intermittent positive pressure breathing).

4.22 Control of pressure gradients by regulated administration of volumes of gas in a cycling pattern (piston-operated resuscitators).

4.23 Respirators which alter external pressure gradients over the entire body or the chest in a pattern that allows gradient for inspiration and expiration.

5. Influence of emotional and psychosocial "voluntary" components on respiratory action persists in disease processes.

5.1 Normal physiological processes require voluntary alteration of respiratory rate.

5.11 Cortical control of respiration defends the tracheobronchial tree from foreign materials.

5.111 Shared pathway in pharynx requires closing of respiratory tree during act of swallowing.

5.112 Reflexes used to assist defecation increase abdominal pressure on rectum by closing glottis and pushing diaphragm downward.

5.113 Respiratory rate is altered during laughing and crying.

5.12 Reflex defenses of the respiratory system itself alter patterns of breathing.

5.121 Sneezing requires forcible pushing of air out of upper respiratory passage.

5.122 Coughing requires forcible movement of air out of lower passages of bronchial tree.

5.13 Somesthetic stimuli alter respiratory rate.

5.131 Increased respiration often accompanies sensation of pain anywhere in the body.

5.132 Rapid external temperature change (as sudden cold) may cause rapid alteration in respiratory rate.

5.14 Emotional stimuli alter respiratory rate.

5.141 Fear, anxiety, and worry increase respiratory rate.

5.142 Alteration of rate may become chronic and reflect pathological emotional conditions (as hysteria).

5.15 Respiratory rate responds promptly to altered metabolic conditions, both normal and pathological.
 5.151 Eupnea: Normal adult rate: 14 to 16/min.
 5.152 Tachypnea: Rapid rate: over 24/min.
 5.153 Bradypnea: Slow rate: under 10/min.
 5.154 Dyspnea: Difficult respiration, and is a subjective sign as experienced by the individual.
 5.155 Periodic breathing results from pathophysiological stimulus to respiratory centers.
  5.1551 Cheyne-Stokes: Period of tachypnea followed by period of cessation of respiration.
  5.1552 Kussmaul: Bradypnea observed in diabetic acidosis.

5.2 Relaxed tidal exchange of gases is essential for well-being of the individual.
 5.21 Even breathlessness of ordinary vigorous activity is attended by some degree of anxiety in the individual.
 5.22 "Air-breathers" must defend their respiration above all other threats from the environment.
 5.23 Intense anxiety accompanies respiratory difficulty and serves to increase the difficulty.

NURSING PROCESS

1. The defense of the individual's patent airway is the most urgent nursing responsibility.
 1.1 Time limit for intervention when gaseous exchange is obstructed is physiologically established by viability of nervous system tissue.
  1.11 Equipment required to aid in establishing patent airway must be readily available and in working order at all times on every hospital unit.
  1.12 Every nurse must know where equipment is kept and how to use it effectively.
  1.13 Every patient must be under continuing observation when pathology or condition suggests possibility of respiratory embarrassment.
  1.14 Even when no suggestion exists of potential threat, every patient must be observed sufficiently to insure his safety from respiratory threat.
 1.2 Knowledge of physiological parameters of respiratory function is essential to judicious intervention to maintain an airway.
  1.21 Frequent assessment of individual respiratory pattern forms a basis for recognition of alterations in it.
   1.211 Quantitative and qualitative knowledge of how the individual patient breathes.

1.212 Recognition of periodic patterns in the individual's respiratory cycle, including respiratory movements during sleep.

1.213 Knowledge of drugs or treatments administered to individual that may have an expected or untoward effect on respiratory pattern.

1.22 Observation of respiratory effectiveness in the individual patient.

1.221 Skin color as an indicator of sufficient oxygenation of tissues.

1.222 Observation of body areas that indicate cyanotic condition first.

1.2221 Mucosa of mouth, lips, and circumoral color changes.

1.2222 Alteration in color of nail beds.

1.223 Behavioral changes that indicate increasing restlessness and anxiety.

1.224 Awareness of expressed difficulty by individual, even when physiological signs are meager.

1.225 Sensitivity to the respiratory sounds as indices of impending difficulty.

1.2251 Wheezing indicates bronchial obstruction.

1.2252 Noise of secretions indicates need for cleansing airway.

1.2253 Complete SILENCE can mean complete OBSTRUCTION.

1.2254 Stridor indicates obstruction at narrow point of larynx.

1.226 Respiratory movements of the musculature may indicate adequacy of respirations.

1.2261 High, thoracic respirations may accompany hypoventilation.

1.2262 Abdominal muscles should move with adequate ventilation of lungs.

1.2263 Retraction of sternum indicates respiratory distress of urgent nature.

1.2264 Strain of neck muscles (especially sternocleidomastoids) and lip-pursing accompany labored expiratory phase.

2. Nursing intervention assures compensatory adjustments for individual whose respiratory function is limited by disease.

2.1 Energy conservation is designed to permit adequate strength for respirations themselves.

2.11 Individual is not permitted to exceed his own limits of tolerance for activity.

2.12 Necessary care is provided when he is unable to use energy for activities of daily living.

2.13 Adequate rest and planning for activities when respiratory rate is threatened by mobility.

2.14 Control of environmental conditions to provide maximum benefit, including temperature and humidity.

2.15 Constant assessment of individual's ability to perform, based on observation and knowledge of physiological determinants.

2.2 Aseptic precautions are meticulously observed to avoid infection in individual whose own defenses are compromised.

2.21 Absolute protection of individual from exposure to all upper respiratory infections.

2.22 Provision for safe removal of respiratory secretions.

2.23 Aseptic technique in the use of all equipment used to remove secretions or assist respirations.

2.24 Good personal hygiene, including frequent opportunities for adequate handwashing for nurse and patient.

2.25 Meticulous and repeated oral hygiene.

3. The individual patient's safety must be guarded at all times when devices are used to supply oxygen, assist respiration, or administer medication by inhalation.

3.1 The physical characteristics of administering oxygen establish the rules that insure patient safety.

3.11 Environmental control includes strict prevention of sources of combustion.

3.111 No smoking signs displayed prominently and observed.

3.112 Electrical equipment used which has no metal-on-metal contacts to produce sparks.

3.1121 Ordinary (electrical source) radios and television sets must be excluded.

3.1122 Therapeutic equipment, including suction machines, used only when constructed so that open sparking is not possible.

3.1123 Alternatives, such as hand-bell, used as call signal when signals have metal-metal switches.

3.113 Patient instructed in safety measures to eliminate fear and promote his own well-being.

3.12 Oxygen equipment tested and in excellent working order.

3.13 Adequate humidification maintained AT ALL TIMES.

3.14 Oxygen delivery at prescribed rate, depending on equipment used and purpose of therapy.

3.15 Removal of secretions stimulated by nasal catheter.

3.151 Nosedrops administered when ordered.

3.152 Nasal catheter changed every 8 hours from one nostril to the other to prevent continuing trauma and irritation to the mucosa.

3.153 Nasal catheter tip placed in correct position in nasal pharynx.

3.154 Nasal catheter taped in position without tension on nose.

3.16 Functional alarm system on oxygen pressure lines, and immediate response when alarm is sounded.

3.2 Use of positive-pressure devices requires knowledge of the function and structure of the equipment being used.

3.21 Setting for pressures established by physician and maintained by the nurse to follow the individual's respiratory cycle.

3.22 Teach individual to cycle respirations with the cycle of the machine.

3.23 Adequate humidification at all times.

3.24 Oxygen precautions when this is the gas used.

3.25 Medication to be administered by inhalation properly measured and placed for aerosol therapy.

4. Emotional components in respiratory patterns must be evaluated and dealt with to assure maximum benefit from treatment of respiratory disease.

4.1 Anxiety that attends respiratory distress requires the reassuring presence of the nurse.

4.11 The individual is never left alone as long as the threat to his airway exists in any degree.

4.12 Constant observation of individual's condition reassures the patient and the nurse.

4.13 Call system should be immediately available to the individual, and response to it prompt.

4.14 Adequate explanation of the necessary use of equipment alleviates the stress of anxiety over complex machinery.

4.2 Physiological alterations in respiratory pattern continue even during respiratory distress.

4.21 Energy conservation includes elimination of emotional stress that influences respiratory rate.

4.22 Prevention of exacerbation of respiratory distress, by providing rest and limiting activity, serves to decrease anxiety created by the difficulty in breathing.

4.221 Evaluation of effectiveness of cough to produce secretions, so that sedative depression of cough may be ordered if necessary.

4.222 Identification of factors that create tension in the environment, so that they may be eliminated or minimized.

4.3 Teaching patient and his family the need for conservation of energy and the use of machines that assist respiration decreases level of anxiety.

4.31 Use of oxygen equipment is often life-threatening to lay public.

4.32 Understanding the purpose of the therapy offers the only reassurance possible to patient and his family.

Vocabulary

alveoli
anoxic
Boyle's law
bronchi
bronchioles
compliance
cough
Dalton's law
dead space
decompressed
emphysema
expiration
external respiration
Henry's law
humidified
hyperbaric
hypoxic
inspiration
internal respiration
intrathoracic
Law of Partial Pressures
parenchyma
pulmonary function
pulmonary insufficiency
pulmonary volumina
respiratory
sternal retraction
stridor
tidal volume
ventilation
vital capacity

General Bibliography

COMROE, JULIUS H., ET AL.: The Lung, ed. 2. Year Book Medical Publishers, Inc., Chicago, 1962.

HAAS, ALBERT: Essentials of Living with Pulmonary Emphysema. Institute of Physical Medicine and Rehabilitation, New York University Medical Center, 1963.

HENRY, JAMES P.: Biomedical Aspects of Space Flight. Holt, Rinehart & Winston, Inc., New York, 1966.

PACE, WILLIAM R.: Pulmonary Physiology in Clinical Practice. F. A. Davis Co., Philadelphia, 1965.

Introduction to Respiratory Diseases, ed. 2. National Tuberculosis Association, 1964.

Articles

BURGESS, ALEX M.: A comparison of common methods of oxygen therapy for bed patients. Amer. J. Nurs. 65:96-99, 1965.

BURROWS, BENJAMIN: Chronic obstructive lung disease. Postgrad. Med. 39:105-112, 1966.

CLEMENTS, JOHN A.: Surface tension in the lungs. Sci. Amer. 207:120-130, Dec. 1962.

COMROE, JULIUS H., JR.: The lung. Sci. Amer. 214:56-68, Feb. 1966.

ELSNER, ROBERT, ET AL.: Cardiovascular defense against asphyxia. Science 153:941-949, Aug. 26, 1966.

FENN, WALLACE O.: The mechanism of breathing. Sci. Amer. 202:138-148, Jan. 1960.

HADLEY, FLORENCE, AND BORDICKS, KATHERINE: Respiratory difficulty: Causes and care. Amer. J. Nurs. 62:64-67, Oct. 1962.

HONG, SUK KI, AND RAHN, HERMANN: The diving women of Korea and Japan. Sci. Amer. 216:34-43, May 1967.

KURIHARA, MARIE: Postural drainage, clapping and vibrating. Amer. J. Nurs. 65:76-79, Nov. 1965.

Respiratory tract aspiration (programmed instruction). Amer. J. Nurs. 66:2483-2510, Nov. 1966.

RODMAN, THEODORE: Management of tracheobronchial secretions. Amer. J. Nurs. 66:2474-2477, Nov. 1966.

SASAHARA, ARTHUR A., AND FOSTER, VIVIENNE L.: Pulmonary embolism: Recognition and treatment. Amer. J. Nurs. 67:1634-1641, Aug. 1967.

SECOR, JANE: The patient with emphysema. Amer. J. Nurs. 65:74-81, July 1965.

STREICH, URSEL: Oxygen therapy and hypoxia. Nurs. Science II:49-57, Feb. 1964.

7 Nursing the Patient with a Disturbance of Homeostasis: Cellular Oxygen Needs

Tissue Oxygenation Depends on Effective Internal Respiration

The delivery of oxygen to the alveolar membrane for diffusion into the circulating bloodstream is the task of the respiratory system. But the major work of respiratory exchange takes place throughout the body at the semipermeable membrane of every cell. Here the functional units of metabolic activity demand the oxygen supply that is essential for the biochemical reactions which ultimately produce the energy necessary to sustain life. Respiratory effectiveness, therefore, must involve all of the body tissues, and, for this reason, the transport system in the blood is extremely important. No oxygen can be brought to the cells in sufficient concentration unless the transport mechanisms are adequate and healthy.

The exchange of gases across the alveolar membrane is the first step in internal respiration. In the alveolar space, the pressure gradients of oxygen and carbon dioxide in the air space and in the capillaries determine the direction of movement of these substances. The Po_2 in the alveoli averages about 104 mm. Hg. In the venous blood of the lung capillaries, the Po_2 is about 40 mm. Hg. There is thus a substantial pressure gradient of 64 mm. Hg, so that oxygen readily diffuses through the alveolar membrane, through the interstitial region, and then through the capillary wall. When this oxygen supply is carried to the tissues, there is a higher Po_2 in the capillary than in the cells, and therefore oxygen moves once more into the region of lower concentration. A revised relationship exists with carbon dioxide; the direction of movement of this gas is out of the cells and into the blood, and at the alveoli the CO_2 freely diffuses into the air space to be removed from the body with the stream of exhaled air.

Approximately 97% of the oxygen diffused into the lung capillaries is immediately associated in loose chemical combination with hemoglobin, forming oxyhemoglobin, and is transported in this form to the body tissues.

The remaining 3% of the diffused oxygen is carried in the plasma as a dissolved gas. All of the hemoglobin is held inside of the red blood cells; thus, successful internal respiration is dependent upon a sufficient supply of hemoglobin carried in an adequate number of red blood cells.

Hemoglobin is a remarkable substance. It is composed of two major fractions, heme and globin. The globin fraction is a protein which is synthesized in the body, using the amino acids available in the diet of the individual. There are several kinds of hemoglobin, but the variation in their chemical structure rests always in the globin or protein fraction. The hemoglobin in the developing fetus, for example, is somewhat different from that which would be normal in the adult. At least one aberrant form of hemoglobin has been implicated in a congenital disease. A great deal of attention has been devoted to this specific form of hemoglobin, because the variation in its globin structure consists of a very minor substitution of an amino acid that differs from the one found in normal hemoglobin. The possibility of influencing the development of the globin portion in such individuals in order to rectify this genetic error is very appealing to molecular biologists seeking evidence that intervention can alter specifically identified mistakes of this kind. Thus far, of course, they have not succeeded, but the details of hemoglobin structure are well identified by the chemist and contribute to understanding of all protein formation in the body.

The heme fraction of hemoglobin is the working portion of this rather large molecule (molecular weight, 66,700). It is this portion that is responsible for the deep red pigmentation that identifies the living warm-blooded animal. The bright-red spot appearing early in the gestation of such animals indicates that red blood cells are manufactured very quickly as the embryo develops. It is an awesome fact that the bright red of animal life and the bright green of plant life arise from substances that are closely related chemical cousins. The heme fraction of hemoglobin is constructed of four members of the porphyrin family arranged around a central iron atom. The same portion of the chlorophyll atom is also composed of porphyrins, but they surround a central magnesium atom. The pathways for their manufacture in plants and animals are also extremely similar. It is the heme fraction of the hemoglobin molecule that is capable of binding oxygen in a loose chemical combination. Four heme fractions are associated with each globin fraction, so that every molecule of hemoglobin has the potential for carrying four molecules of oxygen. The loose bond that makes it so easy for oxygen to join hemoglobin, and, indeed, to leave it, accounts for the effectiveness of this compound as a mechanism for oxygen transport. Blood, treated so that it will not clot, may be poured from vessel to vessel in the laboratory, and, as this is done, the blood becomes a brighter and brighter red. This red is characteristic of oxyhemoglobin, as is apparent in arterial bleeding. Even this casual exposure to air is sufficient to permit the chemical attachment of oxygen to the hemoglobin molecule. The oxygen-carrying capability of each hemoglobin molecule is restricted, however, by its chemical structure. It can handle oxygen at only four sites; thus, it is remarkable that oxygenation of the blood, as it passes through the alveoli, usually results in 90% saturation of the hemoglobin.

The effective function of hemoglobin depends, then, on its heme fraction, and, because the heme fraction is built on an iron atom, the supply of iron to the body must be sufficient to permit the production of sufficient heme. As is so often the case when a substance is essential to the organism's total well-being, the body is remarkably frugal in its expenditure of iron and has effective pathways to save and salvage this important substance. The total amount of iron required to maintain adequate hemoglobin production is relatively small in quantity—there is usually about 4.5 gm. of iron in the entire body. Some 65% of this total amount is bound in hemoglobin. The rest of the iron may be stored in the body, especially in the liver cells, in the form of a large-molecule compound called ferritin. As the red cells mature and ultimately die in their normal life-patterns, their hemoglobin is released and removed from the plasma, and the iron thus freed is also stored as ferritin. Thus, iron is recovered and reused in the body over and over again. There is a very limited loss of iron, principally in the bile and the feces, of about 1.2 mg. in a 24-hour period. The menstruating female loses somewhat more, averaging a loss of about 2.1 mg. Iron is available to the individual only if it can be absorbed in the gastrointestinal tract. Excessive amounts in the diet are not absorbed if the body does not need the iron, but pathological interference with absorption, including diarrhea, may result in an iron deficiency. Under ordinary circumstances, the small amount of iron needed to compensate for the small daily loss is supplied in the diet. Obviously, any blood loss from an acute hemorrhage or a long-term chronic loss of blood carries necessary iron with it, which the body, therefore, cannot conserve. Such losses must be made up by the administration of iron, either in the diet or by medication. Hemoglobin production depends upon an adequate source of necessary raw materials and iron is the central atom upon which the complex structure is built.

The Erythrocyte

The hemoglobin is useful to the organism only when it is properly packaged, however, and this, of course, means carried in the red blood cell. The cell is red because of the hemoglobin; in fact, the depth of its coloration is related to the concentration of hemoglobin carried. The cells constitute an essential proportion of the "formed" elements in the circulating blood. If blood is allowed to stand undisturbed, the heavier, cellular components tend to settle towards the bottom of the vessel, leaving a clear, supernatant, yellow liquid (the blood plasma) on top. When the blood is spun in a centrifuge so that all of the formed elements are pulled to the bottom of the container, the cellular part of the blood constitutes about 40% of the total blood volume. This relationship of formed elements to plasma is called the hematocrit. The normal values vary somewhat in men and women because of the normal loss of blood in the menses; in the male, the hematocrit is 47 (±7), whereas in the female, it is 42 (± 5). The chief value of the hematocrit measurement is to establish the

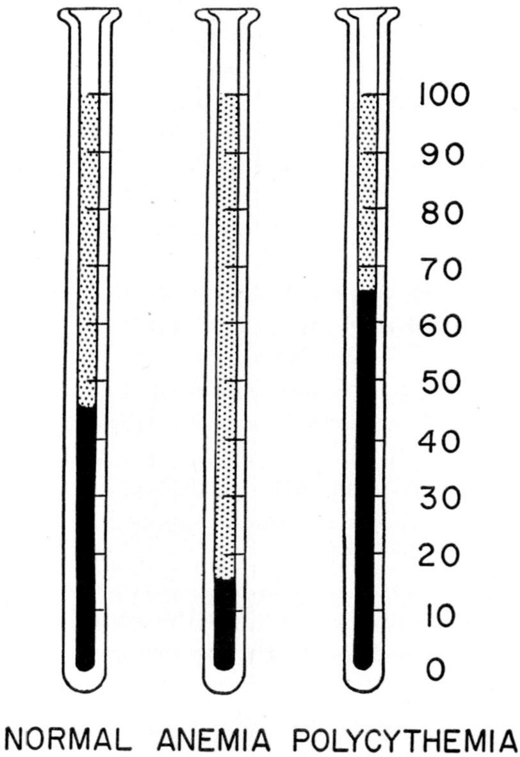

FIGURE 58. The hematocrit is a measure of the relationship between formed elements and the fluid portion of the blood. In certain kinds of anemia, it reflects the decrease in the formed elements, and in polycythemia the relative increase in the number of red blood cells. It is also useful in evaluation of fluid balance, a high hematocrit in this instance suggesting dehydration. (From Guyton, A.C.: *Textbook of Medical Physiology,* 3rd ed. W.B. Saunders Co., Philadelphia, 1966.)

concentration of formed elements to plasma in the circulating blood volume, and the variation is important because it indicates alterations in blood viscosity. A high hematocrit denotes an increased number of cells proportionate to the fluid volume, and this signifies increased viscosity and increased resistance to blood flow. A decreased hematocrit indicates an insufficient number of red cells per fluid volume and signifies a severe interference with oxygen-carrying capacity of the blood. The red blood cell itself is about 34% hemoglobin, a proportion that permits an average concentration of 20 ml. of oxygen for every 100 ml. of blood. This is usually measured clinically in grams of hemoglobin per 100 ml. of blood. Once more there is a variation in normal values for men and women. A hemoglobin of 16 gm./100 ml. is normal for the adult male, while the adult female averages about 14 gm./100 ml. It is interesting that the normal concentration of oxygen in the blood averages approximately the same as the concentration of oxygen in atmospheric air at sea level.

Each of the 4,500,000 to 5,000,000 red blood cells circulating in the vessels of a normal adult represents a "package" of hemoglobin, and each package is constructed for its task with a fidelity to its purpose that is remarkable, even among the many astonishing tissues through which it flows. The mature red cell has no nucleus and therefore no means of replicating itself, so that, once it has reached maturity, it enters a "life-span" during which it is active, and at the termination of which it is destroyed. The average life-span of a normal red cell is 120 days, and in that time it passes through many tissues and many vessels in the body. Some of the vessels through which it must pass to continue its oxygen-carrying journey are tiny, microscopic capillaries, because it is there that the major work of gaseous exchange must take place. The cell is able to adjust its configuration for passage even through tiny vessels that are of lesser diameter than the cell itself. This ability is a function of its size, its shape, and the plasticity of its membrane. The cell is shaped as a biconcave disc 8 microns in length and 2 microns at the widest point on each end of the biconcavity. The central portion of the disc is 1 micron wide. This shape permits the cell to bend and fold on itself as it enters the very tiny capillaries that are narrower than a red cell. The bending places no stress on the plastic membrane of the cell because of the shape, and the cell can therefore be squeezed through the tiny capillaries without being disrupted, owing to the tension of its altered shape. As the cell grows older, the membrane loses some of its plasticity; it is theorized that the cell is ultimately disrupted in a tiny vessel because of its aging membrane. Some cells are thus constantly being disrupted in the body (although younger cells have taken their place), and when the contents are discharged into the circulating blood, the reticuloendothelial cells of the capillary walls

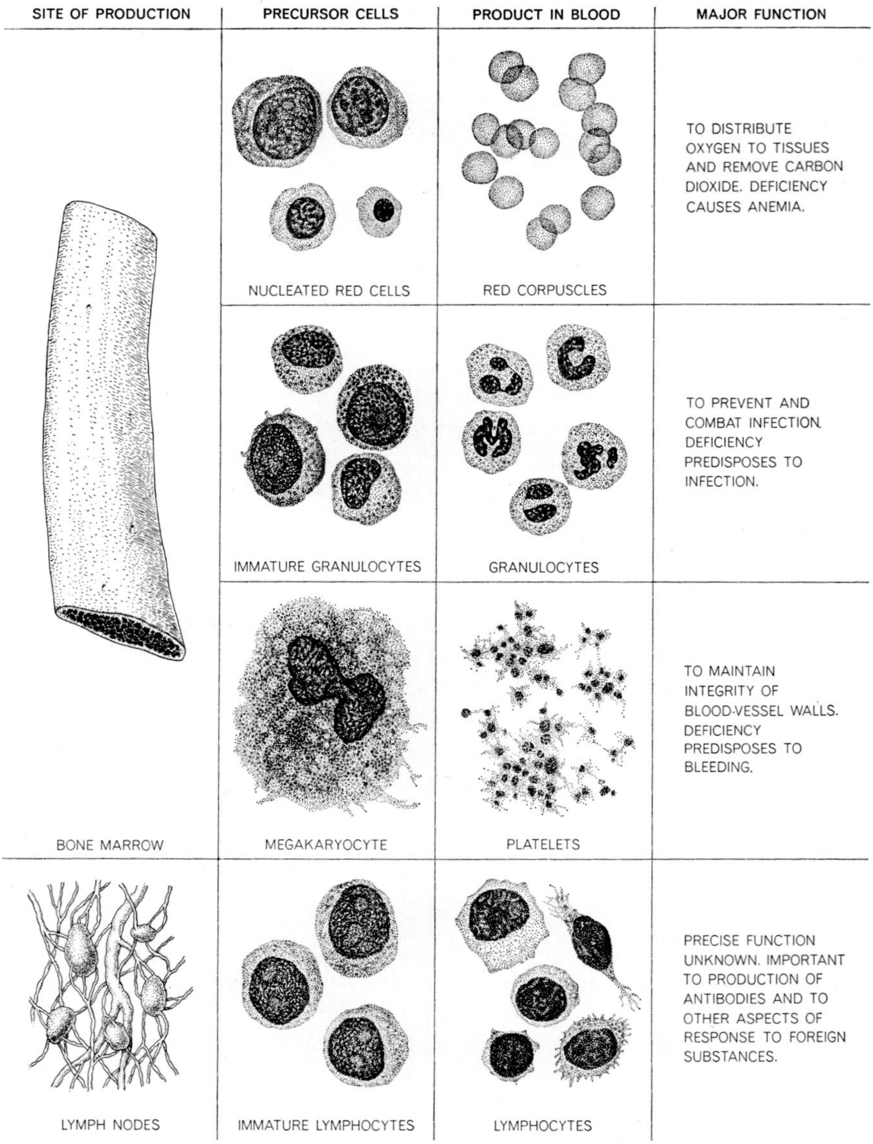

FIGURE 59. The formed elements of the blood possess a structure and function that are identified by the various kinds of cells which constitute the blood. The enlargement here is about 1000 diameters. (From Frei, E., and Freireich, E.: "Leukemia." Copyright ©1964 by *Scientific American, Inc.* All rights reserved.)

sweep up the hemoglobin and enter it into the iron-conserving pattern described above. The other fractions of hemoglobin are degraded, primarily in the liver, and eliminated, chiefly in the bile. It is, in fact, the degraded pigments of heme which give color pigments to the bile. Normally these same pigments provide the usual color of the feces. Any obstruction to the removal of bile from either the liver, the gall bladder, or the intestinal tract results in an excessive build-up of color pigments in the blood, and this is manifested clinically as jaundice—a yellowish coloration of the skin and mucosal surfaces of the body.

The non-nucleated, and therefore nonreplicating, red blood cell must be created anew in the body every day as the aging cells are destroyed. This process takes place in the bone marrow in tissues called hemapoietic (to form blood), and the essential function of these tissues is emphasized by the fact that they are protected and encased in bone. Such a rigid protective framework is characteristic of only one other kind of tissue in the body, that is, the nerve tissue of the central nervous system, and it indicates a priority of importance in the maintenance of life functions. The presence of hemapoietic tissue within the bone marrow space emphasizes, too, how expertly engineered and utilized is the available space within the body structure. In the child, in whom growth places a constant demand on hemapoietic tissues, the long bones are the principal site of hemapoiesis. As the individual matures, only enough functional marrow must retain this property to allow replacement of the normal attrition of red cells, and hemapoiesis is therefore limited, after the age of twenty, to the bones of the rib cage, vertebrae, and the base of the skull.

The mature red cell is not immediately produced in the marrow. It evolves through a series of stages beginning with a primordial cell called the hematocytoblast. There are several stages of immaturity, during which the cell possesses a nucleus, necessary to the gradual change it undergoes. Under usual conditions, immature red blood cells, i.e., those containing nuclei, are found in very limited number in the circulating blood. When the number of immature red cells increases in the circulating blood, it indicates a very active and rapid hemapoiesis in response to the body's demand for red blood cells. Such a demand is usually mediated by a disease process. The reticulocyte is an immature red cell normally found in a concentration of only 0.5% in the blood. This count increases markedly in response, for example, to chronic blood loss, and indicates that the hemapoietic tissue is being forced to function at a high rate, and that proportionately more immature cells are being released into the circulating blood. The immature cells, however, do not perform the function of the mature erythrocyte.

The red cells, as the principal "formed elements" in the circulating blood, are regulated in the normal function of the body so that the viscosity of the blood is held to a physiological balance. Increased viscosity, of course, increases resistance to flow, which, in turn, requires an increased force (blood pressure) produced by increased cardiac action. For this reason, the number of red cells, though sufficient to oxygenate the tissues, cannot increase past the homeostatic limits without the danger of serious interference with circulatory action. Apparently the stimulus to red cell formation is the oxygen tension in the tissues. The mechanism of stimulation is complex and only partially understood, but hypoxia seems to be the basic condition that stimulates red cell production. This feedback, dependent upon the oxygen-transporting capability of red blood cells themselves, is evidenced in a number of physiological as well as pathological situations. Individuals adapted to high altitudes, for example, have a proportionately higher count of red blood cells in their circulation. This adaptation, in fact, takes place over a period of weeks in individuals who are not regular inhabitants of such altitudes, but who remain there long enough for the alteration to occur. Athletes, who demand of their tissues the increased metabolic activity of skeletal muscle action, display a higher red blood cell count than, for example, individuals who live a far more sedentary life. Prolonged bedrest results in a decreased red blood cell count too, and this is further indication of the importance of mobilization, even when the individual must remain in bed for a period of time.

The Pathophysiology of Anemia

Erythrocytes influence the health of the entire organism through the fundamental process of oxygen transport, but the factors regulating their effectiveness include their size, shape, numbers, and longevity. Disease processes that interfere at any of these essential points result in the symptoms of anemia (without blood). It is immediately apparent that anemia is not only a disease of the blood: it involves, in a most fundamental manner, every tissue in the body. The physiological balance between the production of erythrocytes and their normal destruction is the measure of effective red cell activity. Any factors interfering with either the production or the normal life-span of the red blood cell result in a clinical condition of anemia.

As a packaging device, the red cell encloses a specified volume of hemoglobin. This, of course, represents still another factor in the presence of anemia in the individual, since the red cell is effective only because it can carry hemoglobin. A red cell of normal size with its normal complement of hemoglobin is described as normochromic (normal color) and normocytic (normal-sized cell). A large red cell is called macrocytic (large cell), while a small red cell is called microcytic (small cell). If a cell contains more hemoglobin than normal, it is described as hyperchromic (more color); if it contains less than the normal pigmented hemoglobin, it is called hypochromic (less color).

The most obvious cause of a deficiency of red blood cells is the loss of blood during an acute hemorrhage. The total blood volume is quickly restored, once such hemorrhaging is terminated, by an increase in the blood plasma, resulting in a dilution in the concentration of red blood cells. Recovery by the production of red blood cells takes place over a period of time, but during the interval when the total red blood cell count has been reduced after an acute blood loss, the red blood cells are unchanged. They are therefore described as normochromic, normocytic; thus, the anemia is not characterized by alteration in the size, shape, or amount of hemoglobin in individual red cells, but only by the total number of red cells circulating in the blood. The rationale of therapy that prescribes transfusion of whole blood is thus aimed not only at restoration of total blood volume, but also at the restoration of oxygen transport in the circulation. When the blood loss is a slow and chronic process, however, the problem is compounded by a lack of dramatic symptomatology that calls attention to the loss before alteration of the red cell effectiveness has already been accomplished. Chronic blood loss carries red cells away, and with them the essential supply of iron usually conserved by the body. The production of hemoglobin is restricted by the loss of iron, and the red blood cells produced are smaller in size than normal. Such individuals therefore develop a microcytic, hypochromic anemia. Obviously, they will benefit from whole blood transfusion, but dietary factors of a long-standing nature are also required to initiate full recovery. The red cells of such individuals may carry as little as 15% hemoglobin, in contrast to the normal concentration of 34%.

Alterations in the size and shape of red blood cells are often related to genetic defects that mediate their production. Any cell that is unable to move without damage through the tiny capillaries will not survive the usual life-span of the normal erythrocyte. A cell that is too large will be disrupted under the pressure of its movement through the capillary, at least in part, because the membrane of the enlarged cell is more fragile than that of its normal-sized counterpart. A cell that is not a biconcave disc will also be disrupted as it bends its way through a tiny vessel. A spherical-shaped cell cannot be subjected to the stress of bending without breaking its membrane and spilling its contents. Thus, any cell that is not biconcave and capable of withstanding such tensions is doomed to a very limited existence. Individuals who are unable to manufacture red blood cells of normal size and shape suffer anemias characterized by excessive red blood cell destruction. These are very serious diseases which cannot be cured, and which can be controlled only by devoted clinical interevention. Some individuals are benefited by surgical removal of the spleen, which plays an important role in red blood cell destruction, but nothing can yet be done to alter the individual's ability to manufacture red cells of normal shape.

Obviously, any interference with the ability of the hemapoietic tissues to make red blood cells will result in a serious deficiency of these essential constituents of blood. The hemapoietic tissues are extremely active, and, even though they are protected by the bone within which they reside, they respond promptly to any forces interfering with the rapid mitotic behavior that characterizes them. The forces that alter the replicating abilities of cells are those capable of interefering with the orderly processes of cellular reproduction. In the atomic age, the most notorious enemies of cellular reproduction are the tremendous energies carried by radiation of all kinds. Such assaults on rapidly reproducing cells result in a radical alteration of their function, and thus effectively stop such activities. The real terror of the effects of the atomic bomb rests with the damage perpetrated on hemapoietic tissues. Exposure to x-rays can produce the same results, and, in fact, exposure to radiation sources over a long period of time inevitably results in destruction of hemapoietic tissue. Many industrial chemicals can achieve the same dire result, particularly aromatic organic compounds. This danger thus exists in drug administration, and many drugs have been implicated in damage to hemapoietic tissues. Cancers are also frequently responsible for destruction of the body's blood-cell-making mechanisms. Injury to hemapoietic tissue results in an aplastic (without shape) anemia. It is threatening to the organism to have its source of red blood cells cut off, but, in addition, the hemapoietic tissues also produce other cellular elements in the blood, including those that are essential to defense of the individual against infection. When the hemapoietic tissues are destroyed or very limited, the production of leukocytes is also limited, and this includes the white cells responsible for antibody formation in the body defense against all kinds of inflammatory stimuli. The most immediate danger in aplastic anemia is the suppression of these defense elements, and the individuals are gravely threatened by pathogens of all kinds. In fact, they may even be threatened by the ordinary microorganisms which do not usually act as pathogens because the defense mechanism keeps them under control. An aplastic anemia is, therefore, an event of great urgency, requiring extremely cautious medical and nursing intervention.

The manufacture of red blood cells by the hemapoietic tissues presupposes a ready supply of essential raw materials. The complex manufacturing process depends to some degree on the dietary supply of critical

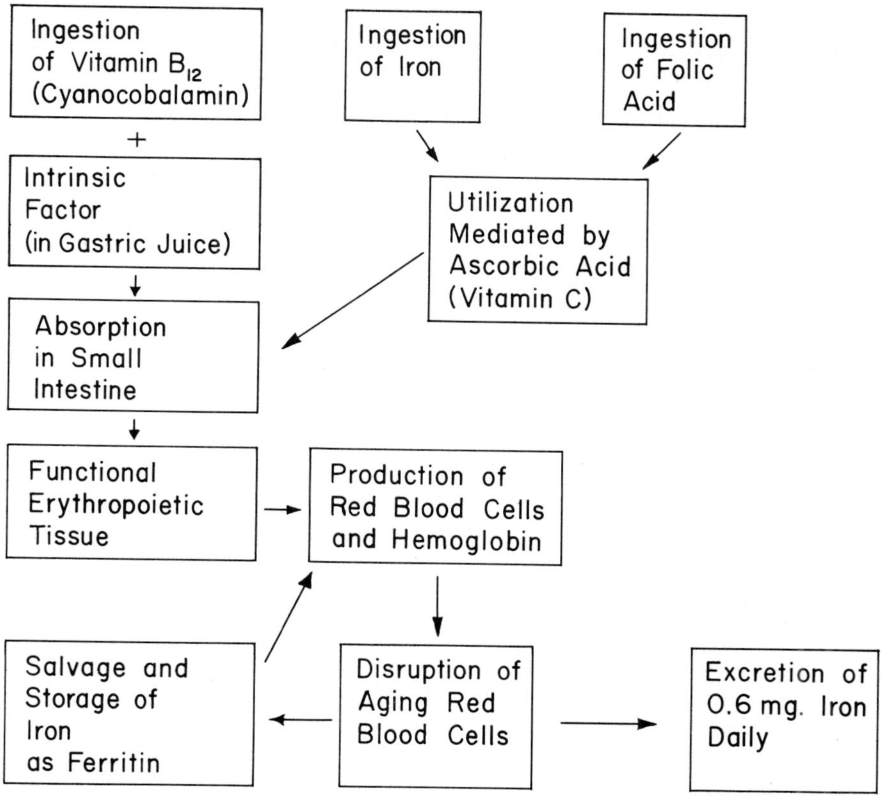

FIGURE 60. Adequate cellular oxygenation results only when normal red cells are available in adequate quantity. The manufacture of the final product depends on many variables, and interference at any of the essential steps in the process results in a variety of clinical forms of anemia.

substances, but the ability of the body to utilize these substances does not rest entirely in the bone marrow. The most obvious deficiency, of course, would appear to be that of iron, and yet such anemias occur in males only as a result of blood loss. Iron deficiency anemia is common, however, in women, largely because of the loss of blood during the menses. The demands of a pregnancy may also compromise the iron supply available to the mother. Strict dietary deficiency of iron may accompany the development of anemia from other causes, but it is very rarely the sole responsible agent even though women maintain an iron balance with considerably less stability than men. The use of iron as a supplement to diet is often irrational when the medication is proprietary in nature; unfortunately, an astonishing sum of money is spent every year for "tonics" that purport to correct just such (largely nonexistent) deficiencies. Iron is absorbed from the gastrointestinal tract only in an ionized, ferrous form. There is some evidence that ascorbic acid (vitamin C) is necessary for the reduction of the ferric compounds ordinarily found in foods to ferrous compounds that can be absorbed from the gastrointestinal tract. A mildly acid pH is necessary for this chemical change to occur, and it apparently does not take place in the absence of gastric juice. The ingestion of absorbable iron in normal individuals does not add to an already sufficient iron storage in the body, although iron is absorbed readily in individuals who are deficient in the total body iron. The question raised so energetically by Popeye and other spinach-eaters is largely an academic one, since a real iron deficiency often requires medication supplements; only if it is very minimal does it respond to diet alone. Many of the tonic mixtures claimed to "strengthen" the blood contain other drugs that are mildly stimulating, and thus contribute to the sense of well-being that is so widely advertised. The individual who treats his own blood, because he believes it to be "tired," may be masking or ignoring very serious symptoms that require medical intervention.

The nutritional deficiency of necessary raw materials for the manufacture of red cells is, nevertheless, very real. The problem, however, focuses on a vitamin known as B_{12} or cyanocobalamin, a substance absolutely necessary for the maturation of the red blood cell. Since this is a substance that the human body cannot manufacture, the entire supply is dependent upon ingestion of the vitamin and upon its *proper absorption* from the gastrointestinal tract. Vitamin B_{12} is the only water-soluble vitamin that is not manufactured in the cells of plants and higher animals. It is produced or synthesized by bacteria, and the high concentration of the vitamin in the tissues of sheep and cows is apparently related to the bacterial growth in the gastrointestinal tracts of these ruminants. But even the ingestion of sufficient amounts of vitamin B_{12} is to no avail unless there is an adequate supply of gastric juice in the individual's stomach. One of the constituents of gastric juice is a substance known as the intrinsic factor, a mucoprotein which, in the acidic pH of the stomach, combines with the ingested B_{12} and thereby renders it absorbable. In the absence of gastric juice, there is no intrinsic factor, and thus this important vitamin cannot be utilized by the body. It is for this reason, among others, that complete gastrectomy is not performed unless it is absolutely essential. Many pathological processes interfere with gastric juice production, including, most notably, cancers of the stomach. Severe anemia accompanies such changes because of the lack of intrinsic factor. A very severe type of anemia is associated with gastric achlorhydria. This anemia is called "pernicious," because the long-term effects include severe damage to the nervous tissue and consequent permanent crippling of the individual so afflicted. In 1926, the treatment of pernicious anemia with liver was first attempted, and, though this required the daily ingestion of liver (a dietary modification that few individuals could welcome), it had a definitive effect on the progress of this very severe disease. Eventually parenteral solutions of liver extract were made, but it was not until 1948 that the vitamin itself was isolated and identified. The individual with pernicious anemia develops a very characteristic lemon-yellow pallor of the skin and is usually prematurely gray-haired. The development of neurological symptoms often begins with paresthesias, or sensations of "needles and pins" in the extremities. Early treatment is extremely urgent, since neurological loss cannot be reversed, and the prevention of nerve damage is therefore a primary goal in treatment. Characteristic beefy lesions of the tongue and mouth (glossitis) are found too, and indicate widespread inflammatory changes in the lining of the gastrointestinal tract that are also manifested by other symptoms, including epigastric distress and flatulence. It must be emphasized that pernicious anemia does not develop from dietary deficiency alone. Its etiology is not known, but it can be very successfully treated by the administration of vitamin B_{12}. The daily administration of the vitamin is, however, as essential to the continuing well-being of the individual as is insulin to the diabetic. The individual must retain a lifetime dependence on cyanocobalamin in order to keep the symptoms of pernicious anemia under control.

Another dietary constituent essential for red blood cell production is folic acid. This substance is apparently a coenzyme of vitamin B_{12} and, in this way, is essential for erythropoiesis. Unlike the case of vitamin B_{12}, however, a frank dietary deficiency of folic acid may cause severe anemias. This may occur rather quickly when dietary intake is reduced, but it also occurs when absorption in the gastrointestinal tract is prevented because of severe diarrhea. Gastrointestinal infections, often accompanied by diarrhea, may add to the folic acid deficiency because the microorganisms compete with the body cells for the available folic acid. Although mechanisms of anemia development are quite distinct in the deficiencies of cyanocobalamin and folic acid, concurrent deficiencies of both of these substances is not uncommon. Rather dramatic response often results when the substances are administered to the individual. Folic acid, in addition, is dependent upon an adequate ascorbic acid supply for the chemical mediation of a usable form of folic acid. This may be significant when ascorbic acid deficiency accompanies a minimal or subclinical folic acid dietary intake and is enough to precipitate a serious anemia.

The competent production of erythrocytes is thus a process that depends upon a delicate balance of factors both within the organism and without. The most immediate response of the entire body to a limitation of oxygen-transporting cells, regardless of the cause, is an increased demand on cardiac work. This compensatory system attempts to overcome the hemoglobin deficiency by speeding the passage of blood through the tissues. In a severe anemia, the cardiac output may be doubled, and this vastly increased work load on the heart cannot, of course, fail to have serious implications for the well-being of the individual. The development of primary anemias, such as pernicious anemia, is in itself a serious clinical problem. But the readiness with which many pathophysiological changes elsewhere in the body create secondary anemias is even more compelling as a common clinical problem.

Care of the Anemic Patient

The Conservation of Energy

Since oxygen is so vital to the metabolic activity of all body tissues, it is obvious that deprivation of oxygen through a failure of the transport mechanisms will quickly result in a slowing and insufficiency of metabolic activity. Even muscle cells, accustomed to a constant degree of hypoxia, are overwhelmed, so that they are unable to continue to function without the development of profound signs of fatigue. Characteristically, the anemic patient presents the picture of an individual who fatigues quickly with minimal activity, and in whom even rest does not completely restore well-being. The first consideration in nursing such patients is clearly related

Table 12: Blood Flow to Different Organs and Tissues Under Basal Conditions*

	PER CENT	ML./MIN.
Brain	14	700
Heart	3	150
Bronchial	3	150
Kidneys	22	1100
Liver	27	1350
Portal	(21)	(1050)
Arterial	(6)	(300)
Muscle (inactive state)	15	750
Bone	5	250
Skin (cool weather)	6	300
Thyroid gland	1	50
Adrenal glands	0.5	25
Other tissues	3.5	175
Total	**100.0**	**5000**

*Based mainly on data compiled by Dr. L. A. Sapirstein. (From A. C. Guyton: *Textbook of Medical Physiology*, 3rd ed. W. B. Saunders Company, Philadelphia, 1966.)

to maintaining a level of activity which will not place undue stress on an already compromised metabolism, and thus conservation of energy is a crucial nursing responsibility. Oxygen utilization is directly related to activity, and oxygen demand can be limited only by restriction of activity to that which is essential for the individual's well-being. Nursing intervention of this kind cannot insure an increased hemapoiesis or improvement of hemoglobin concentrations per se. But it allows the individual to spend his energy wisely and restricts the demands placed upon vital tissues. The compensatory change involving cardiac function is reflected in an increased energy expense even when the individual is at rest. The measure of the potential difficulty that is created by increased cardiac output secondary to anemia is highly individualized. It depends to a large degree on the source of the anemia itself. Obviously, when cardiac disability already exists, such compensatory changes in the cardiovascular function may exact a high toll in the individual. It is not unusual that secondary anemia accompanies a long-standing decompensation of the heart, and such a precursor would increase the urgency of protecting the patient from unnecessary energy utilization.

Anemia may produce rather startling clinical symptoms, but in most instances the development of secondary anemia is covert, and the recognition of the symptoms of this complicating condition requires sensitive and alert observation. Bedrest alone may result in a lowered red blood cell count and the development of compensatory response to anemia. The presence of nutritional failure from any cause is another frequent contributor; often the combination of bedrest, dietary restriction, and dyscrasia is concurrent. Gastrointestinal infection, especially that accompanied by diarrhea, is another frequent precursor of anemia. The clinical evidence of anemia is always present when there is a history of recent blood loss, either acute or chronic in nature. It is well to assume that every individual who has had major surgical procedures will display some sign of hemoglobin deficiency. This accompanies not only the blood loss during surgery, even when it is minimal, but also the frequent period of starvation which is a requisite of postoperative surgical care in many kinds of procedures. Kidney pathology of many kinds is almost a guarantee of anemia, because the kidney apparently elaborates a substance that stimulates erythropoiesis, and this function may be depressed in kidney disease. Anemia is not infrequent in aging individuals, as much from dietary failure as from the presence of chronic diseases of many etiologies. Any pathology that alters the function of the hemapoietic tissues, even though primarily directed at other formed elements such as the leukocytes or the platelets, has a definitive effect on red blood cell formation too. The nursing care of any person who has had a long-standing illness, or a very severe one, must be oriented to the possibility of hemoglobin deficiency. The weak patient, the individual with a marked weight loss, the immobilized, and the bedridden—in all of these, the possibility of anemia and its effect on their well-being must be a continuing nursing consideration. And, of course, attention should be directed to the loss of blood in the menstrual flow in patients who may be hospitalized for reasons in no way related to this cyclic function. Evaluation of the nature of the menses may contribute significant information about the patient, though the menstruating woman frequently ignores this regular event and, unless it is attended by unusual blood loss, will not ascribe importance to it at all. Such a loss of blood, however, superimposed upon a surgical procedure—even when replacement therapy has been adequate—may emphasize how precarious the hemoglobin balance is in the female during the menstrual years.

Since the basic demand for oxygen does not decrease, and in fact, increases as a result of increased cardiac function, the care of the anemic patient must emphasize conservation measures gauged to the individual's tolerance for activity. How this is accomplished is a very individual matter, and in fact, tends to vary considerably even in the same individual. In some patients, the fatigue that accompanies nursing activities may be best minimized by performing these functions as rapidly as possible so as to limit the total time during which the individual is required to participate. In other patients, allowing periods of rest and planning in advance for necessary activity may be more useful. The restriction of physical activity will be altered as the patient regains his hemoglobin concentration and is capable of increased activity as a result. Since the cardiovascular system responds so promptly to a decreased hemoglobin concentration, frequent measurement of the quantity and quality of the pulse rate contributes important information *to the nurse* as a parameter of the individual's energy expense. The physician requires that the pulse rate and, of course, the coordinated respiratory rate be recorded at regular intervals, and often nurses do not realize how essential this information may be in what the nurse proposes to do with and for the patient. The surgical nurse who is ambulating a patient early in his postoperative course learns quickly that the individual's tolerance is ascertained readily by changes in his pulse rate and quality as his position is changed. This same information is available to the nurse whenever the issue of the patient's energy utilization is an important aspect of his care.

Control of the external environment is another facet of providing the individual with an optimal situation for energy conservation. If it is important that he be given the opportunity to rest, and even to nap, then it is equally essential that the external surroundings permit this. The control of noise, distraction, and tension in the hospital ward is a first prerequisite to a restful environment. Satisfaction of essential needs, such as provision of toilet utensils, may also contribute to an environment in which rest is possible.

When dietary management is clearly indicated in the treatment of secondary anemia, the food selection and consumption by the patient are essential aspects of the total therapeutic plan. Very real issues may arise in reference to food intake, since the development of secondary anemia is often related to the food pattern. The surgical patient, of course, has had little wilful control over this specific area. But the interest in the diet may be difficult to muster in many patients, and the ingestion of the specific foods that will benefit him most may be resisted. When the anemia is clinically significant, the individual is often given drugs to supplement his iron intake. The oral drugs most commonly used for this purpose may cause gastrointestinal symptoms. Many patients complain that the pills cause diarrhea, and they refuse them for this reason. Such problems should be promptly reported to the physician, since drugs that are effective may be substituted for those that cause the unpleasant side-effects. Adequate dietary management must involve knowledge on the part of the nurse of that portion of his meal that the patient actually consumes. If he is not able to take his diet, or is failing to take an adequate one, this must be reported to the physician.

Any factor that places additional demand on the energy resource of the anemic patient must be avoided. This certainly includes infections of any kind, and particularly those that are easily transmitted, such as upper respiratory infections. The surgical patient is always zealously guarded from wound infection, and, in the presence of gastrointestinal infection, very careful asepsis is instituted to prevent cross-contamination. It is often difficult to regulate the external temperature so that the anemic patient is comfortable. Such individuals often feel "cold" even in moderate temperatures and will require extra blankets and perhaps a warm robe when they are up and about.

The Conservation of Structural Integrity

Protection of cardiac function by limiting energy expense in the anemic individual also serves to conserve the structural integrity of the overworked heart. Continued excessive demand of cardiac output leads inevitably to cardiac enlargement and the danger of decompensation and failure. Essentially, the correction of the anemia is a prior consideration in the prevention of structural cardiac alteration; thus, every effort in the therapeutic plan directed at improving the hemoglobin concentration is also helpful in minimizing cardiac involvement.

The fatigue and weakness apparent in the severely anemic individual create an urgent necessity for providing for his safety and for the prevention of injury. If the individual is permitted to ambulate, the nurse must be thoroughly familiar with his ability to do so with safety. He may, for example, be allowed to go the toilet, and it is a nursing responsibility to be certain that he is able to do so without becoming dizzy or fainting en route. If he is allowed to remain in the toilet by himself, the nurse must be certain that he can manage alone and that he knows how to summon help if he should require it. Often the individual denies—even to himself—that ambulation is difficult. His behavior may tell the nurse more than he is willing to verbalize. In fact, the nurse must constantly be alert to patients who propel themselves painstakingly down the ward, holding onto bedsteads and articles of furniture, or tending to move towards the wall for support as they walk. Such behavior indicates that the individual should not be permitted to move about without assistance; a failure to detect this kind of behavior is often responsible for the injuries sustained by falling or fainting during hospitalizations. Such individuals, of course, must never be permitted to bathe without assistance, either in the tub or in the shower. It is never prudent to assume that an individual can mobilize himself without danger of injury unless the nurse has positive evidence of his ability to do so. Many more patients will attempt to move independently than will demand assistance when they no longer require it. The incidence of serious injury, including head injuries and broken limbs, in hospital wards, is appalling and can be eliminated only by the most conscientious attention of the nursing personnel to the individual's ability to navigate without help. It is true that some individuals will attempt to get out of bed in defiance of the physician's wish that they remain there. But even in these instances, the patient may indicate his intentions in subtle ways which the nurse must learn to recognize.

The individual with anemia does not heal as readily as the one well supplied with oxygen-transport cells. This in itself emphasizes the importance of the therapy designed to improve tissue oxygenation. But often the patient who develops secondary anemia is also the one who has other evidence of nutritional failure. He must be zealously guarded from pressure sores and the possibility of decubiti. Frequent positioning in bed is essential here too, in addition to meticulous hygienic practices.

The therapeutic diet that is prescribed to combat anemia contributes to the patient's structural integrity, as well as to his energy supply. If his general nutritional status can be improved, the benefits of adequate protein intake are as marked for him as for other individuals. His own sense of convalescence may accurately reflect the change in his blood picture, and this in itself will influence his willingness and ability to accept his diet.

The anemic individual must frequently have blood samples taken for laboratory analysis. When these procedures must be carried out at regular intervals, the individual often fears for his structural integrity, even though he has no realistic reason to do so. Patients who must have blood removed will often express the fear that this process is depriving them of blood they can hardly spare. The prospect of the introduction of a needle into the vein is usually interpreted as an encroachment on his integrity that the patient would willingly dispense with, and still it is essential that the laboratory profile of his blood be repeated as a guide to the therapeutic plan. Although 10 ml. of blood represents only a tiny fraction of his supply, to the patient the large syringe used to withdraw the blood may seem gigantic. The most cautious aseptic technique, of course, must be used when the procedure is performed. Often, through no fault of the technician, but because of altered capillary fragility or other factors related to the anemia itself, there is some extravasation of blood into the soft tissues surrounding the site of injection of the needle. The resultant hematoma, or bruise, may alarm the individual because it appears to be a structural change of some moment. There may also be localized discomfort related to the pressure of the extravasated blood. Such patients may frequently display these obvious signs of their contribution of blood, and do so with considerable affect. They can readily be reassured that the blood loss is not a significant one and that the bruising is not a permanent alteration. The individual may, for example, be encouraged to drink a little more water so that he can feel he is replacing his "lost" blood. Replacement actually occurs very promptly, although the removal of 10 ml. of blood barely influences the total circulating blood volume anyway. If, however, drinking a glass of water afterwards is comforting, and if he is permitted oral fluids, there is no reason why this cannot be suggested to him. A severe hematoma at an injection site may be made more comfortable by the application of local heat, but this must be ordered by the physician. The individual may also complain of pain at the injection site if he is given essential replacement drugs parenterally. The injection of liver and iron extracts into the muscle is painful, and when it must be repeated daily, the patient may with great justice resist the treatment. The injection of any substance into a muscle must be done with extreme care to avoid injury to nerves in the area. In addition, the placing of a volume of liquid into the muscle creates a localized area of pressure, and the diffusion of the medication is rarely instantaneous. Thus, the patient may have many areas of localized pain and discomfort in the muscles where the injections are given. This may create discomfort enough to warrant concerted nursing intervention. The local application of heat or cold to minimize the discomfort may be done, however, only with a physician's express order, specifying the type of application, the length of time it is applied, and the precise area where it may be placed. Serious nerve injury has accompanied intramuscular injection, and the complaint of pain by the patient should not be shrugged away by the nurse. When injections must be made frequently, there is an increased possibility of localized infection too, and such infections may cause a great deal of discomfort, as well as sloughing and necrosis at the site. The threat thus posed to the structural integrity of the individual is obvious.

The Conservation of Personal Integrity

The effect of hypoxia on the central nervous system frequently results in irritability and irascibility quite inappropriate to the precipitating situations. The very serious primary anemia, pernicious anemia, is often accompanied by behavioral changes so marked that the individual is frankly psychotic. It is significant that this can be entirely reversed as the anemia is improved. The individual with secondary anemia will not display behavior as marked as this, but he will often demonstrate a behavioral pattern that challenges the nurse's desire to help him. A physiologically determined behavior is one over which the individual cannot exercise much control. His irritation and disaffection are undoubtedly as upsetting to the individual as to those who care for him, and it is sometimes extremely difficult to make the necessary adaptations in his care that will satisfy him. Hostility and anger aroused in the nurse by irritable and frightened patients rarely achieve a nursing goal worth-while to either of them. The irritability that may be stimulated by tissue deprivation is further aggravated by the extreme weakness and ready fatigability of the anemic patient. It is rarely possible to differentiate, in the individual's behavior, between those factors arising from tissue hypoxia in the nervous system and those fostered by his feelings of inadequacy and incompetence. Second only to respiratory distress, the inability of an individual to move through the activities of his daily life without exhaustion is a frightening and forbidding experience. His relative well-being at rest quickly gives way to helplessness, when the energy it takes to simply walk across the room leaves him physically fatigued. Since secondary anemia frequently accompanies other disease entities, it is perhaps wise to assume that irritability in a patient reflects physiological mechanisms he cannot control, as well as the disaffection that arises from his emotional response to restricted freedom of movement. Sometimes the effect associated with this kind of helplessness results in withdrawal, depression, and absolute compliance on the part of the individual patient. Although this creates an individual who gives the nurse little trouble, the danger signals of an inappropriate response are there and deserve recognition.

The individual who greets the laboratory technician with apprehension deserves that his concern be respected. The individual often objects to the removal of blood samples in a half-serious or joking way, and the nurse needs to be aware that such a response may mask a very genuine concern in that individual. His behavior may appear childish, or churlish, but in either instance the nurse only reinforces his fear if she treats him either as a recalcitrant child or as an unwilling but captured victim. The tremendous importance of the blood as the fluid of life is reflected in the layman's response to it. Almost every young woman can recall the stage, which almost everyone experiences, when the sight of blood is the signal for an exaggerated emotional response. Even though the procedure for removing blood as a laboratory sample is part of even the most cursory physical examination, few individuals face it with complete equanimity. The young child fears both the discomfort of the needle and the sight of his own blood seeping out, and such a reaction is far from uncommon, even in the adult. The anemic individual quickly realizes that a great deal of concern is invested in his blood sample; his personal fears may easily begin to focus on the laboratory reports that measure his progress. He thus has additional reason to dread the procedure itself, and when he suggests, ever so casually, that he cannot spare the blood that is being removed, he may be expressing a fear fundamental to his entire view of himself. While an expert technician can perform the procedure with a minimum of pain in a minimum of time, it is never entirely without discomfort. When a vein has been entered repeatedly to withdraw blood, inflammation may cause a thrombosing or closing of the vein, so that its use for subsequent withdrawals is impossible. In individuals whose veins are readily palpated or visualized, it may be quite simple to remove the blood quickly without much pain. But in individuals in whom this is not the case—and not only obese persons have veins that are difficult to locate—the relatively simple procedure may become a very tortured experience. If the technician cannot locate an appropriate vein in two attempts, the task probably should be delayed, and perhaps even turned over to another technician. It is cruel and unnecessary to repeatedly puncture the individual's arm, hands, or legs to find a usable vein unless doing so is a matter of genuine urgency. When such a difficulty exists in an emergency situation, the time wasted on frequent attempts is often better spent on a surgical incision into the superficial tissues to locate a vein by direct visualization. This procedure, called a "cut-down" in the jargon of the hospital, is justified when the issue is sufficiently urgent. In any event, a promise that the procedure is painless is a falsehood, and the individual will respond far more positively if the possibility of discomfort is acknowledged. To be meaningful, such an admission must recognize that the relative discomfort of the procedure is offset by the importance of the knowledge that it can give to the physician. But there is probably no phrase found on a patient's chart that is more demonstrable of useless anguish and discomfort than a laboratory report that says, "quantity insufficient to test." If the individual is helped to understand the reason for the examination and not censured for his reaction to the dislocation and pain it may create, he is far more apt to accept it, and the results of the procedure are more certain to be satisfactory.

When the anemia is susceptible to dietary management, the individual must be taught how to select foods which will supply the necessary elements for hemoglobin production. It is apparent, however, that not all anemias will respond to this single approach; before the nurse can assure the individual that dietary modification is useful, she should be certain that this is true in the individual instance. The selection of a well-balanced diet for all persons is not the same thing as choosing a diet that is therapeutically aimed at improvement of a nutritional-deficiency anemia. The frequency with which the public media have emphasized the importance of dietary iron is not proportionate to the number of individuals whose anemia has arisen because of other pathophysiological changes. A realistic approach to the question of diet does not mean that dietary instruction is avoided, even when modification of the anemia cannot be entirely dependent upon the diet. It is particularly important that women recognize their precarious balance of iron, which might easily be tipped in one direction or the other by their food selection. It is also essential that the individual understand that the promises of the manufacturers of "tonics" are rarely kept, and that, in any event, this kind of self-medication depends once more on self-diagnosis, and this practice is always fraught with danger.

The individual who is receiving oral hematinics (blood-stimulating drugs) should be warned that his stool color will change. The iron compounds ordinarily given by mouth will produce a "tarry" stool. This change may be alarming to many individuals but especially to those who have experienced gastrointestinal bleeding and recognize this as a symptom of such bleeding. This change in the stool also makes it necessary that such drugs, as well as red meats, be withheld from the individual when a laboratory examination of the stool for the presence of blood is planned. Since covert bleeding in the gastrointestinal tract is so commonly a cause of iron-deficiency anemia, such an examination is not at all unusual, unless the cause of the anemia has already been definitively determined. Changes such as these cause alarm and dismay in individuals who do not anticipate them, and patients should be instructed in the effects of the drug in order to prevent such an event.

The dependency created by fatigue and weakness can be gradually relieved as the individual becomes capable of more and more independence in his own care. Such a weaning from dependence is accomplished when the nurse evaluates the individual's progress from day to day. In the care of the patient with anemia, essential laboratory values should be part of the nurse's knowledge about the patient and should be used as a guide for permitting increasing independent activity. His personal integrity is best supported by physical well-being, but during the time when his body is responding to the treatment, the nurse's recognition of his limitations and of the feeling tone created by his disease is essential to his concept of himself.

The Conservation of Social Integrity

The social exchange so important to this aspect of the individual's integrity cannot exist in a vital fashion unless the individual has the energy required. The astronomical cost of blood tonics as a cure-all for fatigue and tiredness probably reflects the desire of many individuals to maintain a satisfactory social exchange. The anemic individual, incapable of sustained physical, emotional, or mental involvement in life, must create family situations in which the disaffections grow out of the limits that anemia places on participation. It is relatively easy to rationalize fatigue when an individual has spent his day in a productive and active way. But when that same degree of fatigue develops from minimal activity and fatigue itself is the prime complaint, it is equally simple to shrug it off as a personality disturbance. The knowledge that iron has a salutary effect on lassitude and fatigue is as ancient as the practice of medicine. The mystical association of the strength of iron with its effect on the body is a folkway that persists to this day. Even the ancients recognized that when patients with a marked pallor were given drinking water in which old swords were allowed to rust, the entire feeling tone and appearance of the individual gradually improved. If modern man seeks to drink a fluid only slightly less magical than that which held the rusty swords, it is because the association of vigor with iron has an unquestionable physiological base.

On the other hand, the well established knowledge of dietary effects on the health of circulating blood has not succeeded in limiting dietary extremism. In young people, the conformist pressure of adolescence frequently creates dietary restrictions that are eminently capable of creating iron deficiency anemias. The very definite problem confronting the adolescent girl in maintaining a positive iron balance is ignored when the diet is selected according to social determinants rather than physiological need. Because the menses is a recurrent physiological function of the body, the effects of this monthly blood loss are usually overlooked or simply never understood by the adolescent youngster. In addition, the search for information relating to the menstrual function is rarely undertaken. The relationship of this bodily function to sexual activity has served to perpetuate the reluctance to discuss menstruation, even with professional people who are well informed. Few youngsters are sufficiently informed to be able to recognize a normal menstrual flow, and, in any event, changes in the menses are apt to be greeted not only with apprehension but with guilt. In efforts being made to introduce sound scientific sexual knowledge in the public educational institutions, emphasis on the importance of dietary support of hemoglobin production should always be made to young women. For this group in the population and for the pregnant woman, iron in the diet is essential to good health, and such knowledge should be widespread.

Dietary problems related to anemia are also frequent in the aging population. There is a natural attrition of hemapoietic function in the older individual, and it may be further compromised by chronic disease. For older individuals, particularly those living alone and preparing their own meals, the diet may be markedly deficient in iron; this, added to the other factors, creates a true iron-deficiency anemia. Older people, for economic reasons and sometimes simply because they do not have adequate dentures, often skimp on the protein foods that offer the best sources of iron in the diet. This is the same age group in which the distinction between fatigue justified by activity and that stimulated by anemia is difficult to determine. And, of course, it is to this group that geriatric tonics and elixirs are promoted as the answer to the problems of increasing weakness and fatigue. Unfortunately, this is the same population beset with chronic gastrointestinal bleeding, kidney disease, and sometimes chronic congestive failure—all anemia-producing syndromes. In addition, the changes of aging may decrease gastric juice production and thus initiate the severe anemia that attends the inability to absorb vitamin B_{12}. The proprietary preparations sold over the counter are "shotgun" mixtures and may actually mask important symptoms. For example, folic acid may hide the developing symptoms of pernicious anemia, including the neurological changes which cannot be reversed. Regular medical care and information and assistance in dietary planning are important to the aging population for many reasons. The prevention of anemia is certainly one of them.

The vagueness of a complaint of "fatigue" discourages the seeking of medical attention when anemia is a factor in producing the symptom. Secondary anemias, unless they are very severe, rarely produce a symptomatology that is definitive enough to encourage medical help. The feeling of tiredness is stimulated by so many other conditions that mere tiredness is rarely a reason for medical care. Such complaints are often ascribed to the emotional complexities of life; even physicians have occasionally been guilty of paying too little attention to this complaint when the patient does present himself, apologetically, for care. The laboratory definition of inadequate hemoglobin is so precise, and the technique for determining it so simple, that every patient should at least have the benefit of this procedure as part of his physical examination. The individual is ill-served if his complaint is ignored or rationalized when it has a reasonable basis in his hemoglobin concentration.

The social interaction which is part and parcel of the hospital environment can just as readily reflect impatience and ignorance when the patient's chief complaint is his sensation of helpless fatigue. An alert nursing staff expects secondary anemia as a complication of many other disease entities, and with it the behavioral manifestations of tissue hypoxia. While pallor and weakness accompany many bouts with disease, wherever they exist, the individual is entitled to a blood profile to rule out the possibility of anemia. Once a diagnosis of anemia is confirmed and made part of the patient's history, every nurse caring for that patient has a responsibility to recognize its presence and its influence on the individual's behavior. Many a disgruntled patient, confronted by an impatient nurse, is a victim of his hypochromic red blood cells.

There is probably no area of nursing care in which the physiological influence is more demanding in understanding and evaluating behavior than in the treatment of the anemic patient. There is evidence here that not all disease is startling in its manifestations and dramatic in its treatment. The struggle just to keep functional in the face of ill-defined symptoms creates anxiety and distress; recognition of the struggle is often buried in an approach to patient care that emphasizes psychosocial needs at the expense of pathophysiological change. The balance that must be struck in these areas of nursing care is precise and unequivocal in the care of the patient with anemia.

Family members must be helped to understand that the individual is not retreating behind his complaint of fatigue, and that his feelings of helplessness are justifiable and real. They must understand how to select foods that will benefit the anemic individual. If medication is prescribed when the patient is discharged, the importance of taking it faithfully must be understood as well. If long-term parenteral drugs must be given, then either a family member must be taught how to do it, or arrangements must be made for a visiting nurse to come to the home to administer the drug. The family and the patient must be helped to understand the need for energy conservation for as long as such restriction of activity is essential. They must also realize that good personal hygiene and protection from infection are essential.

Lacking a dramatic impact and the tremendous sums of money invested in research in more "exciting" diseases, the incidence of anemia in both the primary and secondary forms presents a major clinical problem to the physician and the nurse. While recovery may be prompt, it also may be very prolonged; for the suffering individual, anemia restricts and restrains his participation in daily activities for as long as the deficiency persists. In most instances, the anemia itself is readily identified by relatively simple and inexpensive laboratory analysis. Discovering its cause and promoting recovery may be a far more painstaking task. But, by sheer numbers, the victims of anemia demand the devoted attention of the nurse.

Model VII: Local Application of Heat and Cold

OBJECTIVES

1. To understand the influence of physical principles that govern thermal energy exchange.
2. To understand the therapeutic intent of application of heat or cold to the body surface.
3. To understand the effects of thermal energy on the viability of living tissues.
4. To recognize the physiological effects that measure the effectiveness of the application of local heat or cold in the absence of more specific measuring devices.
5. To understand the implications of folk attitudes on the use of local application of heat or cold.
6. To understand the function of devices used to apply heat or cold to the body surface so as to insure the individual's safety and comfort during such therapy.

ESSENTIAL SCIENCE CONCEPTS

1. The physics of thermal energy is based on the kinetic molecular theory.
    - 1.1 Heat is the energy of molecules in motion.
        - 1.11 An increase in the average kinetic (moving) energy in any system results in an increase in the total heat in the system.
        - 1.12 A decrease in the average kinetic energy in any system results in a decrease in the total heat in the system.
        - 1.13 The temperature of a system is a measurement made by utilizing acceptable conventions as scales.
            - 1.131 A thermometer "records" the average kinetic energy (heat) in a system.
            - 1.132 A thermometer is a system that responds by alteration of its kinetic energy within an arbitrary scale, easily interpreted by the observer.
                - 1.1311 Fahrenheit scale is based on the temperature of an ice-salt mixture and that of human blood.
                - 1.1312 Centigrade scale is based on freezing and boiling point of water.
                - 1.1313 Conversion scale between two systems necessary because the arbitrary intervals are mathematically different.
                    - 1.13121 $9/5°C + 32 = °F$
                    - 1.13122 $(°F - 32) \times 5/9 = °C$
    - 1.2 Heat is transferred from one source to another only when a gradient

(difference in temperature) exists, and always from the higher to the lower temperature (second law of thermodynamics).

1.21 Radiant heat (from the sun) is the ultimate source of all heat on the earth's surface.

1.211 Radiation is the transmission of energy by waves to surrounding bodies of lower temperature.

1.212 All systems of higher temperature radiate heat to environments of lower temperature (including the human body).

1.213 "Room temperature" means that objects in an environment are in equilibrium with surrounding temperature.

1.22 Conduction is a form of heat transfer requiring contact of surfaces with a temperature gradient.

1.221 Heat is conducted by molecular impacts which impart increased kinetic energy from a rapidly moving molecule to a slower one.

1.222 Conductivity varies as a physical characteristic of all substances.

1.2221 Metals (good electrical conductors) are generally good heat conductors.

1.2222 Gases (including air) are poor heat conductors.

1.23 Convection is a form of heat transfer dependent upon moving currents.

1.231 In a still environment, warm air tends to rise (because of increased molecular motion) and cold air to fall or settle.

1.232 Moving currents of air of lower temperature remove heat from the surface of a body that is at higher temperature.

1.24 Evaporation is a form of heat transfer requiring the change of a liquid into a vapor from the surface of a heated body.

1.241 The "heat of vaporization" is specific for each substance, and is a measure of the energy required to change it from a liquid to a gas.

1.242 Effective heat loss by evaporation depends upon the vapor content of the surrounding environment.

1.243 Evaporation can occur only into a gaseous environment of lower humidity.

2. Heat regulation in homeothermic organisms permits adaptation to a broad range of environmental temperature conditions.

2.1 The organism sustains its internal homeostatic temperature by metabolic processes that provide constant energy.

2.11 The metabolic rate is a measure of the rate of oxidative chemical change designed to maintain heat (energy) production in all environments.

2.12 The range of body temperature establishes the effective range of enzyme action and chemical interaction necessary to physiological function.

2.13 An increased heat production in the body represents a speeded metabolic rate (measurable at 7% increase in rate per Fahrenheit degree rise in temperature).

2.2 Internal constancy of the body temperature is maintained by physiological interaction with the external environment.

2.21 The living organism is a thermal system which continuously exchanges heat with its immediate environment.

2.211 70% of heat loss from the body is by radiation.

2.212 25% of heat loss from the body is by evaporation.

2.213 Heat loss by conduction is minimal to external environment, but principal means of heat transfer is the internal environment.

2.214 Body heat is dissipated at the rate of 300 to 2000 British thermal units (BTU) per hour with ordinary activities of daily life.

2.22 The central nervous system mediates the control of body heat by regulation of heat loss from the body surface or retention.

2.221 Metabolic rate influences temperature control in the thalamus and vice versa.

2.222 Regulation of size of the bed of peripheral (capillary) vessels on the body surface influences heat exchange with the environment.

2.2221 Vasodilatation results in increased heat loss.

2.2222 Vasoconstriction results in increased heat retention.

2.223 Regulation of fluid loss (by perspiration) represents interaction between organism and the environment.

3. The effects of thermal energy on living tissues is limited by cellular response and viability within homeostatic limits.

3.1 Heat source above homeostatic limits alters structure, and therefore function of affected tissues.

3.11 Regional effects reflect organismic defense against localized changes in the temperature gradient.

3.111 Local heat source produces vasodilatation of capillary bed with observable erythema of affected skin surface.

3.112 Highly localized erythema at one site on the body surface produces measurable increase in skin temperature at far distant and unaffected sites on the body surface.

3.12 Damaging heat source alters chemical structure of tissues, resulting in death of affected cells.

3.121 Proteins are denatured by heat above homeostatic limit.

3.122 Vesiculation (blistering) reflects damage to surface tissues.

3.123 Excess heat exposure subjects tissues to oxidative change (burning) with destruction and charring of tissues affected.

3.124 Increased external heat source causes increased metabolic rate (and oxygen consumption) in tissues immediately affected by increased temperature.

3.2 Cold source below homeostatic limits alters structure, and therefore function of affected tissues.

3.21 Local application of cold causes vasoconstriction and blanching of affected surface, as well as skin temperature change in distant and unaffected sites.

3.22 Prolonged vasoconstriction due to local cold source interferes with adequate circulation of nutrients to affected tissues, with possibility of cell death.

3.23 Lowered temperature in a local area reduces metabolic rate and oxygen consumption of affected tissues.

3.24 Temperatures below freezing point of body fluids cause ice crystal formation within cells, with disruption and death of cells.

4. Therapeutic uses of thermal energy manipulate the organism's temperature-regulating systems by external alteration of the body's heat exchange with its immediate external environment.

4.1 Sensory perception of changes in temperature of external environment allow the organism to adapt or seek safety.

4.11 Warning sensation of pain accompanies alterations above or below safe thermal limits at the body surface.

4.12 Pain perception at body surface to changes in thermal environment is lost when stimuli are prolonged.

4.121 Excess heat or cold alters function of local nerve cells and fibers.

4.122 Application of heat in excess of 90°F (radiant source) increases local tissue metabolism more than it increases circulation to the part.

4.123 Excess cold may be used as anesthetic to relieve pain.

4.1231 Viability of tissues protected by limitation of exposed area and length of time of exposure.

4.1232 Where tissue viability is already lost, continuous exposure of affected area provides good pain relief.

4.124 Local heat effectively relieves local pain within an optimal temperature range of 91.4°F to 95.0°F.

4.2 Alteration of peripheral (capillary) blood flow by changes in local thermal environment.

4.21 Vasodilatation by controlled heat source improves circulation in affected tissues.

4.211 Maximal increase in blood flow to extremities occurs in an external temperature range of 80°F to 85°F.

4.212 If circulation cannot supply nutrients for increased metabolic rate accompanying heat exchange, benefits are lost and further damage may result.

4.22 Local heat enhances circulation to inflammatory area so that resolution and localization of infection are speeded up.

4.3 Selection of appliances used to alter local thermal exchange depends on therapeutic intent.

4.31 Direct-contact appliances function by conduction of heat to or from the body surface affected.

4.311 Contact of skin surface with appliance requires use of conductive medium suitable to the task.

4.312 Dry application of heat or cold reduces thermal exchange because of poor conductive qualities of the air blanket that intervenes.

4.3121 Pressure of appliance (related to its weight) decreases air space and increases thermal exchange.

4.3122 Cloth covers used on appliances at skin surface slow thermal exchange.

4.313 Wet application of heat increases thermal exchange because of conductive properties of water.

4.3131 High specific heat of water prolongs effective exposure to heat source.

4.3132 Wet-surface contact with tissues may cause local maceration when exposure is prolonged, and especially if weight of appliance is producing pressure on affected surface.

4.314 Maximum temperature of 105°F is limit of safe heat application.

4.315 Application of local heat or cold may cause systemic response so that individual is aware of environmental discomfort.

4.32 Radiation appliances regulated for effectiveness by intensity of heat source, distance from affected area, and length of time of exposure.

4.321 Ordinary light sources require regulation since a 50-watt bulb produces 140 BTU/hr (conversion factor: $2.8 \times \text{wattage} = \text{BTU/hr} \pm 10\%$).

4.322 Non-light sources regulated by time and distance according to predetermined safety charts.

NURSING PROCESS

1. Effective therapeutic use of local thermal exchange must be regulated by observation of physiological effect on tissues.
   - 1.1 Knowledge of therapeutic purpose is essential to effective nursing intervention.
     - 1.11 Relief of pain at localized site is determined by patient's evaluation of effectiveness.
     - 1.12 Improvement of circulation to a part is assessed by subjective response of individual patient and observation of evidence of improved circulation.
       - 1.121 Color of skin surface with assessment of degree of erythema produced.
       - 1.122 Temperature of skin surface.
       - 1.123 Evidence of localization of inflammatory process, including quantitative evaluation of drainage.
   - 1.2 Frequent observation of the patient so that intervention insures therapeutic goal.
     - 1.21 Prevention of marked systemic response by manipulation of external environment.
       - 1.211 Adequate covering of bedclothes if cold application induces sensation of chilliness.
       - 1.212 Knowledge of thermostatic reading on appliances utilizing this regulatory system to maintain consistent exchange as prescribed by the physician.
       - 1.213 Control of room temperature and humidity, and of air currents whenever possible.
     - 1.22 Use of specific appliance indicated by disease process on precise local area specified by physician.
       - 1.221 Localized application of heat and cold where precise thermal exchange is necessary.
       - 1.222 Application of heat or cold to regional areas when specified and essential to adequate therapy.
     - 1.23 Renewal and repetition of local application as ordered by physician and as required by disease process to insure continuity of effect desired.
     - 1.24 Observation and recording of condition of local area before and after treatment, with special emphasis on change induced by therapy.
2. The safety of the individual must be guarded by nursing technique in the absence of precise measurements involving thermal exchange.
   - 2.1 Precision of physician's order is based on desired effect and safety to exposed tissues.
     - 2.11 Only precise region included in order to be exposed to appliance used.

2.12 Specific temperature regulated when possible by measurement with thermometer or checking of thermostatic control.

2.13 Appliance used as ordered by physician with no substitutions.

2.14 Length of time of exposure specified in order and observed by the nurse, including time limit when appliance is removed or renewed.

2.2 Comfort of the individual is a parameter of safety when thermal appliances are used.

2.21 Preparation for the treatment considers degree and length of relative immobilization that may be required.

2.211 Essential nursing care completed before treatment is instituted, if possible.

2.212 Sufficient explanation to individual so that he understands restriction of activity and length of time.

2.22 Immobilization limited, where possible, by applying treatment so that the appliance is well anchored or supported and does not require the individual's active maintenance of it in position.

2.23 Ascertainment of functional and safe equipment to preclude injury.

2.231 All electrical devices carefully checked before being brought to the bedside.

2.232 Electrical equipment checked at intervals during usage.

2.233 No leakage of fluid from appliances utilizing water as source of thermal exchange (includes melting ice in ice bags).

2.234 Use of proper coverings to prevent local tissue damage —dry when ordered dry, moist when ordered wet.

2.24 Proper use of equipment to insure therapeutic goal without injury.

2.241 Weight of appliance regulated by proper filling with sufficient water to maintain temperature as required.

2.2411 Hot-water bottles partially filled and excess air expelled.

2.2412 Wet applications moist without soaking, and removed after 30 minutes to prevent maceration of skin surface.

2.242 Distance of radiant source carefully measured and maintained by frequent observation.

2.243 Thermostatic control set at temperature ordered, as in aquamatic pads and electric heating devices.

2.25 Control of environmental situation to insure privacy and comfort to the individual.

2.251 Proper draping when application requires removal of bedclothes.

2.252 Loincloths when bed-cradle is used.

2.253 Limit air currents that alter effective use of appliances.

2.3 Aseptic precautions scrupulously observed when application involves open area of the skin surface.

2.31 Surgical asepsis when wet dressings are used on open area, since liquid medium provides for transmission of microorganisms.

2.32 Airtight outer coverings must be sterile to prevent movement of bacteria into the wound.

3. Folk ideas about the use of external heat and cold influence the patient's perception of this kind of therapy.

3.1 Widespread use of local heat and cold indicates frequent substitution of self-treatment for medical consultation.

3.2 Familiarity with therapy of this kind predisposes individual to cherished ideas about its use.

3.21 Lay applications of heat often employ temperatures that are hotter than safety allows.

3.211 Limitation of temperature in hospital may create complaints that application is not hot enough.

3.212 Use of electric heating pads at high temperatures produces unsafe levels of local heat.

3.22 Folk medicine is heavily endowed with counterirritant measures such as "horse liniments" and mustard plasters.

3.3 The purpose of the prescribed therapy should be explained to the individual in terms he can understand.

3.31 Emphasis is placed on importance of keeping appliance at the site prescribed by the physician.

3.32 Prompt renewal or removal of appliance serves to emphasize its therapeutic intent for the individual.

3.33 Provide means so that individual can participate by notifying nurse when appliance needs attention or untoward symptoms develop.

3.34 Safeguard his comfort and safety by proper technique and observation of effects.

Vocabulary

anemia
aplasia
aplastic anemia
chlorophyll
cyanosis
erythrocytes
fatigue
fragility
hemapoietic
hematinic
hematocrit
hematocytoblast
heme
hemoglobin
hyperchromic
hypochromic
isolation
jaundice
macrocyte
microcyte
negativism
pallor
pernicious anemia
porphyrins
proprietary drug
psychosis
reticulocyte
syncope

General Bibliography

ALLEN, EDGAR, BARKER, NELSON, AND HINES, EDGAR: Peripheral Vascular Disease, ed. 3. W. B. Saunders Co., Philadelphia, 1962.

DEGRUCHY, G. C.: Clinical Hematology in Medical Practice, ed. 2. F. A. Davis Co., Philadelphia, 1964.

GOODALE, RAYMOND H.: Clinical Interpretation of Laboratory Tests, ed. 5. F. A. Davis Co., Philadelphia, 1964.

COHN, HOWARD D.: Hemostasis and blood coagulation. Amer. J. Nurs. 65:116-119, 1965.

LAKI, KOLMAN: The clotting of fibrinogen. Sci. Amer. 206:60-65, March 1962.

LEVEY, RAPHAEL H.: The thymus hormone. Sci. Amer. 211:66-67, July 1964.

PERUTZ, M. F.: The hemoglobin molecule. Sci. Amer. 211:64-76, Nov. 1964.

Recognizing early signs of internal hemorrhage (programmed instruction). Amer. J. Nurs. 65:119-138, Dec. 1965.

UNGLAUB, WALTER, ET AL.: Recent experiences in diagnosing and treating pernicious anemia. Postgrad. Med. XXIX:399-407, April 1961.

ZUCKER, MARJORIE: Blood platelets. Sci. Amer. 204:58-64, Feb. 1961.

ZUCKERKANDL, EMILE: The evolution of hemoglobin. Sci. Amer. 212:110-118, May 1965.

8 Nursing the Patient with Disease Arising from Aberrant Cellular Growth

Cell Replication Is Dependent upon the Activity of Genetic Materials

The mystery and miracle of life are summarized in the word "growth." From the inception of a new being by the combination of germinal cells from its parents to the gradual process whereby a 7-pound, 18-inch newborn develops into a 170-pound, 6-foot adult, the wonder of growth is a pervasive influence on all human awareness. There are an orderliness and integrity in the changes mediated by the growth process of such dimensions that it is safe to predict—and expect—at what point the process will be at almost any time in the life-span. The expectation of growth patterns has a predictability that is consistently supported within highly specific patterns of change. Extremely basic social and economic values arise fundamentally out of such expectations with a consistency so reliable that the focus of the educational objectives of every culture is keyed to the physiological progress that is called "growth."

Experience alone has fortified societies throughout history with the certainty of such knowledge, but it is only within recent historical time that knowledge of the dynamics has been developed. The initial scientific studies of growth in the individual centered on the hereditary influences as they evolved, and the indices that allowed prediction of the nature of unborn generations were described. But such study had serious limitations. Although it was possible to predict with some accuracy the characteristics of the unborn, it soon became apparent that the pattern was never precisely duplicated. Years of tedious observation led to inescapable conclusions. Certain characteristics of the individual always recurred in subsequent generations, but some recurred only within a precisely restricted mathematical statement of probability. And occasionally there was a marked change in a characteristic which could not possibly have been predicted. This, of course, was the science of genetics. Dominant characteristics reappeared in subsequent generations consistently, whereas those that reappeared in specific percentages of individuals were identified as recessives. Radical changes were known to be mutations, but how and why these occurred could not be explained in rational terms.

An expanding technology, and most specifically the development of more and more powerful microscopes, made it possible to identify some of the cellular landmarks. In some instances, changes that regularly recurred in those landmarks helped to identify their function, but many such alterations remained mysterious. The research ultimately led to the identification of chromosomes in the dividing cell and finally to genes as discrete units of germinal material. The mitotic behavior of the cell was thoroughly explored, and it became apparent that self-replication always involved a division of the germinal material so that each daughter cell was similarly endowed. The endowment, it must be emphasized, was only similar, because unique differences continued to be demonstrated by individual organisms. The observation of the activity of the cellular landmarks was not sufficient to identify the dynamics involved.

Students of cellular behavior could visualize the active cell, but the research was soon directed towards an analysis of the contents of the cell itself and the structure of the microscopic organelles that seemed to be involved in replication. As early as 1869, a substance named "nuclein" was identified as a cellular constituent, although it was not until 1924 that it was established as a substance concentrated in the nucleus of the cell. In 1940, the technical means for analysis of cellular materials had improved sufficiently so that nuclein was identified as deoxyribonucleic acid, now widely known as DNA. It was also possible to determine that the quantity of DNA in the nuclei of specific cells was remarkably consistent for that cell. For the first time it was possible to ask the question, "Is DNA the essential constituent material of the genes?"

Researchers extracted DNA from one strain of bacterial cells and substituted it in another strain; thus, for the first time, human intervention had made it possible to alter the hereditary pattern of a living organism. It was no longer in doubt that DNA was the carrier of genetic information. Now the biochemist took his place in the vanguard of cellular research. A whole new avenue of understanding of life was traveled for the first time, and the science of molecular biology gained its first foothold in biological research.

In 1953, Watson and Crick described the chemical structure of DNA, for which astounding feat they shared the Nobel Prize with Wilkins in 1962. The achievement of this remarkable elucidation of the structure of DNA rested on research that was intricate, complex, and beautiful, and it answered many of the questions first raised in the monastery garden where Gregor Mendel watched his peas grow.

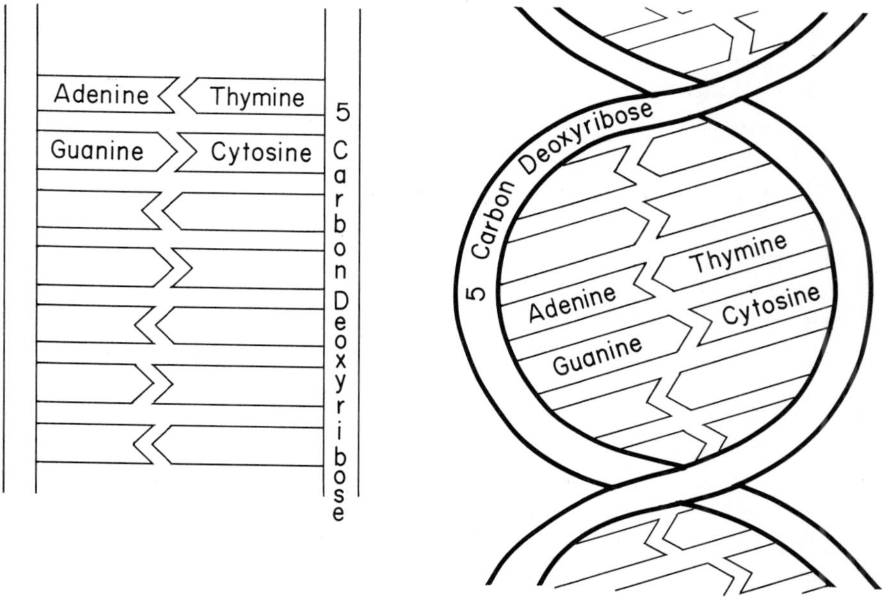

FIGURE 61. The rungs of the "ladder" of the DNA molecule are twisted in the shape of a double helix. The rungs themselves always consist of regularly paired nucleotides: adenine with thymine and guanine with cytosine.

The DNA molecule is a double helix chain much like a spiraled ladder, turning upon itself with rungs that remain stiff and straight, thus holding the elastic sides apart. The twisting sides of the ladder are composed of sugars (5-carbon deoxyriboses) and phosphate groups. The rungs are composed of nitrogenous bases—combinations of nucleic acids that are specifically aligned in the molecule in distinctive arrangements unique for each species of living thing. In the human cell, there are four nucleic acids: adenine and thymine, guanine and cytosine. They are found in complementary pairs in just that twin arrangement—an adenine always paired to a thymine, and a guanine always paired to a cytosine. These four substances occur in the DNA molecule in a specific pattern, and their place on the rungs of the twisting ladder identifies the specificity of that particular DNA molecule. They thus constitute an alphabet, but one capable of limitless arrangement of constituent parts whereby thousands of characteristics of the organism are spelled out, just as letters are rearranged in the familiar word game that children play. Thus, the four nitrogenous bases of the DNA molecule establish a pattern, or template, for the transmission of characteristics to individual organisms by the way in which they are arranged in the rungs of the vital ladder. Genetic information is coded in the sequence of the nitrogenous bases. The genetic code is slowly being translated by the research scientist so that its messages —identifiable by alterations in the molecular structure of DNA—can be understood by the biologist.

The gene transmits its heritage to subsequent generations because it is a template upon which are formed the enzymes required by the cells for the manufacture of proteins essential to life. Enzymes in the body are the organizing systems that guide and direct life processes. An enzyme is an organic catalyst, and each step in protein synthesis is mediated by a specific enzyme. Each gene produces a specific enzyme—one with a discrete role to play in protein synthesis. The concept of one gene to one enzyme was an important step forward in understanding the function of the nucleus. An alteration in the gene, often as simple a matter as the wrong placement of a pair of amino acids, alters the kind of enzyme it will pattern. If the enzyme is changed, it may not function in the expected manner and thus may interfere with the proper construction of the protein. Ordinarily, the double chain of the DNA with the paired nucleic acids along the rungs separates into two single strands during cellular division. Since the nucleic acids are complementary, as the single strands are reconstituted, they re-form precisely as they were before separation. The strands do not completely separate all at once, but open much like a zipper, with gradual and progressive replication of the new second strand. Thus, every replicated DNA consists of one half of the original molecule plus a second half newly constructed to exactly duplicate the original in complementary pairing of its nucleic acids.

It has been possible to pinpoint precise genetic abnormality with some disease processes. A very definitive abnormality in a precise gene has been known for a long time in individuals who are mongoloids. It is now possible to demonstrate the chemical alteration in that peculiar-appearing gene, and the molecular biologist looks forward to a time when intervention will make it possible to alter the aberrant gene, thus reversing the symptoms that arise from it. This is a mechanism that can be demonstrated in nature. Viruses exert their effect on cells by substituting their genetic code for that of the cell they have invaded. They utilize the nutrients available in the cell, but, having enslaved its nucleus, force the production of viral protein. When the cell is exhausted, it is disrupted, and many newly manufactured viruses are then freed to begin the cycle again in other cells. In addition, many physical agents can alter the structure of the gene by substituting or forcing the substitution of inappropriate nucleic acids or by simply knocking off a portion of the molecule by high-energy impact. Radioactivity is probably effective in altering the genetic code in this way, and the concern for the health of germinal cells rests squarely on the fact that such alterations are frequently not compatible with life.

These exciting research findings are being vigorously pursued in laboratories all over the world. The focus on basic research must continue, and with it the fruitful exploration of disease processes which seem to be related to cellular function. Cancer research has received a tremendous stimulus from molecular biology. The dedicated scientist shares with the layman an intense desire to find a cure for this most cruel of human afflictions. But the scientist also knows that such knowledge comes painstakingly slowly in the laboratory; each newly fitted part of the puzzle is celebrated because it leads to further study and reinforces the hope for final understanding.

The ability of the cell to replicate itself is the fundamental basis for all growth processes. Mere reproduction of the cell, however, is accompanied by a number of complex and interacting variables. During embryonic development and throughout the rapid-growth periods of infancy and childhood, much of the energy of replication must be consistently devoted to the creation of new tissues. When the growth period has been stabilized in the adult, cellular activity continues to maintain and replace cells as required by the organism. There is a tremendous difference in the rates of replacement, with some tissues being re-formed and replaced rapidly and continuously and others incapable of being re-formed at all. The tissues, for example, that are under constant stress from the environment, such as the skin, mucous membranes, and lining of the gastrointestinal and respiratory tracts, are capable of constant and fast replacement. Other tissues, such as the neurons of the central nervous system, are fully supplied at birth and can never be replaced, once they are lost. Thus, cells are not only highly differentiated in their function but also in their ability to replace and duplicate themselves.

Under ordinary circumstances, the replacement of tissues following normal attrition or moderate injury takes place in an orderly fashion. New

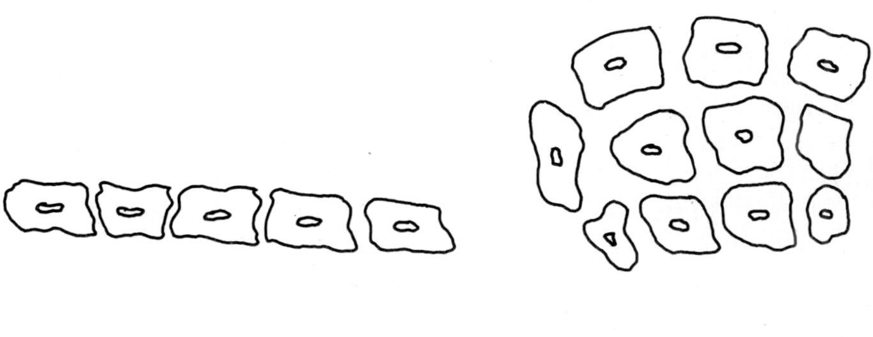

FIGURE 62. The orderly restraint that characterizes replication of normal tissues is replaced by anarchy in tumor growth.

epithelial cells replace those worn off at the surface of the body—but only enough are re-formed to exactly replace what was lost. Once the replacement takes place, *growth stops*. In this way, tissues formed of the cells remain discrete and separate. Epithelial cells do not encroach upon muscle cells which lie underneath them. The entire process is one of order and restraint dictated by specific need.

The limitation of growth imposed by replicating tissues upon themselves is not well understood. Many theories have been offered to explain the restraint that is normal in tissue repair and maintenance. This somewhat academic problem, however, is a vital community issue because such growth limitation and restraint are not operative in the case of malignant cells. The problem of cancer is the problem of aberrant cellular growth, of disorder and anarchy in the usual patterns of cellular reproduction.

The knowledge that now seems to be within reach may someday explain why certain cells begin a growth cycle that goes on independent of the organism's needs. Every type of cell in the human body is capable of entering this anarchic growth pattern. Quite commonly, the cell that is normally highly active (such as epithelial tissue) exhibits the kind of runaway growth that is, ultimately, harmful to the total organism. Such neoplasms (new growths) are categorized as carcinomas. Neoplasms that arise from other kinds of tissues are called sarcomas. The neoplasms found in children often tend to arise from the rapidly growing tissues of their embryonic forebears and are, for that reason, of a rapidly progressing type. The remarkable fact is that such phenomena do not occur more often than they do. It is estimated that in the 100 trillion cells of the body, nearly a billion cells per minute are undergoing mitotic change. With such a range of probability, it is not difficult to imagine that mutations occur with fair regularity. But why some mutations allow anarchy and some apparently do not has not yet been determined. When it is, the secret of malignant neoplasms will be known.

Aberrant Cellular Growth and the Space-Occupying Neoplasm

There is no doubt that malignant growths begin with a single cell, capable of reproducing itself in spite of the normal mechanisms of the body to restrain and restrict tissue growth. By the time such a mitotic tumor has reached the diameter of one centimeter, it is estimated to involve 500 million cells. A "critical colony size" has been postulated for such growths, which suggests that the tumor may remain dormant or even disappear unless the critical point is attained. When the critical size is reached, however, uncontrolled growth takes place. Even an infinitely

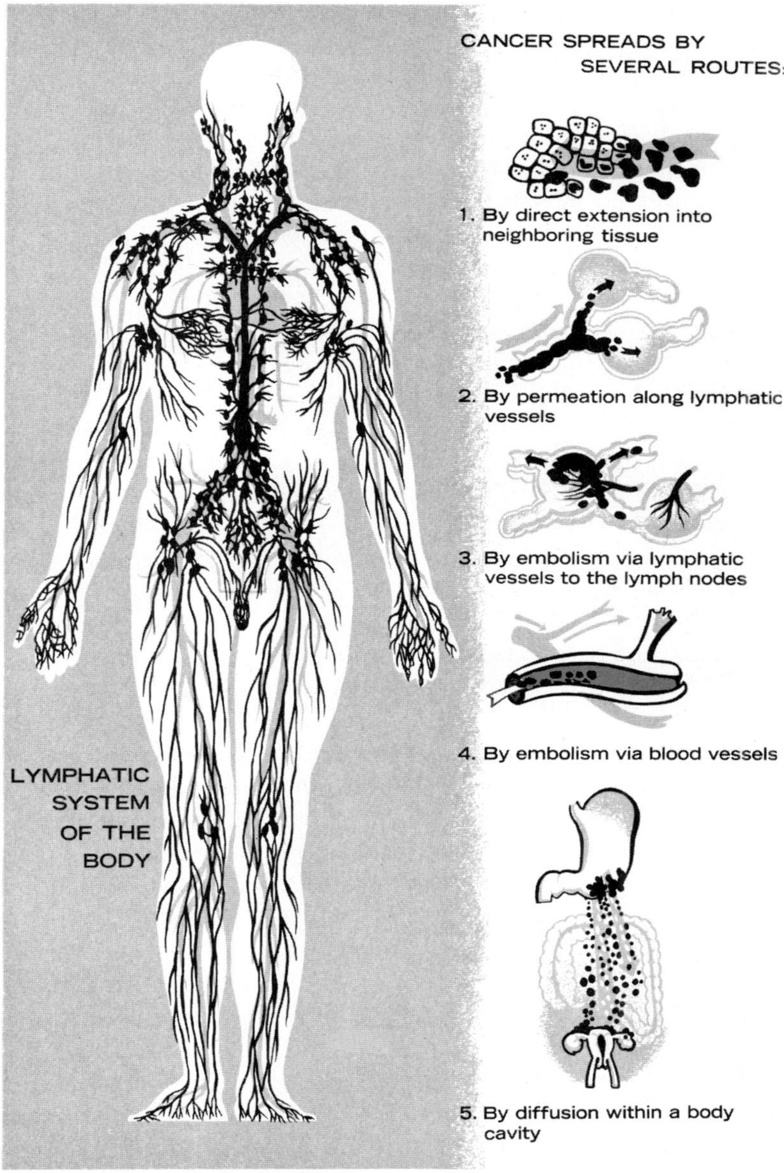

FIGURE 63. The sinister behavior of malignant cells is best evidenced by their ability to invade, infiltrate, and spread to all parts of the body. While the usual transport systems are often the carriers of malignant cells, transmission by other routes is also possible. (From *Cancer Source Book for Nurses*. Courtesy of the American Cancer Society, Inc.)

small tumor mass may wreak irreparable damage long before it is discovered. Very small tumors are, in fact, discoverable only if they are close enough to the surface of the body to be detected by ordinary means. This is the crucial issue in the clinical approach to mitotic neoplasms. If they can be discovered early enough for removal, then the individual may, indeed, be "cured." But even very small new growths have the potential for creating widespread damage before they are large enough to be detected.

The most potent factor that threatens the organism is that malignant cells, in their anarchy, are capable of invading other tissues. The cluster of malignant cells do not remain in a definitive pattern as do normal cells. They tend to break away from the body of the neoplasm itself. The tendency for these aberrant cells to break away rather easily must be related to membrane dynamics in some way, and one theory suggests an alteration in calcium metabolism. Until the membrane function at a cellular level is much better understood, this will remain a puzzling question. Also, in addition to their unquestioned ability to free themselves from the parent cell aggregate, many kinds of malignant cells possess ameboid motility. They can travel, and some of them have actually been clocked at specific rates of speed. Whether they begin their undisciplined journey under their own power or are simply hitchhikers in the usual transport systems of the body, such as the bloodstream or the lymph channels, they are capable of reaching distant sites in the body and of establishing new growing clusters of malignant cells. This transfer of tumor sites distant from the original, or primary, site is called metastasis. Metastasis can take place very early in the development of a primary neoplasm; therefore, early identification and localization of the tumor are an urgent clinical necessity. Only surgical removal before daughter tumors have been established in the body can be successful in controlling the disease. The insidiousness of this invasive capacity, however, leaves a cloud of doubt over all surgical treatment of mitotic phenomena, and, because the surgeon can rarely be positive that he has removed every single malignant cell, surgical excision is never described as an out-and-out cure. Instead, the surgeon talks of patients with "five-year" and "ten-year" cures—reference to survival times of such individuals without evidence of recurrence. Even this is not a guarantee that symptoms will not once again develop, or, in fact, that the individual may not begin the process all over again with a new and unrelated anarchic growth in another tissue.

The invasive property of neoplasms establishes the pathophysiology of this disease wherever it occurs, because it always involves encroachment on healthy tissues. The symptoms of the disease frequently arise from the fact that these space-occupying lesions mechanically interfere with the function of essential systems. It is not uncommon that early

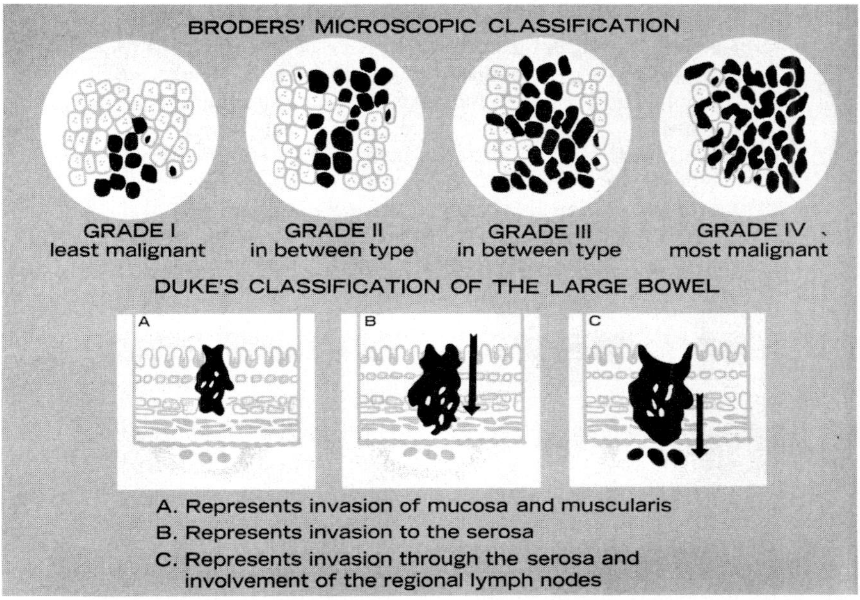

FIGURE 64. The "severity" of a malignant invasion is best determined by pathological examination of the tissues, although the establishment of a "grade" of malignancy does not always indicate the severity of the clinical manifestations of the tumor. (From *Cancer Source Book for Nurses.* Courtesy of the American Cancer Society, Inc.)

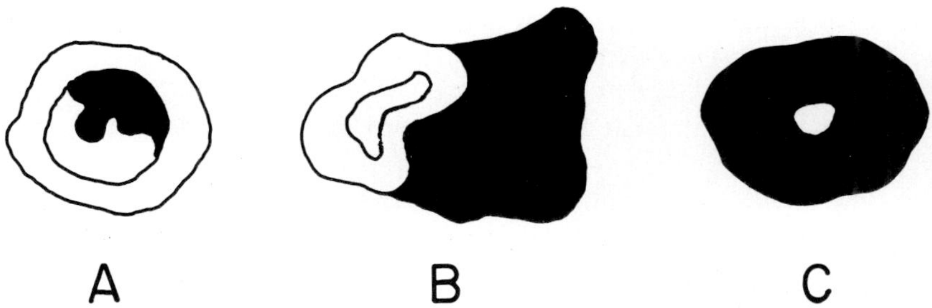

FIGURE 65. Encroachment on the patency of tubes often produces the first symptoms. (A) narrowing of the lumen by the presence of an encroaching tumor; (B) pressure on the outside of the tube causing constriction of the lumen; (C) annular lesion thickens the walls, constricting the lumen.

signs are manifest by invasion of patent tubes in body systems—tubes that must remain patent in order to assure physiological function. Mechanical interference with the lumen of the tube may be established by an actual invasion into the tube space itself by pressure from adjacent tissues where the tumor is growing. If the tumor is within the walls of the organ, it may constrict the lumen by an annular (ringlike) pattern that gradually reduces the patency of the tube. Such interference is common in the gastrointestinal tract, the urinary tract, the lungs, the blood vessels, the lymphatics, and the drainage channels of the cerebral system. Invasive destruction of the occupied tissues often results in erosion of large blood vessels with attendant hemorrhage. And the pressure of tissue destruction involving nerve tracts produces pain that is extremely difficult to manage clinically. Loss of nerve function is also common.

One of the most striking clinical problems in individuals with malignant neoplasms is the evidence of widespread metabolic failure, especially as the disease progresses. The typical wasting of body substance in individuals with an advancing malignancy is called cachexia (poor condition). Much attention has been paid to the nutritional failure so apparent in the awful wasting seen in cachectic individuals. The utter malnutrition is associated with a very severe anemia. Efforts to pinpoint the dynamics of nutritional failure have failed thus far, although the competitive demand of the aberrant cells as they rapidly reproduce and extend their influence certainly must have some bearing on the problem. Not even force-feeding will help the wasting individual or improve his nutritional state. The totality of metabolic failure in such patients is one of the most crucial areas for research. The parasitic independence of the tumor cells, seizing nutrients and making every body function subservient to their destructive need, is somehow related to the anarchic path they choose in the first place. The analogy with the behavior of viruses at the cellular level suggests that, if the viral process can be unraveled, real progress will be made in the war against malignancies.

The Issues of Cancer Control

The order, constraint, and compelling wisdom in the pattern of cellular growth and replication is sacrificed for utter, complete, and senseless destruction by malignant cells. To meet that confusing wilderness of uncontrolled and undisciplined cellular behavior in a controlled and disciplined way presents a therapeutic problem of considerable dimensions. In the first place, to understand the *loss* of control, it is essential to define clearly the mechanisms of control. The knowledge is growing, but it is far from sufficient as yet. There are numerous areas of concern and research devoted to reaching a sufficiency that will allow rational therapy.

The first exciting knowledge rests clearly in understanding the language of the gene. Not only are the words in that language becoming known, but there is now a dictionary that has already allowed some of the secrets of replication to be identified. The molecular biologist also seeks better understanding of the environmental factors long implicated in mutative change. Some chemicals are villains; clinical observation has persistently involved them. Substances found in food, in cigarettes, and even in polluted air have stimulated aberrant cell replication often enough to be described as carcinogens—cancer producers. Long before the cell could be explored, the clinician described malignancies that were instigated by "irritation" of tissues. As study moves forward, more and more such substances are being identified, even though their specific role in cancer formation cannot yet be pinned down. The action of high-energy radiation is another malignancy-stimulating source in the environment. The increasing attention to radioactivity follows sadly the man-created sources of such high-energy contaminants. And while the onus of culpability is unquestionable, the limits of safety and the means of control are far from known. Political issues compound the problem, and the tribal boundaries that have isolated men are crumbling in the face of radiation that cannot be stopped by any kind of wall, no matter what it is made of. Finally, under the electron microscope, the scientist has watched the virus subjugate the cell and has recognized that this kind of assault must have broad implications within the environment of mankind.

It is certain that the mechanisms of control exist within a cell, but only in relationship to many other cells. The replicating cell is a *functional*

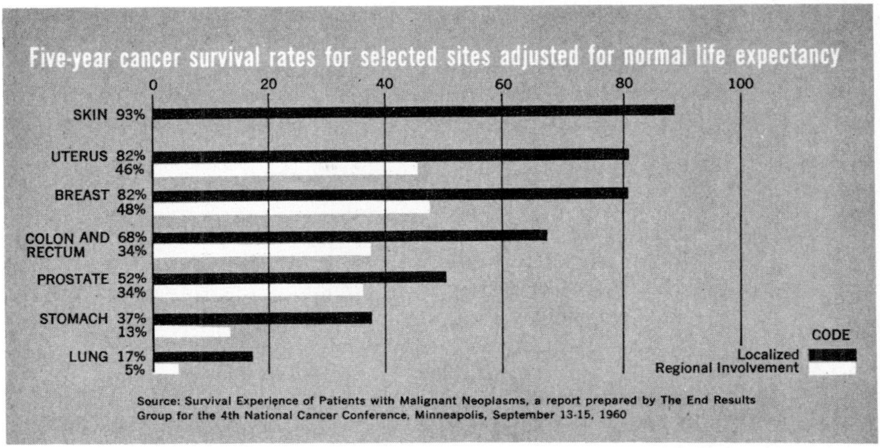

FIGURE 66. The likelihood of survival five years after the original diagnosis of cancer is considerably enhanced if the diagnosis is made when the lesion is still localized. Once regional areas are involved in the disease, the chance of survival is considerably lessened. (From *Cancer Source Book for Nurses.* Courtesy of the American Cancer Society, Inc.)

entity. It does what its predecessor did. In general, the more highly specialized it is, the less likely it is that it can produce others of its kind. In addition, many kinds of cells are joined to form a functional organ. The parenchyma requires a supportive structure in which to operate and service tissues, such as blood vessels and nerves, to integrate its function with the rest of the organism. Where the structure is a complex architecture, even normal healing processes tend to alter some of the relationships that existed before the disease occurred. This is constantly a clinical issue in disease affecting such organs as the liver or the kidneys, for example. The ordinary cell, however, does not interfere with the pattern in a system. A glandular cell produces its specific hormone. There is no competition between cell types, no invasion of other cells, no interference with growth or structural pattern. The malignant cell defies every one of these rules, and, until the rules are spelled out, the defiance will go unchecked.

Thus, the therapeutic goal has two main facets. First, the anarchy must stop. Secondly, the damage wrought must be, somehow, corrected. Until positive assurance is a clinical reality, it will not be prudent to predict a cure. The enemy is microscopic, and perhaps, even with the sophisticated instruments available, submicroscopic. Terrible dilemmas are born of this certainty. The questions must be asked, and somehow the confidence of the answers must continue to be painstakingly sought.

1. Will an attack by radiation or antimetabolite drugs—now the best hope of therapy in some kinds of malignancies—eliminate *every single malignant cell* in the body?
2. Is the malignant cell susceptible to such treatment, and what will be the effect on the normal cells in the immediate vicinity?
3. Can the anarchic tissue be excised completely by surgical means, and, if so, can the organ or system be restructured so that it continues to function adequately?
4. How can one determine that surgical excision has, indeed, removed *every* cancer cell? Just one remaining cell means a potential for renewed growth.
5. What effect does handling or manipulating the tumor mass have on spreading the malignant cells which might not break loose if the tumor were not handled?
6. Does the surgical procedure involve such a radical removal of tissue as to permanently alter the structure of the individual's body, and to what degree is the gain worth such disfigurement, along with the risk of subsequent recurrence of the tumor?
7. How does one decide whether or not radical surgical procedures to prolong life are "worthwhile"?
8. How radical should palliative procedures be?

9. How intensively should treatment be pursued in the individual with a far-advanced malignant disease?
10. How justifiable is the use of experimental drugs, treatments, or surgical procedures on a human subject with a malignant disease?

The nursing issues in the care of the patient with malignant disease are compounded of the therapeutic dilemmas and the intense human need of the victim and his family. They are not susceptible to easy solution.

The Dying Patient

There is a "survival rate" in the treatment of malignant neoplasms. The rate of "cure," in fact, is rising, but the number of people who succumb to cancer every year has remained essentially unchanged. Improved diagnostic measures, the wide dissemination of the "seven danger signals" of cancer, expanding therapeutic efforts, and the excitement of new understanding of the dynamics of malignant change offer hope where there was

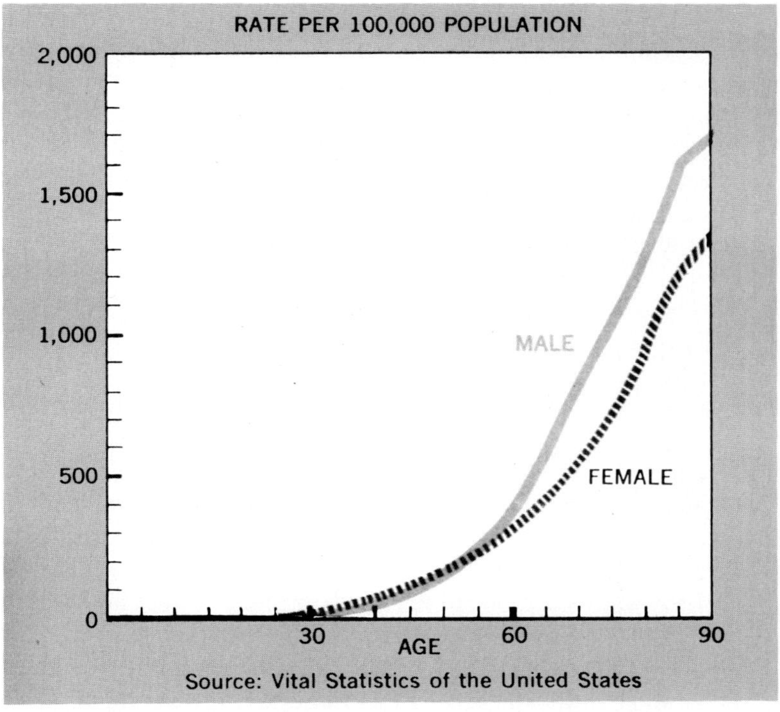

FIGURE 67. Cancer death rates by age and sex—United States, 1959. The death rate has remained remarkably stable in spite of improved diagnostic and therapeutic methods. (From *Cancer Source Book for Nurses.* Courtesy of the American Cancer Society, Inc.)

little before. But the statistics demand recognition of the fact that the real triumph over this disease is yet to come.

All living beings are confronted with death. In every culture and in every time, men have sought to face the inevitability of death in their own way. There is comfort to be gained in the sharing of ideas and ritual associated with death that arises in the social group. But for every human being, the confrontation ultimately becomes terribly private and lonely. Unfortunately, one of the last places where the full drama of the loneliness of this confrontation can take place with dignity and honesty is the ward of the modern hospital. No doctor or nurse seeks a life of service because he is willing to give in meekly to death. These are the professions of lifesaving, and to them come individuals strongly motivated to bring aid and comfort, wisdom and well-being to the sick. When death intervenes, the initial response of the professional person is almost always one of sorrow and guilt. Their own tenacious desire for health and well-being is translated by physicians and nurses into an intense concern for the human beings entrusted to their care. In a day of wondrous knowledge and fantastic technology, the losing bout with death is even more painful to the practitioner. The desire to protect himself from the heartache and despair of a lost battle is as important to the professional person as to any other human being. Individual solutions may be sound and successful ones, but the collective tendency to establish social patterns in the hospital, which support denial and withdrawal when death intervenes, is a professional issue that demands attention.

It is only in very recent years that insight into human behavior has helped the professional members of the hospital staff to face squarely the problems aroused by a dying patient. The importance of grief behavior for the subsequent emotional health of involved individuals is established by careful study of the effects of the death of a loved one on the surviving family members. The recognition of the behavior of individuals who witness the anguish of dying has helped to bring understanding where superstition and fear once resided. The specific problems in the hospital environment are those that necessarily involve many human beings whose relationship to the event is only peripheral, some of whom are witnesses only because they, too, are hospitalized. The strong feeling, entirely justified, that other patients on the ward must be spared the experience of watching the dying must persist. But a means to satisfy the human needs of the dying patient and his family, while still protecting the rights of other patients, must be found. Often the dying patient is hidden away in a private room, carefully screened from the sight of others. Indeed, the individual himself would want it this way. His relatives, sometimes grieving and upset, are dispatched to areas where they cannot be observed, out of consideration for them as well as for others. This is all perfectly reasonable and sensible, but it has the potential for creating an atmosphere of rejection and indifference which the members of the family cannot fail to feel. The vigil over the dying is an activity from which family members can rarely escape. In the modern hospital, it is a vigil from which staff members ought not to escape, no matter how they rationalize their need to do so. The ultimate measure of true professional interest and compassion derives from the human interactions which transcend the technical skill and use of knowledge that are hallmarks of competence. Professional competence must be assessed in human terms.

It is not easy, and often not even possible, to satisfy the overwhelming desires of family members who are witnesses to the death of a loved one. Much of the anxiety and grief they are experiencing is projected into the activities that surround the bedside. There is, of course, much variation in the way in which families react. It is safe to assume, however, that for all of them—whether well contained or not—the experience is compounded of terror and heartache. Extreme emotional reactions are difficult to handle, and they test the individual nurse or physician to recognize his own reaction to the situation. Many resources may be available, including the assistance of the religious advisor. While some families request this kind of help, others are grateful if it is suggested by the nurse. Frequently, family members are upset by the behavior of the patient, and evidence that the nurse is meeting every need of the individual will help to calm and comfort them. In any event, the nurse's sympathetic concern for the patient and the family can lighten the difficulty they face, even though it cannot be wiped away.

There is never a substitute for the nurse's continuing awareness of the individual worth and integrity of the patient, and there are few times in professional practice when this is more important than when that patient is facing death. Concern and interest, realistically offered, protect the nurse as well as those she cares for, because within such human relationships are the seeds of genuine maturity. Death, like birth, is a life experience, and every human being is entitled to approach it with dignity and honesty. No one can predict how he will face the crucial moments himself, but the reality of life offers to the practitioner of nursing the opportunity to test her own faith and the strength of her own purpose by the devotion and kindness she can offer another human being. If it is personally rewarding to contribute to renewed health and vigor for the patients whom one is blessed to help towards recovery, then it should be equally gratifying to have the privilege of reaching out one's hand to the dying and to add to the dignity and solemnity of that inevitable moment for another human being.

Care of a Patient with a Malignant Neoplasm

The Conservation of Energy

Every resource of the individual with a malignant neoplasm is involved in the body's struggle for control of energy production. The autonomous cells of the neoplasm are rapidly metabolizing tissues that seize the nutrients necessary for energy production at the expense of all other body functions. Such an extraordinary and irrational demand on the energy-producing systems in the body ultimately brings about the failure of energy production, which results in the termination of the life of the entire organism. During the therapeutic process that seeks to destroy, by one means or another, the anarchic cells, the problem of energy conservation in the individual patient requires a protective and supportive alliance between the inherent energy capability of the patient and the skill of medical and nursing intervention. In those stages of the disease that precede the total subservience of the body's processes to the parasitic demands of the malignancy lie the only present hope for recovery, however limited or tenuous it may seem.

The nursing needs of the individual who has passed the point where the energy production of his body is devoted to its own well-being will be discussed later. The struggle against cancer must take place before this failure occurs and in large measure consists in either preventing it, if possible, or prolonging the time during which the balance remains in the patient's favor. Success is measured in direct proportion to early diagnosis and the possibilities thereby opened for vigorous treatment. The most desirable approach is prophylactic, and this is the motivation that has stimulated the search for carcinogenic agents. The best treatment for any disease is prevention. The powerful tradition of the effectiveness of this approach is bound up in the control of infectious disease in the last century. Before the discovery of the causative pathogenic organisms, the incidence and disaster associated with infectious diseases were every bit as difficult a social, economic, and medical problem as malignant disease is to modern populations. It was not an all-at-once victory, even when the responsible organism had been clearly identified. Years of laboratory and clinical research led painstakingly towards the development of vaccines and drugs that would eliminate the outside invaders without damage to the host's own tissues. This historical pattern continues to be an enticing approach, particularly because it succeeded. The outcry against vaccination for smallpox must have borne considerable similarity to that which has been raised against the certain implication of smoking with the incidence of lung cancer. But it was easier to establish the validity of vaccination by active participation of individuals who sought the protection than it is to convince millions of individuals to give up a habit they pursue for a million different reasons. The carcinogens produce malignant change in laboratory animals and, by implication, in human populations where the statistics support an endemic factor. Prevention of exposure to them is, however, much more complex than the prevention of exposure to infectious agents. The complex variables in the environment, many of them man-made, render the issue of preventive control unbelievably difficult. The catastrophes of the atomic age almost demand that the individual fortify himself with disbelief, because the threat is so massive that it forbids individual involvement. Cancer prevention is aimed at a catastrophic reality, so vast in both dollars and human suffering that only individuals who are personally touched by the disease can appreciate the danger it promises. Defense against carcinogens is further complicated by the fact that some sources can be controlled only by political structures. Air pollution, for example, from automobile exhaust and the waste products of industrial processes, is a source of carcinogenic activity that is formidable, indeed, in the face of the widespread social change that would be required for its control. The individual is helpless in the face of it. Control of radioactivity extends the interaction to nations and is, obviously, far beyond the power of an individual. When it is widely advertised that flame-broiling of foods deposits carcinogens on the barbecued hamburger, the effort of an individual to protect himself becomes almost more than the spirit can fathom.

Early discovery of a neoplasm depends almost entirely on its appearance close enough to the body surface to allow its palpation. The only alternative is a regular medical examination designed to uncover such disease before the symptoms have become distinct enough to be recognized by the individual. Unhappily, however, the "physical examination" with which many individuals seek to protect themselves is only rarely comprehensive enough to uncover possible tumor growth. For many years, a very

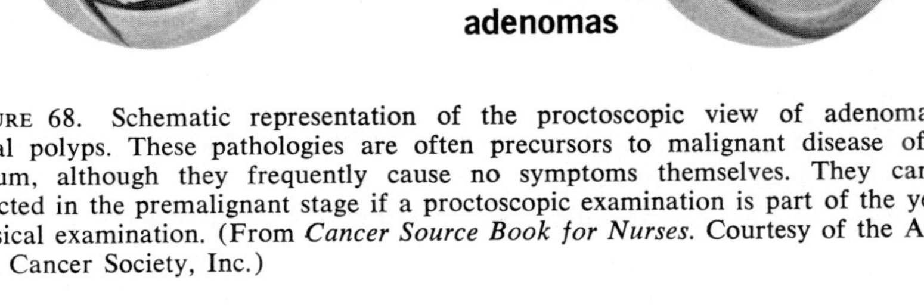

FIGURE 68. Schematic representation of the proctoscopic view of adenomatous rectal polyps. These pathologies are often precursors to malignant disease of the rectum, although they frequently cause no symptoms themselves. They can be detected in the premalignant stage if a proctoscopic examination is part of the yearly physical examination. (From *Cancer Source Book for Nurses.* Courtesy of the American Cancer Society, Inc.)

simple test of the uterine cervical cells has been widely available, but not all physicians include such a test in a routine physical check-up. The incidence of premalignant lesions in the rectum is high enough to suggest that proctoscopic examination be a part of all physical examination routines—but it is not always done. The beginning tumor is so small—even though it is lethal—that x-ray examinations do not always reveal it. And even if the physical examination is very thorough and considers every possible diagnostic test to rule out the presence of malignancy, the likelihood that a nonpalpable beginning tumor will be missed continues to be very high. One of the most difficult clinical problems associated with malignant neoplasms is that early diagnosis is urgently necessary but often impossible with the tools available to the physician or the laboratory technician. The concentration of effort to find such diagnostic aids is tremendous, and, from the clinical point of view, as essential as basic research into the etiology of these diseases.

The very nature of the disease, then, produces a situation in which the victim appears for treatment only when the disease has taken sufficient hold to have wrought serious changes in his physiological function. The symptoms often involve interference with a systemic function, such as an altered bowel pattern, and only rarely are accompanied by a great deal of pain at the onset. By the time the symptoms have involved an observable blood loss, or the creation of severe pain, the spread of the disease is already considerable. Almost all of the patients who present themselves for treatment have had a recent history of unexplained weight loss. This very typical effect of the malignant neoplasm is, of course, entirely related to the metabolic competition established by the autonomous cell growth. By the time this effect has been manifested, the individual's loss of his energy resource is already quite marked. Conserving what he has left depends upon the success of eliminating the competitors.

Ordinarily, attention to the supply of raw materials for energy production and a sensible expenditure of the energy produced are enough to assure conservation for the individual. But another factor influences this process in the patient with a malignant neoplasm. That, of course, is the awful demand made upon the energy-producing systems by the diseased cells themselves. Proper nourishment of the individual is predicated on his own needs, but the competitive struggle for nutrients in his body makes this a frustrating battle. Although the magic formula for proper nutrition under such circumstances continues to elude the clinician, efforts to nourish the patient must continue, even in the face of these defeating odds. This is one time when dietary restriction needs to be carefully examined. If the patient expresses a desire for certain foods, and if they are not absolutely contraindicated by his condition, every effort should be made to obtain them for him. Later, this becomes a matter of his personal comfort and wish, and allowing a permissive diet is then mainly a question of sympathy and consideration. But during that phase of the disease when he is being robbed of an energy resource he desperately needs to protect himself against the disease, the diet he wants and can consume should be provided for him.

Dietary problems are compounded by the frequency with which anorexia accompanies malignant disease. Involvement of the gastrointestinal tract may make the ingestion, the passage, or the absorption of food impossible. However, the issue of nourishment is a primary one, and it is sometimes desirable to employ drastic measures for the single purpose of providing nourishment. The surgical creation of a direct opening into the stomach is one of these measures. This procedure, called a gastrostomy, allows the introduction of highly nutrient foods directly into the stomach when the individual is not able to take them by mouth. Any lesion that interferes with swallowing may require such a procedure to support nutrition during the time that other therapy, directed at the diseased tissue itself, is being carried out. Very-fine-caliber plastic nasogastric tubes, sometimes hooked up to gentle pumps, may also be used to force nutrient foods past an obstructive point and permit continued nutrition. When foods are given by these measures, the principal concern may be with the nutrient value. A measurable fluid intake is also assured by this procedure. It is extremely difficult to nourish an individual by intravenous feedings, although this is an excellent means for controlling fluid and electrolyte intake. The importance of protein foods in the maintenance of the energy production systems in the malignant neoplasm patient, however, is so compelling that whenever there is interference with oral ingestion of food over a long period of time one of the alternative methods must be employed. A severe and protracted anorexia may also be handled clinically by the use of tube feedings. It is obvious that the importance placed on this aspect of care requires that the individual receive his feedings at the intervals prescribed by the physician. The nutrient liquids given must be fresh and that may require refrigeration. The individual's tolerance for them must also be carefully observed. Some nutrient mixtures may cause diarrhea or abdominal distress, although usually, if they are given slowly and carefully, such events will not occur. It is obvious that, if the food is not properly absorbed, it will not benefit the individual, and therefore the appearance of diarrhea will compound his problems. The effects of the nutritional regime may be assessed to a degree by the individual's own evaluation of returning strength, in addition to the behavior assessed by the nurse. The real measure of success, however, and the only one that really indicates that the therapy is swinging the balance in the patient's favor is his weight on a scale. If he continues to lose weight, the treatment is not succeeding. If, however, his weight is maintained or even increased, then the evidence that he is benefiting from his nutrients is considerable. A daily weight is not necessary and, in fact, may create much discouragement, but the weight should be recorded weekly.

The expense of energy to fulfill the requirements of his daily activities may also be conserved. This includes the effort that must be spent in personal hygiene needs. The nurse assesses the individual's participation in these activities by careful observation of his ability to perform them without tiredness and fatigue. It is best to allow him to retain his independence if this can be accomplished without putting undue stress on him.

Attention to bowel and urine function may also be necessary as a means of limiting energy expense. This emphasizes the need for the nurse to identify the usual bowel pattern in the individual patient. This pattern varies considerably from one individual to another even during health. Long-standing illness, especially if the patient is spending long hours at bedrest, is invariably accompanied by an alteration in the bowel habit. The inactivity associated with recumbency, and the nonphysiological position demanded often by the use of bedpans, may result in a retention of the stool that results in much discomfort to the patient. A fecal impaction results when the stool is retained in the rectum over a long period of time, having become progressively dried and difficult to move. If the individual is weakened by his illness, the effort required during a bowel movement may be too great to permit him to completely empty his rectum. The presence of a fecal impaction is rarely signalled by a complete absence of bowel movements. In most instances, there may be a small movement, and even several such movements in a day. But the source of discomfort remains. Any individual who does not have the strength to empty his rectum without a large expense of energy should be closely watched for signs of fecal impaction. The use of gentle cathartics or enemata, where indicated, will lessen the difficulty of the bowel movement and conserve the individual's strength. Only daily observation and knowledge of the individual's habit, however, can forewarn of difficulty before it becomes a reality. Attention to the bowel habit is naturally focused on individuals with a gastrointestinal involvement, but this is a problem for all patients, whether the disease is located in the tract or elsewhere.

The individual treated by surgical means requires the particular nursing care that assists him to withstand the procedure and the process of healing that follows it. The degree to which his energy resource is compromised is highly individualized by his preoperative condition and the nature of the surgical procedure itself. Extensive surgery is extremely demanding, and surgical procedures for malignant lesions often tend to be extensive in nature. Fluid and nutritional support are essential, and the progress of the individual in the healing of the wound is an important measure of his energy utilization.

The nonsurgical therapies available for the treatment of the patient with a malignant neoplasm are often as demanding of his energy resource as the surgical procedure. The goal of destruction of the anarchic cells is assisted by interference with their metabolic activity, and this is frequently accompanied by some insult to the metabolism of healthy tissues. Radiation therapy is sufficiently developed to exclude damage to healthy cells to a very large degree, but since radiation is almost always aimed at internal tissues, some healthy tissue will be involved in the energy exchange. It must also be emphasized that the destruction of tissues within the physiological systems of the body requires the defense mobilization of the body itself. The substitution of the tumor for an area of inflammation is the first level requiring energy expense on the part of the organism, and finally there must be the energy of healing used in the formation of scar tissue to replace the destroyed tissue. The external application of radiant energy to a specific site on the body demands that the entire organism be mobilized in the response of the tissue to this energy source. There is almost always some systemic manifestation of reaction to radiation. Interference with food intake is common, and includes nausea and vomiting, as well as a rather marked anorexia. Such interference, at a time when nutrition is an essential aspect of treatment, makes the necessity to conserve the individual's energy even more urgent.

A number of drugs are also part of the battle against cancer. These chemotherapeutic agents function by a selective interference with the metabolism of the aberrant cells. The most desirable drug would be one that was entirely selective, with no effect whatsoever on normal tissues, but such a drug is yet to be found. The extremely rapid rate of metabolism characteristic of the aberrant cells renders them more susceptible to interference during the metabolic process than is true in the normal mitosis of cells. The rapidity of their mitotic change is the basis for chemotherapeutic agents of all kinds; in fact, some researchers hope to find a means to stop mitosis in all other body cells during the therapeutic period, so that only cancer cells would be affected by the chemicals used. Since the rate of mitosis is related to the rate of metabolic activity, it is also apparent that those cells which are normally very active in the body would also be the ones most likely to be affected by the drugs. This is especially apparent in the hemapoietic tissues, as well as in the gastrointestinal lining. Thus, chemotherapy involves a calculated risk of damage to these tissues during the course of therapy with the drugs. The assault on the cancer cell by chemicals therefore often includes an assault on the very tissues in the body that are the primary source of the individual's defense—the blood-making organs. A severe anemia is often part of the picture of cancer in any event, and in the competition for nutrients and energy production, the body comes off a poor second. Further inhibition of hemapoietic effort creates a problem in providing defense against microorganisms and pathogens in the environment, which might gain a foothold if allowed to superimpose themselves upon a system already poorly able to withstand them. The antimetabolite drugs take their toll in the individual's energy too. The body must have energy to heal, and once more the effects tend to include gastrointestinal symptoms that make the ingestion of adequate nourishment virtually impossible. Some effort has been made to restrict the systemic reaction to chemotherapeutic agents by injecting the substance into a restricted portion of the circulatory system. Such regional limitation of the effects of the drug is often accompanied by systemic reactions in any event, although they may be less marked. The treatment to destroy cells within the functional organism definitely adds to the energy drain on the individual and is often attended by an increase in the need for expert nursing care to conserve his energy.

There is no means available to measure the energy cost involved in fear, despair, or pain, but there is no question that it is considerable. One of the specific difficulties in the care of the patient with a malignant tumor is the increase in discomfort and weakness that attends the therapeutic process itself. While there may be, finally, a remission of symptoms and evidence of real therapeutic achievement, it is extremely difficult for the individual to face the increase in discomfort as part and parcel of the treatment itself. The issue of fear is one neatly tied to the diagnosis of cancer and exists in those who know what the diagnosis is, as well as in those who are only guessing at it. The treatment of cancer by the usual methods described above is such common knowledge that the institution of treatment itself may create alarm where none was evident before. Moreover, no individual can be fearful or anxious without using some of his vital energy to respond in this way. What it costs the individual patient must be assessed by the nurse.

Pain always involves energy expense too. Not all cancer patients suffer great pain, but in an unfortunate few, the pain becomes intractable. The goal of analgesic medication is to relieve the pain as much as possible without turning the individual into a vegetating nonentity. Some individuals want to be narcotized to the point where they lose awareness of their surroundings, and this is not difficult to understand in an individual who is suffering a great deal. But the severe pain does not respond to gentle analgesics, and the question of energy resource is therefore tied directly to pain therapy in the patient with a malignant lesion. When the problem of pain becomes urgent, the only useful drugs are narcotics. These drugs, of course, are addicting, and the rationalization that the patient is going to die anyway is not enough to justify their usage beyond ordinary restraint and good sense. The prevention of addiction, even in the terminally ill, is essential, because they might survive for many weeks during which the issue of addiction is simply added to their other problems. But the pharmacological nature of these drugs, as the addictive process takes place, indicates a nursing viewpoint that intimately involves consideration for the patient's comfort. As the individual becomes addicted, larger and more frequent dosages of the drug become necessary to accomplish the same degree of pain relief. Such pain relief, however, should not be withheld. Judicious use of such drugs is left to the nurse, since most orders for pain medication are written as p.r.n.—to be given as necessary within a specified number of hours. Pain relief is made even more problematical by the fact that pain itself is a subjective symptom which cannot be measured by an observer. The individual's behavior is some index of his discomfort, but there are stoics who do not express discomfort even though it is considerable. Certainly, restlessness and obvious discomfort that cannot be relieved by nursing measures should be dealt with by administering pain-relieving drugs. It is important, however, that the patient be observed following the administration of the drug to be certain that he has, indeed, derived the desirable effect from it. The simple administration of a pain-relieving drug initiates the care the individual requires and is never an end in itself.

When the disease has progressed to the point where the patient's well-being cannot be restored, energy conservation becomes a matter of his personal comfort rather than an active therapeutic goal. The cachexia that accompanies the late stages of a malignancy is evidence of the wasting of body substance demanded by the overwhelming activity of the autonomous cells. Force-feeding or, indeed, any form of heroic effort to nourish the individual cannot overcome the disastrous wasting that occurs. His dietary requirements become a matter of individual desire and should be respected if at all possible. Maintaining an adequate fluid balance is also necessary as a measure of comfort, and should be undertaken even if the fluid must be given by parenteral methods. All nursing activities should be designed with the individual's comfort in mind and should always be performed at a pace he can tolerate without difficulty. An environment that is clean and comfortable is important for every patient but especially for the individual whose condition makes it impossible for him to escape from it, even briefly. Attention to bowel needs must be continued. During protracted periods of illness which are leading inevitably towards death, the presence of family members at the bedside involves the energy resource of the patient too. If a family member expresses the desire and is able to do so, it is worthwhile to allow such a person to aid in the care of the patient. This must, of course, be done judiciously, but often it is easier for both the patient and his relatives if they are allowed to feel that they are contributing to the patient's comfort. The futility that even the professional person feels in the presence of such individuals is shared by other witnesses to the event, and there is much solace in physical activity when the emotional tone is one of frustration and despair. The cruel reality of the wasting death that so often results from malignant neoplasms is characterized by the slow attrition of energy resource in the individual. It is this frequent clinical problem that has endowed the diagnosis of cancer with the heartache and fear that surround it. For many individuals who have witnessed the prolonged struggle, death often appears a gentle and deserved reward.

The Conservation of Structural Integrity

The undisciplined destruction of tissue characteristic of malignant growths threatens structural integrity of the body with the first mitotic division of the first anarchic cell. The random invasive behavior of the cancer cell is directed at a self-interest that subjugates all body function to its will and finally even destroys itself by rendering the continuation of life processes impossible. It is this frantic disorganization that establishes the therapeutic problems in the treatment of cancer. Surgical intervention is possible only when the body structure can be restored by such means, and such a restoration must include a structural integrity that will permit continuing and satisfactory function. The effort of the surgeon to restructure and rebuild in the face of wanton damage frequently results in a surgical procedure that is extensive and disfiguring. In addition, the necessity to remove, if possible, all foci in which the cancer cell may be active requires surgical excision that sacrifices much of the surrounding tissue and thus extends the deformity that may result. Radical as the surgical procedure may have to be, however, it rarely approximates the destruction and disfigurement that the tumor itself can produce if it is not controlled or stopped. Only by absolute elimination of the malignant cells can extensive structural damage be avoided, either as part of the pathology or as a result of surgical intervention, and the importance of an early diagnosis is thus underscored once again.

A pathology capable of utter abandonment in tissue destruction will be manifest by the specific areas involved. One consequence of this fact is the broad spectrum of symptoms that may be produced by cancer. Tumors near the body surface may create open ulcerations while those within the body establish symptoms as they encroach on essential body systems. If the tumor becomes large enough, regardless of its position, the blood supply cannot keep up with its demands for nutrition, and the resulting ischemia of the tumor mass results in tissue death, or necrosis. The death of tissue within the body is frequently accompanied by hemorrhaging, sometimes acute and massive, and sometimes slow and chronic. At the body surface, this same pathological progression produces large necrotic ulcerations, from which bleeding is also possible. The hope of healing such wounds without wide surgical excision is virtually nonexistent, but such intervention is not possible if the ulceration has become established over a large area of the body surface. From time to time, a patient is admitted to the hospital with such a lesion already well established, and it is almost unbelievable that such a progressive ulcer could have existed without the seeking of medical assistance by the individual. Whatever the individual's reasons for failure to see a doctor, the frequency with which this occurs never quite prepares the practitioner for the shock of witnessing it. A persistent sore that does not heal is always suspect, and even though this is one of the "seven danger signals," patients continue to present themselves for treatment long after the point in time when therapy can offer them any genuine hope.

The necrotic ulceration is usually accompanied by very disagreeable odors, none of which can be very effectively masked. The problem of unpleasant odors is one which is traditionally associated with the cancer patient, and it is a nursing issue of considerable moment. Chemical and electrical deodorizers are often used, although they are far from satisfactory in many instances. Absolute cleanliness and frequent dressing changes to remove soiled dressings will help to control the situation to some degree. Sometimes solutions may be ordered in which to bathe the lesion itself, and this assists in controlling the odors. The patient may be aware of the unpleasantness and may carefully watch the approach of nurses and other persons to the bedside. It is not always easy to control a reaction to a situation that readily stimulates disgust and rejection; such control, however, is required in the patient's interest.

The sight of the ulcerative lesion, especially when there has been extensive destruction of the normal landmarks, may also be extremely difficult for those who care for the patient. But the full impact of such disfigurement can only be measured from the patient's vantage point. This is especially difficult when the lesion involves the structure of the face and head; no nursing situation can test the nurse's commitment to the patient more severely than this. Confronting a pathology that is capable of wanton destruction, the professional practitioner reinforces his determination to eliminate this source of human suffering, and the vigor of the search for means of control grows very naturally out of personal experiences of this kind. The reality of the larger problem of cancer research is based on the personal involvement of the practitioner.

When surgical intervention is possible, the surgical procedure in itself may result in a structural alteration that is terribly disfiguring, but the possibility of plastic repair in the future usually exists. This is even true in radical excision of tissues of the face, and remarkable plastic repair techniques exist that restore the contours of the bony parts. During such procedures, necessarily prolonged because they must be performed step by step, the hospitalized individual may continue to be difficult to nurse because of the alteration in his appearance. But the element of hope exists here, and this is a source of assistance both to the patient and to those who care for him. An individual who must have his larynx removed because of a malignancy can be taught to speak again, using swallowed air which he learns to control so that he can form words and be easily understood. Every large urban area has clubs of individuals who have had this surgical procedure, and who devote themselves to helping each other to adapt to the new form of speech. The ability of some individuals to restore themselves to a fruitful and useful life under such handicaps is truly remarkable.

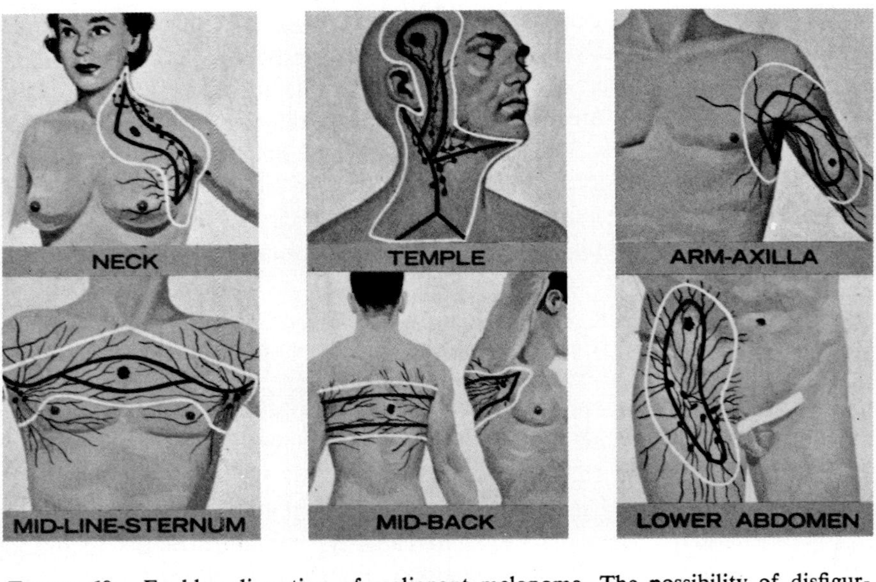

FIGURE 69. En bloc dissection of malignant melanoma. The possibility of disfiguring and extensive surgical removal of tissue must be weighed against the disfigurement and destruction which the tumor itself is capable of causing. Key to illustration: *Black line,* extent of skin excision. *White line,* extent of excision of fascia. (From *Cancer Source Book for Nurses.* Courtesy of the American Cancer Society, Inc.)

Surgical restructuring of body systems may be no less radical in the resulting alteration, but since this does not present such immediate cosmetic problems it is somewhat less difficult to manage. It must be emphasized, however, that such problems continue to be very grave from the individual patient's point of view, and he will require much assistance in learning to adapt his life to the new demands. One common restructuring procedure, for example, must be performed in treatment of malignancies of the lower bowel, sigmoid colon, or the rectum. The lifesaving surgical procedure called a colostomy brings the colon to an opening in the abdominal wall. When this is a permanent colostomy (and it usually is when a malignancy has made it necessary), the individual will empty his bowel through the artificial opening. It is entirely possible for him to control the bowel movement so that he is able to lead quite a normal social life, but it takes a lot of learning to accomplish this, and the individual requires much help from the professional personnel who care for him. In the beginning, this alteration of physiological function requires frequent attention, and during this period of time, the fecal discharge must be removed and the dressings replaced as often as required. Keeping the dressings clean contributes a great deal to the individual's faith in ultimately controlling the function. A number of appliances are available which are preferred to gauze dressings; often such an appliance is introduced to the patient very early in his convalescence. The individual must be taught to care for himself as soon as he has the physical and emotional ability to do so; the sooner he regains his independence, the sooner he is able to face his return to a social life. This is a matter that varies considerably with every individual, but most patients master the new hygiene required and make an excellent adjustment. Revision by surgical procedure of other patent tubes in body systems is not always as satisfactory. The ureters can be attached to the large bowel, if necessary, but the frequency of ascending kidney infection associated with this procedure renders it something of a risk. In general, the possibility of a revised body structure is considerably lessened if the surgery is undertaken before much tissue destruction has taken place, but even this factor may not make it possible to preclude procedures as extensive as colostomy, for example.

It is not always possible to remove enough of the malignant tissue to give the patient hope of controlling the malignancy, but the possibility of palliative surgery still exists. The encroachment of the tumor, for instance, in the head of the pancreas may block the drainage of bile from the gallbladder and bile ducts. In such a situation, it is not possible to remove the pancreas, but the bile duct may be reintroduced at a site below the tumor mass, so that the bile flows freely into the gastrointestinal tract. Such a procedure is not life-saving, but it insures comfort and relief from symptoms for the individual and is therefore eminently worthwhile. Palliative surgery is sometimes undertaken to eliminate nerve tracts when the individual is suffering from intractable pain.

All surgical procedures that are indicated by malignancies pose a difficult dilemma for the surgeon, and it is almost inevitably a dilemma that the patient must share. Frequently, it is not possible to know the extent to which the surgical restructuring must be undertaken until the patient is on the operating table. One of the most common of these very difficult decisions is almost always present in breast surgery. Until the tissue is excised and examined under the microscope, it is not possible to

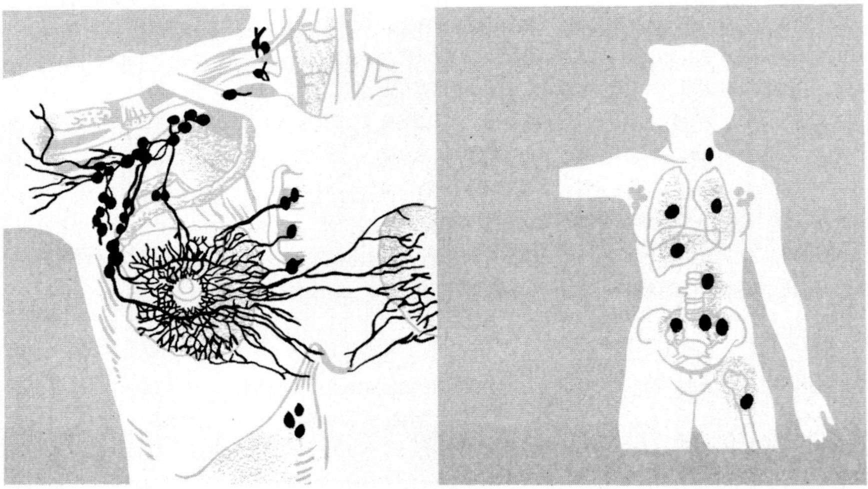

FIGURE 70. Lymphatic spread of breast cancer and distant metastatic sites common with breast cancer. Successful therapy is dependent upon treatment before metastasis has occurred. (From *Cancer Source Book for Nurses*. Courtesy of the American Cancer Society, Inc.)

definitively diagnose it as malignant. In fact, many of the small tumors of the breast are not malignant. When such a tumor is discovered, most physicians feel that an immediate biopsy of the tissue is the only insurance against the risk of malignant progress. The patient is told that the procedure is primarily for the purpose of biopsy, but that, if the tissue is malignant, a much more radical surgical procedure is immediately indicated. When the patient goes to surgery, then, she is aware only that the procedure may be very minor or very extensive and that the decision will be made while she is under the effects of the anesthetic. Such patients wake from the anesthetic with much apprehension, demanding to know, before they are sufficiently awake to understand, whether they had a cancer or not. Since breast amputation is major surgery, there is considerable difference in the postoperative problems when contrasted with a simple biopsy. The preoperative preparation of such patients is extremely difficult, since it is impossible to be entirely reassuring and realistic at the same time. Many nurses share the patient's intense desire for a more definitive statement on what may be expected, but it is foolhardy to be certain when no certainty exists. Measured against the anguish that this method produces in many women, some means of improved preoperative diagnosis is badly needed.

It is terribly important before surgery is undertaken that the patient and his family understand the alternatives available to the physician. They should know that the possibilty always exists that nothing at all can be done. They should know that surgical restructuring may result in a radical change in the body image and perhaps in the cosmetic appearance of the individual. They should have some voice in deciding how radical the surgical intervention should be. This is not a problem susceptible to easy solutions. The professional judgement of the surgeon must be respected and trusted. And yet patients are often operated on and subjected to radical surgery for which they are not properly prepared. It would, perhaps, be foolish to suggest the possibility of a colostomy if there is a chance that it will not be necessary. But the same issue of minor versus major procedures is inherent in the problem of breast tumors, and the method described above is still widely employed. Many individual patients do not have the emotional stamina to face the decisions required in the operating room. But many more do have this inner strength and are never given the opportunity to employ it. Surgery in itself is a threatening prospect, but no patient should be subjected to a radical procedure without prior knowledge of the risks involved and some idea of what that alteration is going to mean to him. It is equally important that the nurse understand exactly what the patient has been told by the surgeon. The patient will ask many uncomfortable questions of the nurse, but the privilege of responding to the patient is limited by what his physician has deemed it necessary that he know. When a patient is obviously confused and uninformed, the nurse should bring this fact to the doctor's attention, and with it the suggestion that the patient needs to understand more than he does. Many physicians are glad to know that this is a problem and will respond to it in a sympathetic and useful way. The same consideration is owed to the family, and their questions should also be directed to the physician if there is any doubt in the nurse's mind as to what they have already been told. The same cautious explanation, couched in language they can understand, should be undertaken after the surgery is completed.

It is not only surgical procedures that create dilemmas in therapy, because the treatment of patients with malignant tumors may also involve many nonsurgical procedures. The question of how vigorously to treat the individual so afflicted may be very difficult for the physician; it is a decision that he must share with the patient himself, if possible, and certainly with the members of his family. Once more, issues arise that have no easy answers. The expense of hospitalization is a great burden for many individuals; hospitalization characterized by expensive therapy, and thereby prolonged, may wipe out a family's resources. In a losing fight for life, the wisdom of such a choice must be questioned. Furthermore, if the individual is already very ill, the decision to employ uncomfortable and trying therapies is one which should be shared with the other human beings involved. Some families insist that everything possible be done to the very last moment; others are content to provide the individual with comfort and relief of pain rather than expose him to disturbing treatment that cannot promise genuine relief. This very crucial social and medical issue has been widely debated and doubtless will continue to be. With research bringing new answers to old problems all the time, the desire to prolong life, in the hope that some truly curative procedure will be found, is understandable from both the physician's viewpoint and that of the family. When the patient is a young person, the desire to mark time is even more compelling. Each instance has to be decided on its own merits, but each instance must also be grounded in the integrity of the human life that is threatened.

The cachectic patient requires the skill of nursing care that prevents the development of structural insult arising from bedrest. Excellent personal hygiene and frequent position change are essential to prevent bedsores. Protection from superimposed infection is also important to save the individual from additional injury, when he is already beset with a wasting disease. All open lesions must be treated with exacting aseptic technique, especially since necrotic tissue provides an excellent medium for bacterial growth. The necrosed ulceration that becomes infected can rarely be controlled satisfactorily, because such patients are also anemic and their own defenses are weakened. Healing requires nourishment to promote it, and the cachectic patient is not able to heal.

The Conservation of Personal Integrity

The diagnosis of cancer is widely interpreted by the layman as a "death-sentence" diagnosis. The long, wasting course of the disease, often accompanied by intractable pain and suffering, has identified it in the public mind as a cruel and unrelenting disaster. Even the most sanguine individual cannot face the reality of malignant disease without calling all of his inner strength to the task. The success of early treatment notwithstanding, by far the most pervasive attitudes towards cancer are compounded of anguish and despair. A threat of such magnitude involves every aspect of the individual's approach to life, and his integrity as an individual is sorely tested.

In large measure because doctors and nurses share with all other members of the social group the attitudes and apprehensions that characterize their view of life and death, the diagnosis of cancer is not one which is easily handled. Human fallibility does not disappear with professional knowledge. When a diagnosis of malignant disease must be made, it is the humanity of the physician and the nurse that creates for them the ability to recognize the terrible threat confronting the patient and his family. The first question is whether or not the patient should be told the truth about his diagnosis. Only the physician can do this, and he must decide, on the strength of what he knows about the individual, whether or not such information can be safely offered to him. Every physician handles this problem in his own way; inevitably, it is a reflection of his own personal beliefs and philosophy of life. It must be emphasized that the decision is the physician's alone. However, the nurse is often placed in an uncomfortable and compromised situation, because her contacts with the patient are conducive to the asking of unbearably difficult questions which she may not freely or honestly answer. It is unlikely that any really comfortable solution will be available to the doctor, nurse, patient, or his family until such time as the prognosis of cancer is considerably improved.

The personal integrity of the individual clearly rests with his own feelings of personal worth. Such worthiness arises from physical well-being, as well as from a sense of participation and usefulness. The experience of debilitating disease quickly challenges personal integrity, and the evidence of progressive wasting cannot easily support the continued integration of an independent spirit. Because gradual weakening accompanies the progress of the disease, few individuals who are not "told" their diagnosis fail, finally, to recognize it in themselves. The suspicion may have been well founded even before they approached the doctor with their symptoms. When treatment is instituted that is widely recognized as that employed in the care of the cancer patient, the individual becomes suspicious, even if his preliminary thoughts were not centered on the possibility of cancer. The subtle exchange with other individuals, particularly those members of his family who are most deeply concerned, may create suspicion in an individual when the physical signs are not particularly convincing to him. And sometimes the individual senses, in his physician's attitude towards him, the inevitability of the diagnosis he dreads. If decisions must be made, and inevitably they must be, that involve his very life, every human being is entitled to the dignity of participation. If he is not told his diagnosis, his participation is denied him, or he is expected to participate in a dishonest fashion. There are those few persons who prefer not to know, but the question they may be afraid to ask directly is often asked in a thousand hidden ways. Their discomfort and pain may be a direct outgrowth of the nagging anxiety they are protecting in themselves. Their dissatisfaction with their care, with their diet, or with a dozen insignificant aspects of hospitalized existence may all rest on the single unasked question. The difficulty of nursing such individuals so that their integrity as human beings is conserved is almost intolerable, because it is beyond the nurse's power to restore to them the decision-making prerogatives they are being denied. Not all human beings are fortunate enough to have the opportunity to prepare themselves for the inevitable moment of death. If an individual is facing death but is denied the knowledge, he is being deprived of his right to make his wishes known, and perhaps even to institute the preparations he chooses for the disposition of his personal belongings. The spiritual preparation for death is also a very personal privilege which should not be denied by the decision of another human being. And finally, the patient often wants the freedom to share his thoughts and feelings with those he loves; when the game of "don't tell him he has cancer" is being played, the family members are unable to allow him to participate in this necessary, although difficult, interaction.

No individual facing the prospect of an incurable disease can do so without a great deal of self-examination. The conclusions that arise out of such an inspection are, unfortunately, often compounded of guilt and superstition. The individual with cancer accuses himself of failure, and if he is not permitted to discuss the diagnosis freely he cannot be relieved of the self-doubt and torture engendered by his feelings of wrongdoing and guilt. Fear thrives on a failure to understand, and denying the patient an opportunity to do so only emphasizes his anxiety and despair. The anxiety that accompanies increasing dependence, unrelenting discomfort and pain, and the prospect of uncomfortable treatment is enough to make the nursing care of the cancer patient difficult. Added to all of the realistic problems he has, the dishonesty of denial and ignorance simply deprives the individual of his personal integrity at a time when he needs the fortification of worthiness more than ever.

Successful treatment is not uncommon, but for the individual who must undergo radical alteration of his body structure, the issue of renewing his personal integrity may be a very real one. The cosmetic damage of breast surgery is easily remedied with appliances that restore the normal configuration, and yet the loss of a breast may have very profound meaning that mere cosmetic camouflage will not hide. The laryngectomee may learn to speak again, but the determination and the will to do so are ninety per cent of the task, and these come only from a deep-seated awareness of one's own integrity. The individual with a colostomy may meet many others who have successfully overcome the disadvantages, but his own effort arises only from his own spirit. The nurse contributes in a substantial way to developing the necessary re-evaluation of his life-style by the patient who has had surgery that restructures his body image. Once more, honesty contributes to integrity. There is no sense in underestimating the difficulties that will face the individual, and recognizing them is far more useful to the patient than denying them. The man who loses a leg can learn to walk, perhaps to dance and run—but he cannot start out that way. The restoration of physical well-being is a painstaking and demanding process in which small success is built on small success, and the goals are realistic and attainable.

There is no kind of nursing intervention in which allowing the individual a voice in his care is more important than in the care of the patient with cancer. This is the strong substance of the nurse-patient interaction, and it allows for reinforcement and support of his personal integrity, even when the nurse has no control over other factors that are denying it to him. Such participation in his daily care emphasizes that his self-respect is reflected in the respect with which he is treated. He may, because of his discomfort, want to be turned in a specific way. He may desire that he be bathed at a specific time. He may have certain requests for his diet which some effort can supply. He may have a pattern for his pain medication that provides him with extended periods of relief. In every instance, adjusting the routine of the nurse to the interests of the patient should always be an aspect of his care, as long as it does not harm or endanger him. He must be permitted to behave without censure. The depressed individual who seeks solace in tears may be allowed this device without being treated as if he were a naughty child. His desire to withdraw may be allowed, and his wish to visit with members of his family should not be denied. It is rarely easy to allow an individual to establish his own routine, but the means to do so are often present if the nurse will seek them.

The individual who has been successfully treated may carry away with him the continuing onus of the diagnosis that he has managed to survive, and even when he has been restored to good health the fear may persist. The importance of follow-up medical care must be emphasized, in any event. He must understand that his continued well-being can be fortified by returning for his regular check-up; he should also know the signals that indicate a need to seek his physician's advice in case the difficulties recur. Realistic appraisal of his condition allows him to make the best adjustment after the treatment has been concluded, but its success depends on his ability to understand what has happened to him.

The less fortunate individual who is not relieved of his symptoms faces the prospect of continuing invalidism and finally a terminal illness. Such patients frequently want an opportunity to express their fears and doubts, and the nurse who is able to listen compassionately may help a great deal, even if the conversation is entirely one-sided. The choice of language used by physicians and nurses within the patient's hearing must be based on an ever-present awareness of his interest in his own welfare. Many clinicians deplore the use of the word cancer because of its lay interpretation. But the "euphemisms" employed may not fool the patient. Individuals learn the jargon of the hospital very quickly, and "ca" means cancer to them as well as to the professional person. They are also acquainted with the scientific terms such as "carcinoma" and "neoplasm," and probably will soon recognize "mitotic phenomena" as another subterfuge for frank naming of the disease. The patient's condition and his diagnosis should not be discussed at all within his hearing, unless he is party to the discussion and permitted to participate. This also precludes such discussion near the bedside of the comatose individual. It is apparent that such individuals are sometimes able to hear what is being said, even if they are not able to respond to it. Caution and good sense should always guide the individual at the bedside of the comatose patient. In fact, it is worthwhile to speak to such a patient while he is being given nursing care. The nurse may not be certain that the patient can hear or understand what is being said, but if he can, impersonal manipulating is avoided by personal involvement that is signalled to the patient.

The nurse can offer the dying patient the physical comfort that derives from perceptive nursing intervention. An approach to the bedside that is warm and considerate, emphasizing the individual and his precise needs, reinforces the technical skill that the nurse may also employ. Caring for such a patient involves all the other human beings who are participants, including the family members. They cannot be ignored or shunted aside, and if the nurse can demonstrate her interest in them, the patient will recognize it as an extension of her interest in him.

The Conservation of Social Integrity

No pathology with the potential for personal disaster as intense as the diagnosis of cancer can fail to have grave social implications. The incidence of the disease alone stimulates much community interest in it, and the emphasis on the causative factors that appear to be identified has repeatedly drawn attention to the social and medical issues created by malignant disease. The likelihood of any individual without a personal acquaintance with someone who has suffered from cancer is remote. Even those not personally touched by it are conversant with the problems confronting public figures whose bouts with the disease are widely publicized. Everyone has a vicarious acquaintance with the problems of cancer, and the interest focused on it will guarantee that it will remain an important public health issue for many years. Not all of the knowledge of cancer is sound, and not all who profess such knowledge are without superstition and folklore. Individuals who have recovered from the disease are often astounded to find that they are feared by poorly informed persons. The myths that cancer is "catching" persist and are unfortunately reinforced by the evidence that some forms do, indeed, seem capable of transmission from one host to another. The stigma of having had cancer sometimes takes the form of social ostracism—a response which hardly fortifies the patient who has struggled to return to a worthwhile life. In spite of the broad attention paid to cancer and cancer research in the public media, sound information is still not widespread; this lack contributes to the individual difficulties of the victims of the disease—both at the time of diagnosis and later when they return to their social environment.

In some ways, the fervent desire of the scientific community to support and encourage research into the etiology and treatment of cancer creates a self-defeating misapprehension in the public mind. The emphasis is often placed on finding a "cure" for cancer. But the truth is that there must be many, many cures as cancer is many, many diseases. The naïve expectation that a cure will be uncovered leads to hopes that are unfounded and to anxiety and concern that might better be spent on creating an environment of comfort and concern for the patient. The problem of communicating scientific ideas to the lay public is a complex one, resting, at least in part, on the semantic difficulties separating these two communities. This is both a social and a personal problem, because it is equally difficult to help patients to understand what they are facing without a shared language.

The diagnosis emphasizes, as do few others, that the patient is a member of a family group. The personal involvement is always multiplied by the individual's role in the family and what his illness means to them. No aspect of their communal life can remain unchanged by a disease which threatens the life of the patient. The involvement of the family is financial; a long hospitalization may threaten their economy for years to come. Their involvement is also emotional; the threat of death only initiates the dynamics of interaction which will finally alter their lives altogether. Their personal concern for the patient must be reflected in the influence of his disease on them. The breadwinner or the homemaker may have to abandon essential roles that bind the family structure together. The specific effect on each member depends on his relationship to the patient and the meanings of the personal involvement for each of them.

There is no way to legislate the behavior of a family group when illness of this kind threatens them. Every group of people will respond in their own way and on their own terms. Nurses and doctors may not always approve of the solutions that families reach under this kind of stress, but it is not their prerogative to approve or disapprove. It is the responsibility of the professional practitioner to recognize that the family of a dying person has a right to participate if they so desire, or a right to withdraw if that is what they must do. Like the patient, the family members and their behavior—collectively and individually—must be accepted just as they are, and offered the same considerate interest and assistance that is the expression of service to the sick.

The family members of the patient with cancer are often deeply involved in the decisions concerning the patient's care. They are frequently told the diagnosis, and participate in the decision as to whether the patient will be told. Sometimes they are able to decide on sensible and worthwhile grounds; at other times the decisions reached are based, instead, on the emotional confusion of the moment. They must be guided to a sensible decision, which may involve considerable effort to educate them to the difficulties they will be facing. Family members must be helped to understand, and teaching them what to expect and how to deal with it will help them in their relationship with the patient.

Subsequent readjustment to family life and the social role is always an aspect of the successful reparative process. The restoration of function in the social milieu is the ultimate goal, but it is reached only with a communal devotion when, for example, the patient has lost his larynx and must learn other ways of communication. The rehabilitative procedures available to the patient who has had reconstructive surgery are considerable, but the success of rehabilitation is a matter of personal interaction with those persons who are most important to him. It cannot be easy for the family members who must care for him to learn to adjust to the colostomy that the patient will have for the rest of his life. And his adjustment is intimately bound up in theirs. A patient who will require care in the home should not be prepared for discharge from the hospital unless a responsible family member has been thoroughly educated to provide that care. It may be necessary to refer the patient to a visiting nurse service, but the ultimate aim is to make him self-sufficient if possible, and often a family member can best achieve this.

The community, conscious of the damage created by cancer in the individual and his family, is prepared to offer many kinds of service to help in his rehabilitation. The local cancer societies not only publish public health materials to encourage early diagnosis and treatment but are often able to supply equipment and materials needed in the home care of patients. The nurse should know the community resources where she practices and recognize the need of individual patients for referral to these agencies.

Cancer nursing requires a dedication and devotion to the welfare of other human beings that can withstand repeated defeat and still bring compassion to the bedside. The faces of tragedy are multiple; even in the most heartbreaking situations, the opportunity for human exchange of interest and concern between nurse and patient must be cherished. Death is not always defeat. If the individual has left behind the touch of his life on others so that they are blessed in remembering him, the full beauty of mortal existence is made complete. The patient may leave this heritage to the nurse, and the nurse is privileged to pass it on to other patients.

Model VIII: The Administration of Medications

OBJECTIVES

1. To recognize the legal specifications of the nurse's role in the administration of drugs.
2. To understand the intent of hospital policy in relationship to the administration of drugs, in reference to the responsibilities of the physician, the nurse, and the pharmacist.
3. To understand the pharmacodynamics of drugs as a basis for intelligent fulfillment of the nurse's participation in drug administration.
4. To understand the importance of observation and evaluation of the individual patient's response to drug therapy.
5. To recognize the nurse's contribution to the effects of drug therapy, as demonstrated by selection of nursing processes which support or potentiate the individual patient's response to prescribed medication.
6. To be aware of the judicious use of drugs and the dangers of self-medication, as a basis for teaching the patient sensible concepts of drug usage.
7. To be aware of the social and economic factors which influence the availability and use of drugs.

ESSENTIAL SCIENCE CONCEPTS

1. The ultimate site of drug action is at the cellular level.
    - 1.1 Effective dosage is dependent upon absorption of the drug at the administrative site.
        - 1.11 Oral administration subjects drug to digestive process.
            - 1.111 Drugs are rapidly absorbed by oral mucosa and thus are not affected by digestive juices at this site (sublingual).
            - 1.112 Rate of passage across gastrointestinal mucosa is dependent on many variables.
                - 1.1121 pH of the contents.
                - 1.1122 Ionization of the drug.
                - 1.1123 Reaction of drug with other constituents (including food).
                - 1.1124 Solubility of the drug.
                - 1.1125 Concentration of the drug.
                - 1.1126 Motility of the tract.
            - 1.113 Drugs absorbed via the gastrointestinal system are shunted through the liver before general distribution in the circulating blood.
        - 1.12 Rectal administration excludes action of digestive tract and liver on drugs.

1.121 Absorption from rectal mucosa is irregular so that dosage must be adjusted.

1.122 Some drugs irritate rectal mucosa and may stimulate defecation reflex, thus eliminating the drug before sufficient absorption takes place.

1.13 Parenteral administration affords most rapid absorption of drugs.

1.131 Subcutaneous administration is restricted to non-irritating drugs.

1.1311 Rate of absorption may be influenced by solvent used for drug.

1.1312 Direct diffusion into capillary bed at site permits rapid establishment of blood level.

1.132 Intramuscular injection permits rapid absorption.

1.1321 Irritating drugs may be safely given by this route.

1.1322 Slightly soluble drugs may be suspended and given by this route.

1.133 Aqueous solutions may be given intravenously for immediate maximum blood level.

1.1331 Some irritating drugs may safely be given directly into the vein.

1.1332 Response to drug is immediate.

1.14 Inhalation of drugs provides rapid absorption via respiratory mucosa.

1.141 Gases and volatile liquids may be given by this route.

1.142 Liquids may be atomized (aerosol) for inhalation administration.

1.143 Dosage is difficult to control.

1.144 Many drugs are irritating to respiratory mucosa.

1.15 Drugs may be absorbed from any mucosal surface.

1.151 Mucosal surfaces of urethra, vagina, conjunctiva, nose, and oropharynx absorb drugs.

1.152 Drugs applied for local action at these sites may cause systemic response because of absorption.

1.16 Intact integument allows few drugs to penetrate.

1.161 Only lipid-soluble substances can be absorbed.

1.162 Some drugs suspended in oil may be absorbed by inunction.

1.2 The preparation of the drug influences effective absorption.

1.21 Dosage is adjusted to the mode of administration.

1.22 Solubility of the drug affects rate of absorption.

1.23 Vehicle in which drug is prepared influences rapidity of absorption.

1.231 Rate of absorption of oral drugs may be modified by a coating soluble at a specific pH.

1.232 Presence or absence of food in gastrointestinal tract.

1.233 Drugs given by intramuscular injection are slowly absorbed in oil solvents.

1.3 Drugs are carried to the tissues by the usual physiological transporting systems.

1.31 The circulatory system is the major transporting mechanism.

1.311 Variations in blood flow affect blood level of drugs.

1.312 Adequate circulation at the absorption site is essential for proper drug levels.

1.313 Direct administration into the circulatory system (venous or arterial) results in most rapid dissemination of drugs.

1.314 Circumvention of the circulatory system is necessary where "blood barriers" exist, as in the blood-brain barrier.

1.32 Distribution to body tissues occurs across semipermeable membranes and into every body fluid compartment.

1.321 Drugs which can diffuse through cell membranes, by active or passive transfer, occupy all fluid compartments.

1.322 Drugs which cannot diffuse occupy limited areas.

1.4 Most drugs, widely disseminated in body fluids, stimulate multiple physiological responses.

1.41 Very few drugs are "specific," i.e., result in a highly discrete physiological response.

1.42 The "therapeutic index" is the balance struck between desirable and undesirable effects.

1.43 The margin of safety for each drug must be individually assessed for the specific patient.

1.431 Variation with age.

1.432 Determination on basis of body weight.

1.433 Sex, and especially the parturient woman.

1.434 Available or desirable route of administration.

1.435 Time of administration.

1.436 Likelihood of sensitivity, allergy, or tolerance, as indicated in history.

1.437 Presence of pathophysiology that would influence distribution and/or excretion.

1.438 Concurrent administration of other drugs.

1.4381 Combined effects may negate therapeutic goal.

1.4382 Potentiation of effect caused by a combination of drugs.

1.4383 Combination of drugs may cause an undesirable effect.

1.5 Mode of biotransformation of drugs influences availability for effective action and ultimate excretion.

1.51 Most biotransformations of drugs inactivate them, although some increase activity.
1.52 The liver is the principal site of biotransformation.
1.53 Cellular enzyme systems cause some biotransformations.
1.54 Individual physiological variations influence biotransformation.
1.541 Young individuals are less able to accomplish these changes.
1.542 Genetic differences.
1.543 Metabolic rate influences rate of biotransformation as measured by body temperature.
1.5431 Increased body temperature and metabolic rate speed metabolic changes of drugs.
1.5432 Decreased body temperature and metabolic rate slow metabolic changes of drugs.
1.544 Nutritional status affects biotransformation rate and capability.
1.545 Pathophysiological conditions influence biotransformations.
1.55 Inactivation of drugs, accomplished by biotransformation, is often essential preparation for excretion from the body.
1.551 The kidneys are the major organs for excretion of drugs.
1.5511 Adequate kidney function is a critical factor in the prescription of many drugs.
1.5512 Urine pH affects excretion of drugs.
1.552 Excretion in bile, following liver metabolism of drugs, may result in elimination with feces or reabsorption for urinary excretion.
1.553 Some drugs may be excreted in perspiration, saliva, or mother's milk.
1.554 Excretion of inhaled gases or volatile liquids obeys the biophysical laws which regulate respiratory exchange.
1.555 Fecal excretion is usually restricted to nonabsorbable drugs in the gastrointestinal tract.
1.6 Toxicity indicates undesirable drug effect.
1.61 Cumulative effect may cause toxic symptoms.
1.611 Some drugs tend to concentrate in specific tissues and be stored, as in depots, thus predisposing to potential overdosage when stores are released.
1.612 Interference with excretion by pathophysiology may result in excessive retention of active drug.
1.62 All drugs may cause a toxic reaction.
1.621 Undesirable drug effects range from mildly distressing to life-threatening.
1.622 The therapeutic and toxic levels of a drug may provide an extremely narrow range or even be equivalent.

1.623 Some undesirable effects of drugs are extensions of the desired physiological response.
1.624 Tissue adaptation to drugs may create prolonged therapeutic problems.
1.6241 Tolerance.
1.6242 Dependency.
1.6243 Habituation.
1.6244 Addiction.
1.63 Drug poisoning requires prompt intervention.
1.631 Use of specific antidotes when available or known.
1.632 Identification of harmful poisons in common household and industrial chemicals.
1.633 Empiric use of survival procedures when identification is delayed or unobtainable.

2. Therapeutic use of drugs is regulated by laws designed to prevent indiscriminate use.
2.1 Federal Food and Drug Administration (FDA) is a part of the Department of Health, Education, and Welfare.
2.11 Original law (1906) established first regulations of purity of drugs.
2.12 Amendments of 1937 strengthened regulations, but left manufacturers free of enforceable controls.
2.13 Durham-Humphrey Amendment (1952) regulated labelling and marketing of drugs.
2.131 FDA single agency to decide which drugs may be sold by prescription only.
2.132 Drug products require an accurate label.
2.14 Kefauver-Harris Amendment (1962) regulated advertising and testing procedures to insure drug safety.
2.141 Honesty in advertising requires generic name of drug in advertisement and on label.
2.142 Rigid controls placed on experimental drugs.
2.143 Manufacturers made solely responsible for safety and purity of drugs.
2.2 Harrison Narcotic Law is administered by Federal Narcotics Bureau, an agency of the Treasury Department.
2.21 Rigidly controls importation, interstate shipment, manufacture and distribution of narcotic drugs.
2.22 Requires strict accounting of narcotic usage, reflected in hospital procedures regulating use of narcotic drugs.
2.3 State and local ordinances control drug distribution and use.

3. The multiplicity of drugs requires standardization for usage by professional organizations.
3.1 "Official" drugs are listed in compendia recognized by the FDA.
3.11 United States Pharmacopeia (USP).

3.111 Revisions made every five years by committee of physicians and pharmacologists.

3.112 Critical evaluations only of drugs proved useful and safe, thus excluding new drugs.

3.12 National Formulary (NF).

3.121 Prepared at irregular intervals by American Pharmaceutical Association.

3.122 Lists "valuable" drugs not included in USP, as well as formulas for drug mixtures.

3.2 Nonofficial drugs are not listed in either USP or NF.

3.22 Council on Drugs of the American Medical Association publishes annual volume, "New Drugs" (formerly "New and Nonofficial Remedies").

3.23 Critical listing of drugs marketed in preceding ten years.

3.3 Hospital formularies list drugs stocked for usage, as determined by local hospital committee of physicians and pharmacists.

3.4 Only licensed physicians and dentists may prescribe drugs.

3.5 Only licensed pharmacists may dispense or compound drugs.

3.6 Dissemination of information to the public from professional organizations to promote sensible usage of drugs.

4. Drug usage is inextricably bound to emotional and psychological determinants in the individual.

4.1 Lay belief in "specific causation" creates unwarranted faith in therapeutic potential of drugs.

4.2 Availability of "proprietary" drugs fosters self-medication.

4.21 Self-medication ALWAYS means self-diagnosis.

4.22 Masking or ameliorating symptoms may allow disease process to reach stage where therapy is difficult or impossible.

4.23 Drug advertisements are misleading to the uninformed, even when legal restrictions are observed.

4.3 Emotional factors potentiate drug action.

4.31 Individual's perception of purpose of drug may influence his response to it.

4.32 "Placebo" effect is based on individual psychological expectations.

5. Socioeconomic factors in drug usage underlie community problems.

5.1 "The Therapeutic Jungle" results from astronomic financial investment in drug manufacture and distribution.

5.11 Nomenclature is disorganized and confusing.

5.12 Economic interests oppose efforts to control manufacture, sale, and use of drugs.

5.13 Unnecessary duplication of drugs by many manufacturers results in fierce competition in marketing of drugs.

5.2 Costs of drugs reflect research and advertising costs of manufacturers.

5.21 Community resources may be tapped to provide drugs when individuals are unable to afford necessary medication.

5.22 Physicians are overwhelmed by literature and samples offered by drug companies.

5.3 Traditional labelling of prescriptions predisposes to errors of administration.

5.4 Formidable profusion of potentially dangerous household, industrial, and agricultural chemicals increases potential for serious poisoning.

5.41 Urban centers have "poison centers" where identification of constituents can be made quickly by phone.

5.42 "Silent" poisoning by environmental chemicals poses serious problems for the genetic welfare of human beings.

NURSING PROCESS

1. The administration of every dose of medication involves the coordinated activity of many persons.

1.1 Safe practice requires a series of written communications.

1.11 Every medication prescription must be written by the physician on an authorized order sheet for the individual patient.

1.111 Specification must be made of drug, dosage, frequency and route of administration.

1.112 Only official abbreviations may be used.

1.113 Each order must bear the physician's legal signature.

1.12 The pharmacist is responsible for providing the supply of drugs as ordered.

1.121 Orders to the pharmacist must be clearly and accurately written on form required by hospital policy.

1.122 Only the pharmacist may label the bottle, clearly indicating drug name and unit dosage.

1.13 The nurse transcribes the physician's orders to forms and cards, as established in the medication administration policy in each hospital.

1.131 Each transcription must exactly reproduce the specifications in the original order, including the date.

1.132 The nurse indicates that the transcription has been made, by initialing or signing as designated on the doctor's original order.

1.133 The medication cards used to guide pouring of individual dosages are kept in a specified place and always returned there.

1.134 Only one drug dosage is entered on a single medication card.

1.135 When the dosage has been administered, the nurse immediately records this fact in the appropriate place on the patient's chart, initialing or signing as required by hospital policy.

1.136 Cancellation of orders requires immediate removal of written forms, and discontinuance recorded on patient's chart.

1.137 No drug may be administered by a nurse without an official written order by the physician.

1.138 The administration of narcotics requires usual written procedure plus recording of required information on appropriate narcotic record immediately following administration of the drug.

1.14 Each new transcription is an opportunity for error, so that checking against all written forms of the order is essential.

1.15 Each participant is responsible for assuring that the drug and dosage ordered are correct and within usual safe limits for the specific drug.

1.16 The patient for whom the drug is intended is identified by correct spelling of his full name and hospital case number; room or bed number is not sufficient for safe identification.

1.17 Written communication of drug orders, as specified by hospital policy, allows continuity of care from shift to shift and day to day.

1.2 Dispensing of individual medications is a nursing responsibility.

1.21 The pharmacist provides stock supplies or individual prescriptions.

1.211 Only the pharmacist may pour medications from one stock bottle to another.

1.212 Only the pharmacist may mix or compound drugs.

1.22 The nurse prepares individual dosages from medication cupboard supply on the ward.

1.221 Only one medication may be placed in each container used to bring drug to the patient.

1.2211 Bottle is always held so that label faces palm of the hand.

1.2212 Liquids are measured by the meniscus at eye level.

1.222 Removal of specified dosage from stock bottle requires conscious reading of the label *three* times: before removing from shelf, before removing drug from bottle, after removing drug from bottle.

1.223 Dosages requiring calculation may be given only by a professional nurse.

1.2231 Calculation which does not require fractional part of stock supply units need not be written (simple multiples of stock unit).

1.2232 Calculations which require fractional part of stock supply unit should be performed in writing and checked by another nurse before and after medication is drawn.

1.224 The nurse preparing medications should be in a quiet environment free of other demands and distractions.

1.225 The nurse is responsible for remaining with poured medications until they have been administered.

1.23 The nurse administers the medication to the patient.

1.231 The nurse who pours the drug *must* administer it to the patient.

1.232 Before administration of the drug, the patient is positively identified.

1.2321 Individual order is checked on patient's chart.

1.2322 Patient is identified by checking identification wrist bands, bed cards, and verbal exchange of his name.

1.2323 If patient is unable to speak, positive identification depends on the nurse: wrist band, or, if necessary, witness of another person.

1.233 Route of administration is observed as ordered.

1.2331 Oral drugs are given with water or fluids as required by nature of the drug.

1.23311 Nurse assists patient as necessary.

1.23312 Nurse witnesses that drug is ingested.

1.23313 Drugs are *never* left at bedside for unsupervised ingestion later unless patient is participating in a "self-medication" project.

1.2332 Parenteral drugs are given with strict aseptic techniques.

1.23321 Careful aseptic preparation of safe administrative site.

1.23322 Aseptic handling of equipment.

1.23323 Subcutaneous or intramuscular injections require specific needle size.

1.23324 Before medication is injected, needle is aspirated to be certain it has not entered a blood vessel.

1.23325 In many hospitals, only physician may give intravenous medication.

1.2333 Rectal medications should be inserted past the anal ring.

1.23331 Nurse uses rubber glove or finger

cot for insertion.

1.23332 Careful handwashing technique is observed before and after.

1.23333 Holding patient's buttocks together for a few moments aids in retention of medication.

1.234 Medication is given at frequency ordered by the physician.

1.2341 Blood level is best maintained when frequency of administration is properly spaced.

1.2342 P.R.N. orders require discriminate judgement of the nurse, but rarely in less than 3 to 4 hour frequency.

2. Following administration of drug, nursing responsibility assumes increased importance.

2.1 Nursing obligation clearly requires continuing observation and evaluation of drug effects.

2.11 Knowledge of the individual patient forms the basis for evaluation of the therapeutic effect of the drug.

2.111 Understanding of the pharmacodynamics of the specific drug alerts the nurse to evidence of desired therapeutic response.

2.112 Attainment of desired therapeutic response may form the basis for modification of physician's regime for patient.

2.113 Expected physiological response may be interpreted to patient to alleviate apprehension.

2.114 Therapeutic effect may signal necessity for adjustment in nursing care plan.

2.12 Sensitive observation may reveal subtle changes in patient's condition that indicate the appearance of untoward reaction to a drug.

2.121 Early observations will recognize response that is discomfiting but not yet dangerous.

2.1211 Prompt report to physician allows his evaluation of therapy and possible modification.

2.1212 Development of gastrointestinal symptoms, such as nausea or anorexia, may require re-evaluation of drug therapy, as well as of nutritional plan and fluid intake.

2.1213 Mild toxic effects may signal achievement of desired physiological response.

2.1214 Expected undesirable effects provide a rationale for nursing care.

2.12141 Administration of anti-inflammatory

drugs requires cautious asepsis to prevent infection.

2.12142 Antihypertensive drugs may cause orthostatic syncope, so that advance planning may prevent accidents.

2.12143 Anticoagulant drugs require prevention of even minor injury, as well as close observation for signs of bleeding.

2.1215 Observation and recording of mild early signs of toxicity provide data for continuing evaluation of drug being used.

2.122 Frequent observation quickly determines the presence of threatening undesirable or toxic effects.

2.1221 Allergic reaction requires immediate withdrawal of medication and necessary countermeasures.

2.1222 Toxic effects may be life-threatening, requiring immediate medical and nursing intervention.

2.12221 Anaphylactic reaction is an extreme emergency.

2.12222 Appearance of early signs of jaundice allows for intervention before reaction becomes irreversible.

2.12223 Early signs of hypoglycemia permit intervention before serious nervous system symptoms appear.

2.12224 Recognition of change in quality and rate of pulse indicates need for prompt medical and nursing intervention.

2.1223 Nursing patient through postanesthetic recovery period demands close observation of vital signs and progress to restored consciousness.

2.2 Concurrent nursing care establishes an environment for effective drug action.

2.21 Drug therapy must be viewed as part of a broad plan for patient care.

2.22 Anticipation of effects of a drug allow for individualization of nursing care.

2.23 Patient's confidence in drug therapy may be enhanced by nurse's ability to inspire confidence in his care.

2.24 Use of nursing processes to promote comfort and well-being may potentiate drug effect, especially with medication for pain or sleep.

2.25 Frequent observation may reassure patient and alleviate apprehension arising from effects of the drug.

2.26 No drug is ever a substitute for nursing care; especially true of tranquilizers and hypnotics.

3. Knowledge of drug action forms a basis for teaching patients sensible usage of drugs.

3.1 Evidence of hearty respect for the benefits and dangers of drug therapy creates a foundation for all teaching of patients.

3.2 Interpretation of drug effects offers patient knowledge as well as reassurance.

3.3 Details of self-administration of prescribed drugs on discharge are frequently taught by the nurse.

3.31 Importance of proper spacing of drug administration may be related to the desired effect.

3.32 Aseptic technique for parenteral administration is taught and practiced, using equipment available in the home.

3.33 Necessity for continued drug therapy must be emphasized when long-term administration is required.

3.331 Emphasis must be placed on importance of regular visits to physician as required, as long as drug therapy is continued.

3.332 Understanding of beginning toxic signs as a clue to notifying the physician.

3.34 Restriction of activities or diet as demanded by specific drugs.

3.35 Danger of concurrent self-medication on the basis of cumulative or antagonistic or nullifying effect.

3.4 Dangers of self-medication should be interpreted whenever possible.

3.41 Encourage skepticism of drug advertisements in public media.

3.42 Emphasis on vagaries of self-diagnosis as a basis for self-medication.

3.43 Recognition of "folk attitudes" and subcultural patterns which influence self-medication (as in use of cathartics).

4. All members of the health team share responsibility for community education and action in relation to drug usage.

4.1 Support of legal restrictions in the distribution and use of drugs.

4.2 Community effort to control blatant drug advertisements in public media.

4.3 Education of public in safe storing, handling, and use of drugs in the home.

4.4 Support of professional organizations seeking standardization of drug nomenclature.

4.5 Personal habits of respect for drug usage.

4.6 Continuing knowledge of new drugs and their relation to drugs already established in clinical use.

4.7 Knowledge of community resources that exist to assist patients to obtain necessary drugs which they cannot afford.

Vocabulary

aberrant
addiction
analgesic
benign
cancer
carcinogen
carcinoma
chromosomes
deoxyribonucleic
dominant
enzyme
genes
genetic code
genetics
germinal
helix
heredity
impaction
intractable pain
lesion
malignant
metastasis
mitosis
necrosis
neoplasm
oncology
palliative
recessive
replicate
somatic
template
tumor
ulceration
virus

General Bibliography

BEADLE, GEORGE, AND BEADLE, MURIEL: The Language of Life. Doubleday & Co., Inc., Garden City, N.Y., 1966.

Cancer Source Book for Nurses. American Cancer Society, 1963.

MERCER, E. H.: Cells: Their Structure and Function. Doubleday & Co., Garden City, N.Y., 1962.

WATSON, JAMES D.: Molecular Biology of the Gene. W. A. Benjamin, Inc., New York, 1965.

Articles

ADAMEK, MARY ELAINE: Some observations on death and a family. Nurs. Sci. III:259-267, Aug. 1965.

ALLFREY, VINCENT, AND MIRSKY, ALFRED: How cells make molecules. Sci. Amer. 205:74-82, Sept. 1961.

BARCKLEY, VIRGINIA: The crises in cancer. Amer. J. Nurs. 67:278-280, Feb. 1967.

BRAUN, ARMIN C.: The reversal of tumor growth. Sci. Amer. 213:75-83, Nov. 1965.

CHANGEUX, JEAN-PIERRE: The control of biochemical reactions. Sci. Amer. 212:36-45, April 1965.

CRICK, F. H. C.: The genetic code: III. Sci. Amer. 215:55-62, Oct. 1966.

DAVIDSON, RAMONA P.: Let's talk about death—To give care in terminal illness. Amer. J. Nurs. 66:74-75, Jan. 1966.

DULBECCO, RENATO: The induction of cancer by viruses. Sci. Amer. 216:28-37, April 1967.

EGAN, ROBERT L.: Mammography. Amer. J. Nurs. 67:108-111, Jan. 1967.

ENGEL, GEORGE: Grief and grieving. Amer. J. Nurs. 64:93-98, Sept. 1964.

FREI, EMIL, AND FREIREICH, EMIL J.: Leukemia. Sci. Amer. 210:88-96, May 1964.

FOX, JEAN E.: Reflections on cancer nursing. Amer. J. Nurs. 66:1317-1319, June 1966.

FULTON, ROBERT, AND LANGTON, PHYLLIS: Attitudes toward death: An emergency mental health problem. Nurs. Forum III:104-112, 1964.

GATES, MARSHALL: Analgesic drugs. Sci. Amer. 215:131-136, Nov. 1966.

GOSS, RICHARD J.: Hypertrophy versus hyperplasia. Science 153:1615-1620, Sept. 1966.

GREEN, DAVID E.: The mitochondrion. Sci. Amer. 210:63-74, Jan. 1964.

HAAGEN-SMIT, A. J.: The control of air pollution. Sci. Amer. 210:24-31, Jan. 1964.

HALTER, HEINZ: How things get into cells. Sci. Amer. 205:167-180, Sept. 1961.

HUGGINS, CHARLES B.: Endocrine-induced regression of cancers. Science 156:1050-1053, May 1967.

KELLENBERGER, EDOUARD: The genetic control of the shape of a virus. Sci. Amer. 215:32-39, Dec. 1966.

KONIGSBERG, IRWIN R.: The embryological origin of muscle. Sci. Amer. 211:61-66, Aug. 1964.

LEWIS, WILMA R.: A time to die. Nurs. Forum IV:7-27, 1965.

MCCAFFERY, MARGO, AND MOSS, FAY: Nursing intervention for bodily pain. Amer. J. Nurs. 67:1224-1227, June 1967.

MOORE, GEORGE E.: Cancer: 100 different diseases, Amer. J. Nurs. 66:749-756, April 1966.

Pain: Part I: Basic concepts and assessment (programmed instruction). Amer. J. Nurs. 66:1085-1108, May 1966.

Pain: Part II: Rationale for intervention (programmed instruction). Amer. J. Nurs. 66:1345-1368, June 1966.

QUINT, JEAN: Obstacles to helping the dying. Amer. J. Nurs. 66:1568-1571, July 1966.

RAPP, FRED, AND MELNICK, JOSEPH L.: The footprints of tumor viruses. Sci. Amer. 214:34-41, March 1966.

ROUS, PEYTON: The challenge to man of the neoplastic cell. Science 157:24-28, July 1967.

RUBIN, HARRY: A defective cancer virus. Sci. Amer. 210:46-52, June 1964.

SPITZER, STEPHEN P., AND FOLTA, JEANETTE R.: Death in the hospital: A problem for study. Nurs. Forum III:85-92, 1964.

TATUM, E. L.: Molecular biology, nucleic acids and the future of medicine. Perspect. Biol. Med. 10:19-31, Autumn 1966.

THALER, OTTO E.: Grief and depression. Nurs. Forum V:8-22, 1966.

UJHELY, GERTRUDE: Grief and depression: Implications for preventive and therapeutic nursing care. Nurs. Forum V:23-35, 1966.

VANDENBERGH, RICHARD L.: Let's talk about death–To overcome inhibiting emotions. Amer. J. Nurs. 66:71-73, Jan. 1966.

WOLFENSBERGER, WOLF: Ethical issues in research with human subjects. Science 155:47-51, Jan. 1967.

WYGANT, W. E., JR.: Dying but not alone. Amer. J. Nurs. 67:574-577, March 1967.

9 Nursing the Patient with an Inflammatory Process

Defense against Injury Is Essential to Environmental Adaptation

The external environment is not friendly. Pulled by gravity and pushed by the weight of the atmosphere, the human organism is bound to the earth's surface. The sun that makes his life possible is also capable of burning his tissues and destroying them. His body fluids freeze at the same temperature as water, and when the ice crystals have disrupted the cell membranes, the tissue dies. His skin is tough and protective, but sharp objects can easily penetrate it. And he shares the earth with thousands of other living things, some of which are microscopic animals that can destroy him if they can successfully invade his body. To survive at all, his body substance must be able to resist invasion, and, if invaded, to fight off the enemy.

The external tissues of the body are excellently adapted to maintaining their integrity and thereby fulfilling their protective function, because they are rapidly replaced when subjected to the ordinary wear and tear as the individual moves through his environment. Even those systems that are "internal" but exposed to environmental stimuli have elaborate mechanisms of protection to keep them free of unwanted invaders. The respiratory system depends on localized tissues and definitive reflex responses to keep the alveoli clean. The stomach contains a highly acid fluid in which few organisms can manage to survive. The movement of mucus out of body openings keeps them swept relatively clear of undesirable visitors. And the complex perceptual systems, which are the mechanisms of awareness and direction, permit the individual to respond defensively to countless confrontations in the environment that have the potential to harm him.

These are, however, the very preliminary postures of defense. They serve to minimize the trauma and insult which would otherwise beset the individual, demanding a continuing expense of his energy to remain alive. Effective as they are, the individual remains vulnerable to countless environmental challenges. The dangers range from minor to catastrophic, and the body's response to them is proportionate. This means that the human organism is capable of mounting a defense suitable to the threat itself and thereby represents another example of the frugality with which life energy is spent. The response to insult or injury is a complex interaction of many physiological functions, some chemical in nature and others on a cellular level. Cannon first used the phrase "the wisdom of the body"; this wisdom is demonstrable in a dramatic way in the priorities established by the organism to insure healing. This is no passive reaction but one which demands energy utilization and therefore the mobilization of all resources available to limit and eliminate sources of threat. For the same reason, it is an organismic function that is restricted in *time,* since prolonged energy expense to promote healing holds the potential for ultimate bankruptcy—a situation often observed in the clinical environment. Thus, the therapeutic goals are predetermined. Medical and nursing intervention are designed to assist the organism in its confrontation by limiting the extent of tissue insult and the time necessary for active physiological defense.

The individuality of every living being is indelibly written in the biochemistry of his body. Except for identical twins, every man possesses his own unique proteins and the capability of quickly distinguishing these from any other kind. The discriminatory talent is coupled with a decided rejection response, so that "foreign" proteins are immediately met by an effort to exclude them. In an environment overwhelmed by microorganisms, this talent of recognition and exclusion defends the organism in both specific and nonspecific ways. It is entirely likely that the individual's precise response to foreign protein is established by his own interaction with the external environment. An organism in utero and immediately following birth does not display this ability to discriminate against foreign proteins. Skin grafted from one species of mice to another within the first week of life grows without challenge from the recipient, and the adult mouse will retain a patch of white fur on his black body. Within less than a month, such an attempted graft is rejected by the recipient, indicating that, in that period of time, the organism has identified its own biochemistry in the environment where it is constantly exposed to that of other individuals. The ability to refuse those proteins which are not innate to the individual organism is called immunity. Furthermore, the ability to develop antagonistic responses to proteins continues throughout the life of the individual, so that, within certain limits, new exposure to strange proteins is met by the development of an immunity response. With so many different proteins available as either potential or actual challengers, at least some of the immunity invested in the biochemistry of the individual must present a broad spectrum of activity. Such is, in fact, the case. The gamma globulins of the plasma, which are large protein molecules (molecular weights of 150,000 to 200,000), act as antibodies, substances able to eliminate foreign proteins in a variety of ways. Some are capable of killing bacteria, and are therefore called *bactericidins.* They maintain a constant "holding action" to restrict any bacterial presence in the circulating blood and thereby preserve its relative freedom from microorganisms. Some are *agglutinins,* which function by causing a clumping or agglutination of bacterial cells. Some are *lysins,* capable of dissolving bacteria, probably by dissolving their cellular membranes. Some function by leading the bacteria to the white blood cells, which are capable of ingesting them; these antibodies are called *opsonins.* And some are *antitoxins,* whose function rests in combining with toxins elaborated by microorganisms and rendering such substances inactive. Any foreign substance that manages to get past the initial tissue barriers and into the circulating blood is called an *antigen.* Antigens are proteins, or combinations of other substances with proteins, and in a broad and nonspecific way, the antibodies of the individual are constantly guarding the integrity of the organism against them. The antibody function of the gamma globulins is an everyday affair, and the full effect of this protective system can be assessed in those few rare individuals who are born with a deficiency of gamma globulins. Before the antibody function of gamma globulins was identified, such individuals did not survive childhood. They do so now with precarious watching and the frequent administration of antibodies in the form of gamma globulins. Without this protection, they are overwhelmed by infection and have no defense when it occurs.

The gamma globulins are capable of confronting and excluding a large number of foreign proteins, but the introduction of highly specific new antigens into the body calls forth a much more specific response from its biochemistry. Such new antigens stimulate the formation of antibodies that are tailor-made to exclude them. This response does not occur immediately, and during the time when it is being elicited, the individual must depend upon the nonspecific behavior of his gamma globulins. Once the antibody formation begins, however, it continues even after the antigen itself is no longer present. The production of specific antibodies to a specific antigen may continue for a year after the stimulant has been removed, and as long as the specific antibodies continue to circulate in the bloodstream, the individual is said to be immune to that specific antigen. This ability to create a defense against new encroachers is the basis for all immunization procedures. Deliberate exposure of an individual to a modified antigen elicits the formation of antibodies and thus serves to protect him from subsequent exposure to that antigen. Immunization with the actual antigen, of course, runs the risk of producing the disease itself, since most such antigens are pathogenic microorganisms. Therefore, immunizing substances are "attenuated" in some way. Some are actually killed pathogens, some are similar strains that produce a milder reaction, while others are similar to the dangerous pathogen, but capable of "fooling" the organism into antibody reactions. The use of "cowpox" to impart immunity against smallpox is one example of this deceptive procedure.

The development of antibodies in the circulating bloodstream is a protective device which remains effective only as long as the antibodies continue to circulate in the blood. This period may be as short as three months or as long as three years. When the antibodies are blood-borne, "booster" dosages of the immunizing factor are repeated at regular intervals in order to insure continuing immunity. Some immunization does last a lifetime, probably because the cells themselves are capable of mounting antibodies to antigenic stimuli. When the antibody is formed within a cell, it stays there, and any subsequent invasion is met with a ready defense. Since viral infections, for example, are intracellular, circulating antibodies in the blood will not protect the individual against them. Therefore, tissue immunity, often in response to viral infection, represents still another facet of the biochemical defense of the integrity of the individual organism.

The biochemical stance of the organism is thus both generalized and extremely unique. The same protective measures, however, have created substantial therapeutic problems in the natural course of some disease entities, as well as in modern therapeutic rationales. These implications will be discussed later. In any event, the ancient Greeks who postulated the theory of humors were not entirely wrong. The humoral nature of defense against tissue insult is a critical factor in the sophisticated science of the twentieth century. And the body's defense does not end there.

The Cellular Defense against Insult

The effectiveness of antibody defense is limited by its presence in the circulating blood or in the tissue cells, and specifically depends upon a previous confrontation with the antigen. Antibody protection takes time; thus, immediate reaction to invasion of the body substance requires a system capable of instantaneous response. This prompt defense rests with the leukocytes, or white blood cells, which are motile and therefore capable of moving to an invasion site under their own power. These cells are formed in the hemapoietic tissues, and thus a ready supply of them is entirely related to the health of these tissues.

From 60 to 80% of the white cells are neutrophiles (so named because of their behavior with staining compounds under the microscope) and are members of the polymorphonuclear leukocyte, or granulocyte, family. The neutrophils are relatively large ameboid cells, 10 to 12 microns in diameter, and possess a large cytoplasmic area that enables them to digest the substances they engulf. They respond promptly to stimuli at the site of an invasive action and are hungry phagocytes. They survive only two or three days but are readily replaced under normal conditions; when they die, they release an enzyme which dissolves not only their own substance but other dead cells and bacteria.

Two other forms of granulocytes are available, though in much smaller numbers. Eosinophils stain a brilliant red under the microscope and are normally present in a concentration of 2 to 4%. This granulocyte increases in number during allergic responses of the individual, but the reason for this is not known. Eosinophils are phagocytes too but are much less effective in this task than the neutrophils. The basophils stain a deep blue-purple in microscopic specimens and are normally present in a concentration of 0.3 to 1% of the white blood cell count. Their exact function is unknown, although they have been shown to contain heparin, a substance that inhibits the coagulation of blood.

Lymphoid tissue in the lymph glands, spleen, thymus gland, tonsils, and gastrointestinal tract produces other white blood cells which are not phagocytic, although they are apparently important contributors to antibody formation. These are the lymphocytes and the monocytes. The lymphocytes constitute from 20 to 30% of the white blood cell count. They are smaller than the granulocytes and appear to have little or no phagocytic ability, but they apparently play an essential role in antibody formation. They are precursors to the monocytes, which normally make up 2 to 7% of the white cell count and are also essential to antibody formation.

In addition to the motile cells normally present in the body, two other forms of moving white cells are seen when an infection or insult has actually developed. One of these, the plasma cell, is observed most often in chronic infectious processes. The other is the macrophage, an unusually large and very phagocytic cell that is derived from the monocyte. The macrophage is the clean-up cell at an infected or inflamed site. Because of its phagocytic abilities, it performs a debridement or removal of tissue debris—an essential prerequisite to subsequent healing. There is compelling evidence that the macrophage may also contribute to the healing process by maturation into the tissues of healing at the site of insult. The macrophage possesses an appetite for any invader—viable or not. It will take on nonviable and relatively indigestible irritants such as silica and talc, or any other substance that stimulates an inflammatory reaction in body tissues.

The leukocytes of the circulating bloodstream are capable of leaving the vascular system and moving into the tissues that are invaded. But there are also, throughout the body, fixed cellular elements capable of phagocytosing invaders. These fixed cells are generally clustered in body areas where the likelihood of invasion is great, generally because of contact with the external environment. There are, for example, phagocytic cells in the liver which are ordinarily so effective that the few bacteria escaping the gastrointestinal tract and entering the portal circulation are removed before that blood passes from the liver into the returning vena cava and the general circulation. These cells, the Kupffer cells, are part of the reticuloendothelial system. There are similar phagocytes in the spleen and bone marrow, and, of course, in the lymph nodes. In solid tissues, the phagocytes are called histiocytes, and they have a localized task of defense.

Thus, an invasion of the body's external barriers is met by a moving army of first-line defenders where the task of exclusion begins. The secondary defenses of the humoral system back up the initial invasion through the nonspecific function of the gamma globulins and, in a few days, by antibody formation against the specific antigen. The initial response, however, is one of localization. The defense is quite simply to restrict the invader to as little tissue involvement as possible, thus minimizing the extent of tissue damage.

The Inflammatory Response: Organization of Defense

The instantaneous response at the site of injury is a vasoconstriction of the local blood vessels, a reaction which lasts only seconds. It is a fleeting instance of the withdrawal of vascularization, as if to limit immediately the insult of the offending source. The prompt vasodilatation that follows at once, however, is characterized by the equally prompt marshaling of the defense elements at the point of injury. As the vessels become actively engorged (hyperemia), they bring leukocytes to the site; almost at once, the white blood cells begin to squeeze through the capillary walls and make their way towards the injured tissue. They are probably directed there by an electrochemical attraction arising from substances liberated by the inflamed cells in a process called chemotaxis. The white cells move by ameboid activity and are drawn to the injured region where they can immediately begin the job of phagocytosis. The substances attracting the white blood cells are probably also responsible for an alteration in the permeability of the walls of the capillaries in the immediate area. It is for this reason that the leukocytes can squeeze out of the capillaries, although there is a movement of fluid out of the vessels as well. The increased fluid escape probably dilutes the toxins in the local area and also acts as

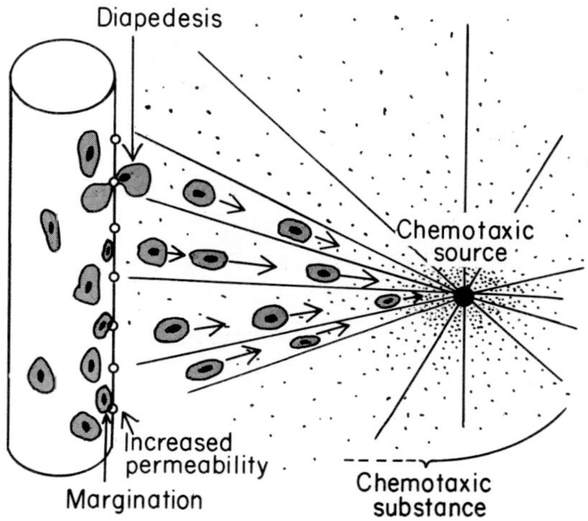

FIGURE 71. The white cells squeeze out of the capillary (diapedesis) and are attracted to the inflammatory site by substances present there. This process is called chemotaxis, and many substances can elicit the response. (From Guyton, A.C.: *Textbook of Medical Physiology,* 3rd ed. W.B. Saunders Co., Philadelphia, 1966.)

a transport medium for the dissemination of other substances involved in the defense against the invader. Very early in the combat, the leukocytes form a limiting circle around the injured site; this border is soon organized so that a ring of fibrin is laid down that is thickly populated by the leukocytes. This is often called a pyogenic membrane, although it is not a membrane at all. It does establish, however, a fence around the area of combat and thus attempts to limit the amount of tissue involvement. Inside of the inflamed area, meanwhile, there is a gradual accumulation of dead leukocytes, cellular debris from damaged tissues, and the fluid exudate brought there by the dilated capillaries. At this stage, the area is acutely inflamed.

Certainly one of the most ancient of man's observations has been that of inflammation. The word itself means "to set on fire," and it is so characteristic of the body's response to injury that it has always been the focus of much medical attention. The "cardinal signs" of inflammation describe the gross appearance of all inflammatory responses, regardless of the provocative agent, and since the first century A.D. the classical description has been taught in the terminology of Celsus. The area is red (rubor) because of the increase in vascularization; it feels warm to the touch (calor) because of the increased blood supply in that localized area. The exudate results in a swelling (tumor), and the area is also painful (dolor), partly from the pressure of the exudate and partly from specific substances in the arena. The fifth cardinal sign, loss of function, was added to this descriptive list by Galen one hundred years later. Before there was any understanding of the dynamics of the inflammatory response, the observers recognized that localization which finally produced pus was a favorable sign in the prognosis. In fact, the production of "laudable pus" was considered essential to the process. The empiric recognition that the individual was in grave danger if localization did not appear characterized the efforts of the medieval physician. The formation of the exudate recognized as pus indicates that the body has walled off the assault, and the discharge of the purulent liquid signifies that the process of healing will take place. If localization does not succeed, an extending area of involvement becomes red, hot, swollen, and painful. Such a spreading of the inflammatory site is called cellulitis. As greater areas of tissue are involved, the escaping inflammant may utilize the transport systems, such as the lymph channels in the region, and streaks of redness may appear, leading away from the site of injury. The lymph nodes, of course, represent still another line of defense, but, in combatting the inflammant, the nodes themselves may become quite inflamed and thus enlarged and tender. Pathogens that invade the circulating bloodstream create a bacteremia; if this cannot be controlled, a generalized septicemia results which then involves all of the body tissues. Therefore, the restriction of the inflammation to a limited place and to defense in a limited time is essential to preventing widespread assault throughout the body. Some pathogens are capable of breaking through the fence of localization. Certain strains of streptococci, for example, elaborate a toxin which forges a path for the invading organism by liquefaction of the substrate tissues in the vicinity of invasion and, unless checked, far beyond.

Once the area has been localized, the process of cleaning-up, or debridement, begins. Ideal healing, of course, would be restoration of the original tissue in its functional form. Such healing is called resolution, and some forms of inflammation do characteristically terminate in this way. If healing is by resolution, there is no demonstrable change in the tissues that were affected. But healing by resolution does not often occur. Most healing requires the development of scar tissue. This is called fibrous tissue substitution. Following debridement, the body replaces the lost tissue by laying down connective tissue. The first response is a friable and very vascular pink tissue that is called granulation tissue. The vascularity gradually decreases, and the fibrous bands become organized in a process called cicatrization. The final scar is virtually avascular; thus, as it matures, it becomes very pale in color. Fibrous tissue substitution is capable of restoring the structural continuity and integrity of the injured part, but it does not restore cellular structure or integrity. It is a tough and excellent "filler" and reinforces the areas weakened by the tissue loss. Where the fibrous tissue substitution has taken place in tissues that are not highly differentiated, it is a very satisfactory substitute for the original. But such scarring may also occur in tissues that *are* highly differentiated; when this occurs, the scarring itself interferes with complete restoration of function of the part. As the scar matures, it tends to contract. Small areas of fibrous tissue substitution on the surface of the body are rarely disabling, even though their position may make them more or less disfiguring. However, large areas of fibrous tissue substitution may cause marked distortion of the body surface because, as they contract, they pull the structure out of alignment. This results not only in disfigurement but often in disablement as well. It is thus apparent that the residual effects of scar tissue may create additional and serious problems for the individual. The importance of limiting the inflammation in space and time is paramount in the care of any patient with an inflammatory process.

Although the central effort of the organism is towards localization, the achievement of this restrictive action depends upon a mobilization of the entire resource. There is a systemic response even to a highly localized injury, reflecting the priority that the organism exhibits in defending its integrity against insult. The vigorous activity at the localized site is characterized by the interaction of many substances, and some of the soluble products of the inflammation are carried away by the circulating blood. There is some evidence that the dissolution of the leukocytes is necessary to produce a substance which directly affects the temperature control "thermostat" in the hypothalamus. If the thermostat is set at a higher temperature, the essential condition is established to speed up the rate of tissue metabolism. The metabolic rate, of course, determines the oxidative processes; when the body is called upon to produce many white blood cells, to provide the materials for the tissues of healing, and to institute antibody formation in the circulating blood, the increased rate of activity demands increased oxygen and nutrients. When the nervous system temperature control is set at a higher point, the effect on the tissues is to rapidly bring the body temperature up to that point. This can be accomplished only by a rapid increase in the rate of energy-heat production. The response may be very rapid, in which case it is characterized by chills. The mechanisms that ordinarily conserve body heat are exaggerated, so that there is an intense vasoconstriction of the peripheral vessels, accompanied by rapid muscular activity which is recognizable as shivering. It must be emphasized that the dynamics of fever accompanied by chilling represent a remarkable increase in energy production, a situation in which the individual is working very hard. As the metabolic rate increases, there must be a compensatory increase in heart and respiratory rates. Thus, a fever is almost always accompanied by an increase in the other vital signs. These measurements indicate the rate of energy production, and the decision as to whether the individual is being helped or harmed thus rests on his unique cluster of needs and on his specific ability to participate so actively in his body's own defense. When the temperature of the blood reaches the thermostatic setting in the hypothalamus, the excessive muscular activity of chilling ceases. The patient no longer feels cold, or for that matter, very warm, even though his body temperature is elevated above normal. Within limits, then, a febrile response to an inflammatory process is part of the defense procedure itself. Since a body temperature over 104°F threatens the cellular integrity, control measures are instituted to prevent a higher body temperature. In some instances, an angry inflammatory site may exist with no evidence of increased temperature. In older and debilitated individuals, such an event is an indication of a faulty defense against the insult. The suppression of the febrile reaction, accomplished by drugs or by local applications of cold, is desirable when the fever threatens the individual, either because it tends to reach higher temperatures than are safe or because the increased rate of metabolism is taxing an already depleted individual past his tolerance of fatigue. The soluble products of the inflammation may also stimulate other symptoms of response of a systemic nature. Anorexia, headache, and fatigue are common. The general sensation of exhaustion that is called "malaise" may, in itself, reflect the priority demanded by the body's defense against the infection. Such a lethargy and withdrawal serve to limit activity and thus to decrease the nonessential demands on the energy production mechanisms of the body. As well-being is restored, the malaise disappears, although the intensity of a severe infection may leave an individual weak for a while longer. Such weakness following an infection is comparable to that which attends hard physical labor, and in a real sense, that analogy is exact.

The Microscopic Enemy

To the layman, being sick frequently means having a "germ." The experience of infection is extremely common; most individuals are hosts to at least one upper respiratory infection every year. The "childhood diseases" are contagious diseases, and few children escape all of them. The variety of "folk medicine" therapies espoused in the cure of infections is an indicator of the tremendous incidence of such events, many of them never brought to the attention of a physician. Even the sophisticated knowledge available to the lay public on the control of pathogenic organisms has not eliminated the naïve faith invested in the "Germ Theory."

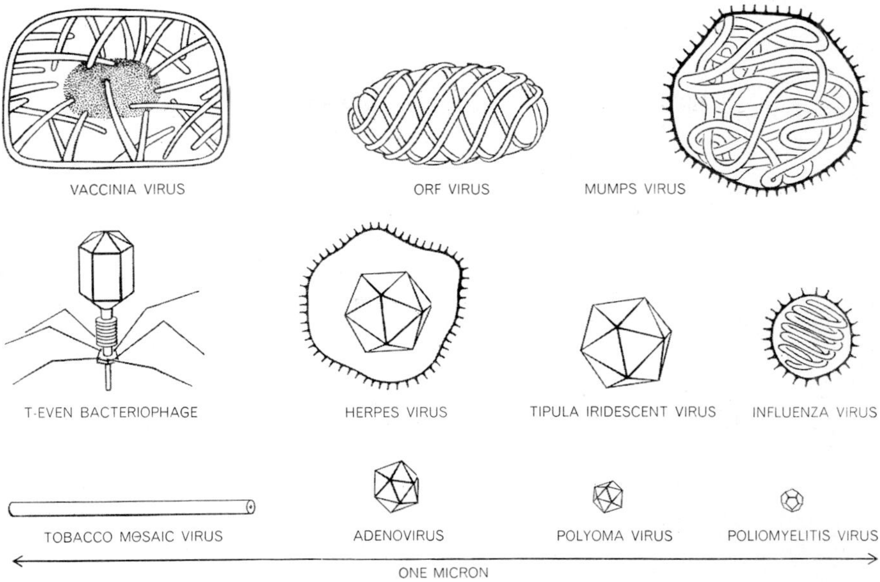

FIGURE 72. Electron microscopes have made it possible to identify the structure of viruses. They are of many sizes and shapes. One micron is a thousandth of a millimeter. It is here enlarged 175,000 times. (From Horne, R.W.: "The Structure of Viruses." Copyright ©1963 by *Scientific American, Inc.* All rights reserved.)

The radical social change that accompanied the identification of microscopic animalcules as the instigators of disease continues to influence attitudes towards all disease, even when the etiology is clearly not related to a microorganism.

The pathogenic microorganisms are always with us. Human infections continue to occur *only* because a human reservoir persists in which the pathogens are happily thriving. Control of contagion can never be entirely relaxed. Although diphtheria, for example, has been a rare affliction since immunization was introduced, a large midwestern city recently suffered an epidemic of this disease in a ghetto population which had not been inoculated. Human infectious disease is transmitted from an infected human being to an uninfected human being—the issue is as simple and complex as that. Many organisms capable of causing diseases are normal inhabitants of the human body; some are abnormal residents but do not create symptoms in their host. Such individuals, often described as "carriers," are, in a sense, infected, but they are not diseased. The potential for disease is present, however, both in the host, where changing conditions in his own body may permit the organism to take hold, and in susceptible individuals to whom he transmits the organism. "Susceptibility" is one of the variables defying control, even though many of its aspects have been identified.

The virus which causes *herpes simplex* seems to be universally acquired in childhood. But the appearance of a "cold sore," or fever blister, in conjunction with another infection is limited to certain individuals. During World War II, there was an alarming incidence of tuberculosis in prisoners of war. The relationship of this fact to concurrent starvation seems reasonable and is substantiated by the high incidence of this infection in alcoholic individuals who frequently do not have an adequate food intake. However, there is also a relationship between the incidence of diabetes and tuberculosis. The persons who suffered whole body radia-

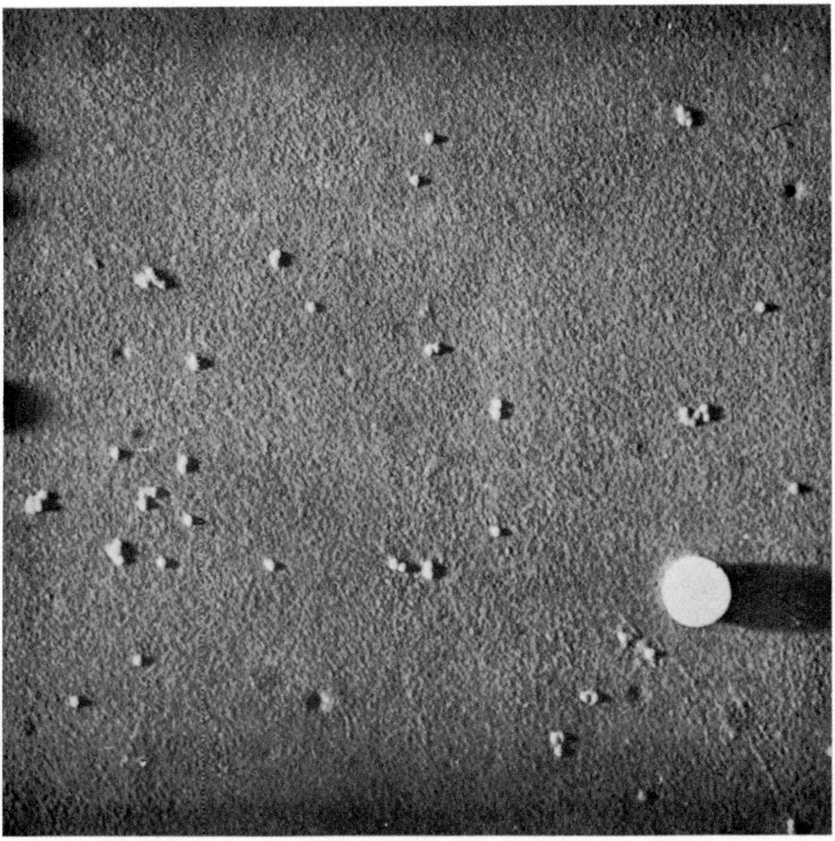

FIGURE 73. The first electron micrograph of human poliomyelitis virus. Each spherical particle is one-millionth of an inch in diameter. Tools such as the electron microscope have vastly increased knowledge of infectious disease. (Bachrach, Schwerdt, and Stanley: Virus Laboratory, University of California.)

tion in the atomic explosions died of septicemia because their defense tissues were destroyed. Individuals receiving long-term antibiotic drug therapy often develop severe fungal infections of the mouth, as well as radical gastrointestinal symptoms related to an altered flora in their digestive tract. Susceptibility, therefore, is a complex condition in which social, communal, economic, psychological, physiological, and nutritional factors interact.

By no means all of the microorganisms that share our environment are carriers of disease. There are many nonpathogenic inhabitants of the human body, some of which exist in an essential symbiotic relationship. Only since the use of antibiotic drugs has become widespread has it been apparent that nonpathogens could become pathogenic. These drugs radically altered the environment in which the organism lives, and certain previously friendly or innocuous organisms became dangerous pathogens as a result. *Escherichia coli* has always been a resident of the lower gastrointestinal tract in man and has occasionally contaminated a surface wound. However, in the revised environment of the antibiotics, this organism has been implicated in septicemia, a situation unheard of before the antibiotics came on the scene.

The word *pathogenesis* means "producing suffering" and, in baldest terms, a pathogen is a disease-producer. But *any* organism which can find a host that permits it to multiply and flourish is capable of being a pathogen. Pathogenicity in itself does not necessarily denote a toxic or damaging effect. It means more accurately that, when an organism can thrive in a host at the expense of the host, it is a pathogen, regardless of its place in the taxonomy. Once more the variables are so complex that the definitions must be left wanting. One of the most important is *specificity*. Most organisms causing human disease do not cause disease in other species. Certain organisms, of course, have a life-cycle during which they consecutively inhabit different species. Malaria is an excellent example of this life-pattern. But many a researcher has fervently wished, without success, for an easy transmission of human disease to laboratory animals. Some diseases have such a high specificity that their investigation is extremely difficult. The spirochete that causes syphilis can survive outside of the human body for only a few minutes and has never been cultured in the laboratory. The persistence of the human reservoir for this disease, in spite of excellent control procedures in the past twenty years, emphasizes the difficulty of eliminating pathogens from human society.

The human reservoir frustrates control because of the asymptomatic carriers of disease. Such transmission occurs in two ways. In the first place, the most infectious moments in a disease process may occur during the initial, prodromal stage, when symptoms are nonexistent or so mild as to fail to attract attention even of the involved individual. During this time, the organism may be widely spread, and recognition of the disease process may be delayed until after the damage has been perpetrated. Some efforts at control are found in quarantine procedures. Individuals are kept under observation for a specified length of time to be certain that the disease does not develop. They also are isolated from others in an effort to limit the spread of a specific disease. This is a particular problem in pediatric hospitals and, of course, quarantine procedures are familiar to international travelers. But even a quarantine depends upon a predictable and specific disease syndrome; when the expectation does not exist, a preventive procedure cannot be instituted. The carriers of disease who are not themselves ill, or about to become ill, represent another unknown quantity in disease transmission. Few carriers gain the notoriety of Typhoid Mary, whose employment as a cook and food handler established a necessary link in the transmission of the organisms she harbored in her gallbladder. The ubiquitous distribution of staphylococci has become threatening because of species mutations in the face of the antibiotic environment, and the presence of such organisms capable of causing disease in certain individuals is uncomfortably persistent. Efforts at control where transmission to susceptible individuals might lead to disaster are evidenced by the requirement of normal throat cultures in individuals working in newborn nurseries or with infants in children's hospitals. Public health laws requiring examination of the stools of food handlers are also designed to close the path of transmission of known disease organisms.

In much the same way as plush teddy bears create an idea that bears are friendly animals, the designation of certain infections as "childhood diseases" obscures their actual danger. It has long been clinically evident that some of these common afflictions strike some individuals with unusual severity. It has also been frequently observed that when an infection is rampant in a population, the first sufferers often have a much milder experience than those who acquire the disease when the epidemic is at its peak. These factors are closely tied to the question of *virulence,* a description of microbial disease which depends upon the effects of the disease on the host. In general, a virulent organism is one which causes severe symptoms of illness. It is immediately apparent that the severity of an infection is related to dozens of other variables, but it can be demonstrated in the laboratory that virulence of the pathogen can be deliberately modified. The epidemic experience of increasing severity of disease suggests that, as the pathogen passes from one host to the next, it becomes more and more virulent. The opposite effect can be created when the pathogen is passed through artificial media in the laboratory. It is this characteristic, in fact, that is often used in attenuating pathogens to prepare vaccines for immunization. The ability of the pathogen to create severe disease by progressive passage through living hosts and to lose this capacity by passage through artificial hosts cannot be entirely explained. There is a suggestion, at least, that the environmental interaction of the pathogen is an essential aspect of such knowledge.

The ways in which an individual responds to a pathogenic organism is frequently summarized in a misused and misunderstood term, *resistance*. A romantic wistfulness, strongly laced with moral implications, invests the idea of resistance with a kind of strength or fight often confused with a demonstration of wilfulness on the part of the sufferer. The implication that an individual can influence the course of an infection by an exercise of his will strongly colors the layman's use of the word resistance. There are, of course, many circumstances that influence the progress of a disease of this kind, over which the individual has absolutely no control whatsoever. The age of the host is certainly one factor; both the very young and the very old tend to be much more susceptible to infectious disease than others in the population. The nutritional state of the individual is another. Concurrent disease is a frequent precursor of serious infection, diabetes being one of the most notable. The cachectic victims of malignant disease often expire because of pneumonia. The environmental conditions in which the individual spends his illness also markedly influence its effect on him. Availability to infection is certainly a factor too. One of the easiest places in which to contract infection is, unhappily, a hospital ward. The combination of geographic isolation and the immunity in a population is another influential modifier of resistance. There are, for instance, a number of descriptions of primitive populations decimated by common diseases such as measles, because the individuals had never been exposed to the disease before the bearers of civilized culture brought it to them. Genetic factors, too, are apparent in some infected populations. The African people afflicted with genetically determined sickle cell anemia live in an area where malaria is a common disease. For reasons not understood, the sickling tendency renders the individual immune to the greater threat of malaria. Thus, protected by their abnormal gene from the local hazard of malaria, the individuals with sickle cell anemia outlive their less fortunate brothers and perpetuate the genetic abnormality they bear.

A rather specific evaluation of resistance is available for certain diseases which produce identifiable antibodies in their surviving victims. The concentration of antibodies can, in some instances, be measured in the laboratory; this alone perhaps should be identified as the individual's resistance. The presence of antibodies is an indicator of the presence of the disease at some point in the individual's lifetime but does not necessarily indicate that he is presently a host to the disease. The titering of antibodies may be useful as a diagnostic test in some infections in which it is not possible to demonstrate the organism itself. This is the basis for most of the complement-fixation tests used as diagnostic tools, particularly for syphilis.

The likelihood that a specific pathogen will cause disease in a specific individual is further influenced by environmental artifacts which may or may not be susceptible to control measures. Sometimes an exposure to a pathogen does not cause disease because the relative "dose" of transmitted organisms is not sufficient to do so. It is likely that a single spirochete can initiate a syphilitic infection, but many organisms must be present in large numbers before they can establish a disease response in their host. The portal of entry for the pathogen will also determine whether a specific exposure will result in disease. Organisms ordinarily entering the body by the respiratory tract may not cause disease if introduced into the gastrointestinal tract, and some organisms are pathogenic only when they can be admitted through the barriers of ordinary protection, such as through breaks in the skin surface.

The response of the body to invasion by the pathogenic organism involves many variables, but the emphatic importance of environmental interaction involving two living systems, their life-patterns, their relative condition of health, and their physiological need influences all understanding of infection and inflammation.

The Granulomatous Response: Defense by Exclusion

The red, hot, angry appearance of an acute inflammatory reaction suggests the expense of effort being mounted by the body to defend itself. But not all inflammation is so obviously vigorous or forthright. Many injuries and ulcerations simply do not heal. They persist as chronic, long-standing lesions which respond very little, even to vigorous treatment. All evidence of the "fight" so obvious in the acute reaction is gone. There is very little redness and virtually no swelling or local heat. A ridge of fibrous tissue outlines the chronic lesion, and there is a fairly consistent necrosing of its central tissues, with some drainage and discharge which may or may not be purulent. Such an appearance is fairly typical of decubitus ulcerations and bears all the indices of a very restricted blood supply to the area of damage. The persistence of a lesion beyond the time expected for its resolution indicates that the failure of the organism to eliminate the invasion finally gives way to a kind of retreat. The area is walled off, the blood supply to it very limited, and the energy of the body no longer wasted on it. By exclusion, the individual organism tolerates the presence of the lesion but invests no further effort to eliminate it.

This retreat indicates very clearly that the purpose of the attack against intrusion is to perpetuate and preserve the integrity of the *entire* organism. When the concerted effort of the organism has failed to eliminate the lesion, there is a withdrawal of effort and no further investment of the body's resource in defense. Only if the encapsulated lesion is capable of further broaching the integrity of surrounding tissues, or if secondary superinfection should reawaken the acute defense processes, does the organism waste any further attention on the persisting lesion.

The acute inflammatory reaction was characterized by an exudative phase which permitted the removal of the invading organism, as well as the debris of its battle with the body tissues. In the chronic inflammatory response, on the other hand, there is a proliferation of granulation tissue and the subsequent organization of this tissue into a fibrous wall isolating the lesion from the adjacent, unaffected tissues of the body. Any number of factors in the afflicted individual might contribute to the development of a proliferative, granulomatous change in an area of inflammation, including the presence of other disease, the age of the individual, his relative debility, and the effectiveness of the local blood supply to the affected site. Each of these factors limits the effectiveness of the acute defense posture and contributes to a prolongation of the inflammation until the time factor intervenes and the proliferative process takes hold.

In addition to the possibility that an acute situation will persist and become chronic, there are certain pathogens that always stimulate this kind of reaction from the body. In each instance, the possibility of an aggressively mounted attack on the pathogen does not exist, and the individual manifests a granulomatous reaction to the pathogen from the very outset. All of the diseases that excite a granulomatous reaction rather than an acute one are characteristically chronic disorders that have proved to be extremely difficult to control, treat, or even describe definitively. Syphilis, tuberculosis, and leprosy are three of the most widespread diseases which are characteristically infectious granulomatous syndromes.

In each of these diseases, the characteristic lesion is an encapsulated exclusion of the offending pathogenic organisms. As the capsule matures in tuberculosis, for example, it may actually calcify but within it are viable pathogens capable of causing the disease. Any factors that result in a disruption of the capsule have the potential for freeing the pathogen, thus allowing it to be transmitted again. The primary lesion of syphilis is remarkable for its lack of the usual angry inflammatory signs, and the lesion heals without treatment. Unfortunately, it is also painless, and therefore frequently ignored by the infected individual. The second stage is characterized by inflammatory reactions more consistent with an acute response, although the probability of some allergic processes in this phase is present. A generalized skin rash, in conjunction with inflammatory processes in the mucous membranes of the nose, mouth, and throat, characterizes the second stage, and the lesions of this stage are teeming with spirochetes. It is, therefore, a stage of grave potential for transmission of the disease. But this phase, too, subsides without treatment and without apparent residual changes in the affected tissue. It is, however, during the third stage of syphilis that the granulomas are developed. They are called *gumma* (pl., gummata) and may appear in almost any body tissue. During the third phase, intense structural damage occurs in the cardiovascular system or in the central nervous system. By the time the disease has matured to this stage, treatment is symptomatic and palliative. Control with antibiotics in the first and second phase had seemed to promise a genuine cure for victims of syphilis, but it has been recently demonstrated that the spirochete survives the treatment within the host's body in an attenuated form. In rabbits, treated and apparently cured of syphilis, large doses of adrenal hormone have resulted in renewed activity by the spirochete. The long periods of infection which characterize the pathogens causing infectious granulomas, including those intervals when the individual is symptom-free, confound the understanding of precisely what is happening between host and invader. None of the finality and definition so welcome in the acute inflammatory response is available here to provide clear-cut evidence of the organismic interaction taking place in these chronic and stubborn infections.

Confronted with infections that remain as inscrutable as these, the validity of the acute inflammatory reaction in the conservation of the integrity of the individual becomes very apparent. Inflammation is not an evil. It is an essential mechanism of protection in a dangerous world. The initial stages of combat that produce the exudate are essential to the subsequent stages of healing that restore the structural integrity to the injured part and thereby to the entire organism.

Autoimmune Response: The Defense That Creates Disease

The proteins that form a part of the vitreous fluid of the eye are different from every other protein in the body. The fluid that distends the eye must allow the passage of light, bending the rays so that they can reach the retinal receptors. Because of the special function of the vitreous fluid and the absence of these proteins from any other tissue in the body, the proteins in the eye fluid are potentially "foreign" to the rest of the organism. So long as the eye is intact, this creates no problem. But when the eye is injured, the increase of vascularity to the site, plus the loss of vitreous fluid which enables its absorption by the circulating blood, sets up a situation in which a foreign protein reaction can occur to one of the body's own substances. For many years, the problem of "sympathetic ophthalmitis" was a dreaded, but unexplained, phenomenon. Injury to one eye resulted shortly in an acute inflammatory reaction in the *uninjured* eye, and frequently the individual lost his sight in both eyes. Knowledge of antigen-antibody reaction has clarified the reason for a sympathetic inflammation in the uninjured, intact eye. As the foreign protein from the vitreous humor is absorbed in the bloodstream following injury to an eye, the response of the body is to produce antibodies to eliminate these "foreign" antigens. As the antibody titer increases, the antigen in the uninjured eye is also attacked by the antibody, and an acute inflammatory battle is waged. The use of anti-inflammatory drugs (hormones) in the good eye has virtually eliminated the appearance of sympathetic ophthalmitis and has substantially reduced the injury by limiting the reaction when it does occur. It is thus apparent that it is possible for the antibody-producing tissues in the body to make a "mistake" and defend the organism from its own protein. And it is also evident that the immune response is a form of inflammation.

The means by which other body proteins become antigens is not clear. The isolation, under normal conditions, of the proteins of the eye establishes those proteins as "foreign" without too much use of the imagination. But immune reactions, characterized by inflammatory cellular response, also occur when this kind of isolation is not apparent. The possibility that the antibody response is elicited by a combination of body protein with another substance has also been suggested. Conjugation of other substances with the body proteins may explain the persistence of an inflammatory reaction in tissues well past the time when the causative organism has disappeared. Streptococcus infections characteristically can cause long-term inflammatory disease in the heart and kidney, even when the pathogen itself is no longer present. The protein conjugate that acts like an antigen probably is composed of one of the products of metabolism of the Beta hemolytic streptococci and the affected organ tissue. A number of disease processes, affecting many different kinds of body tissue, have been implicated in just such an antigen-antibody relationship, which seems to indicate that the inflammatory process in the affected organ is a reaction to the protein found in that organ. For the past twenty years, a group of diseases have been collectively labeled "collagen disease" because they affect the "ground tissue" or connective tissue of the body. Unusual antibody-antigen activity has been demonstrated in the collagen tissue of patients suffering from these diseases, thus encouraging the concept that these are autoimmune reactions.

It is not possible to offer much therapeutic assistance to individuals with autoimmune disease, although the use of the anti-inflammatory hormones has provided relief of symptoms. However, the difficulty with long-term administration of anti-inflammatory hormones is considerable. The initial enthusiasm for their effect on the badly crippled victim of rheumatoid arthritis, for example, has gradually been transformed into wariness and weighing of the risks that accompany extended usage.

There is still another area of concern that emphasizes the need to understand autoimmunity; this has grown out of new therapeutic efforts to transplant tissues, and even entire organs, when the patient's have been irreversibly damaged by disease. The rejection of transplant tissues is another manifestation of the antigen-antibody response, and much therapeutic effort has been devoted to establishing an environment in which the immune reaction is suppressed, in the hope that the transplanted organ will survive. The really successful kidney transplants have involved identical twins, because such individuals share the same proteins and the likelihood of an immune reaction is diminished. But the tragic persistence of the autoimmune reaction has even doomed what appeared to be successful transplants. When the diseased kidney was the result of the autoimmune disease that follows streptococcus infection (glomerulonephritis), the functional and apparently surviving transplanted kidney ultimately becomes diseased precisely as did the original organs in the recipient patient. Thus, even a successful kidney transplant has only a limited lifetime; though the individual gains some years of relative health, the possibility is always present that his new kidney will succumb to the same autoimmune processes that destroyed the original ones. Not every individual so afflicted, of course, has an identical twin. Close relatives may contribute a kidney, but the further the consanguineous tie, the greater the possibility that the immune reaction will reject the foreign protein of the transplanted organ. The clinical effort to suppress the formation of antibodies is fraught with danger to the patient too. The suppression of antibody formation has been accomplished by whole body radiation and by the use of antimetabolite drugs, but in either instance the suppression of the immune response means an absolute removal of the defense mechanism so essential to survival. The danger of overwhelming infection is very real, and even the elaborate techniques developed to protect the individual have not always succeeded in preventing a lethal infection. The philosophical problems of organ transplant are being widely debated by both professional practitioners and the lay public. But it is painfully apparent that the philosophical issues will not be resolved until the physiological aspects are far better understood.

Care of a Patient with an Acute Inflammatory Process

The Conservation of Energy

The "biological priority" evidenced by the body's response to an acute infection and subsequent healing is achieved by a mobilization of energy resource directed precisely at the insult. There is the need to actively engage the invading organisms—that requires an energy expense. There is a need to produce the leukocytes in numbers sufficient to challenge the invader—*that* requires an energy expense. There is a need to increase the local blood flow and to carry the constituent substances to the site—*that* requires an energy expense. There is a need to remove the debris and the soluble products of the infecting organism and the cells confronting it—*that* too requires an energy expense. And finally there is a need to bring the products of repair to the site and to reconstruct the damaged area with new protein in organized tissue—and *that* requires an energy expense. The entire episode is remarkable for the activity and movement, for the rapidly changing characteristics in the localized area, a process of ebb and flow—and all of it performed through the cooperative interaction of all body systems. The lethargy and limitation of physical activity that characterize the behavior of the individual during the acute phase of the inflammatory reaction conserve the energy available for the prior demand made by the infection. No aspect of the energy-producing capability of the individual can be ignored during an acute infection; just as it establishes the pathophysiological focus in the organism, it defines the dimensions of medical and nursing intervention.

In addition, the processes of inflammation and repair are achieved within a time limit. The devotion of energy expenditure in itself limits the period of time in which the organism can focus all of its energy potential on the exclusion of a noxious pathogen. The alternative of granulomatous isolation fulfills the need to restore structural continuity to the body, but it does not restore structural integrity, and the danger of another skirmish remains ever present. It is remarkable how the energy potential of the individual dictates the quality of the body's defenses against such invasion. In the young individual whose general health has not been undermined by long-standing disease, the expectation is always rapid healing. Whatever the instinct that provides solace to the young child when he brings his scratch to Mother for a kiss, the certainty of rapid healing and repair makes such therapy eminently appropriate. The nurse quickly learns to be apprehensive about the presence of infection in any patient who is weakened, debilitated, or malnourished, whether this state of affairs has arisen from chronic disease or from the accumulated insults of aging. And nowhere in the hospital is there more concern and attention to the prevention of microorganism transmission than in the ritualized techniques of the newborn nursery. This, too, is tacit recognition that the ability to establish a priority of energy utilization for anything except the fundamental metabolic demands of the individual does not exist in the very, very young. In a general sense, then, the ability to heal and withstand the assault of infection is directly related to the energy that the individual can muster in his own defense. When the nurse provides care for such a patient, some of the responsibility for defense is invested in her.

Energy conservation in this type of nursing intervention is considerably more than restriction of activity by the individual. This is always true, but the guidelines are unusually clear when the patient has an infected wound or an inflammatory disease. Energy is not being restricted or limited —it must be *directed.* The systemic response itself is characterized by a remarkable increase in energy production to meet the remarkable increase in demand. Except for unusual situations discussed later, it is harmful to the individual to attempt to curb his energy production. The focus of care must parallel the focus of biological intent.

The fifth cardinal sign of the inflammatory process, loss of function, may be obscured when the affected part is already relatively restricted in its movement. An infected surgical wound on the abdominal wall, for example, is locally immobilized, but the muscular activity of the abdomen is limited anyway when the individual is on bedrest. The tendency of the body tissues to splint areas of injury is more apparent when the injury involves the usual skeletal-muscle movements of the individual. The broken bone is splinted by spasm and contraction of the muscles in the vicinity of the injury. The infected finger is splinted by the swelling of the inflammation, as well as by the pain aroused by movement. Perhaps the fifth cardinal sign is better expressed as a *resting,* or even arresting, of the affected part. The limitation of movement has at least two functions. In the first place, such a limitation decreases the mechanical effect of movement of the active cells and their products, thereby limiting the total tissue involvement, or affected space, of the response. In the second place, the restriction decreases the metabolic demand in the unaffected tissues in the vicinity of the inflammation, thereby conserving the nutrients and oxygen supply for the critical need in the area itself. This is a biological determinant; therefore, rest of the part, whether this means bedrest for the entire organism or merely splinting of an affected limb, must also be a nursing determinant. When bedrest is essential to therapy during the acute phase of the process, then all of the conservation measures related to personal hygiene and activity are required.

The systemic manifestation of energy production of an unusual nature is measured by the vital signs, and the frequent febrile reaction accompanying this phase requires adjustment in the provision for the basic nursing needs of the individual. Since the body temperature is regulated by a constant interaction with the external environment, the regulation of comfort, as well as therapeutic effectiveness, involves intervention by the nurse to establish optimal environmental conditions individualized for the patient's needs. Chilling is hard work, and although it finally results in an

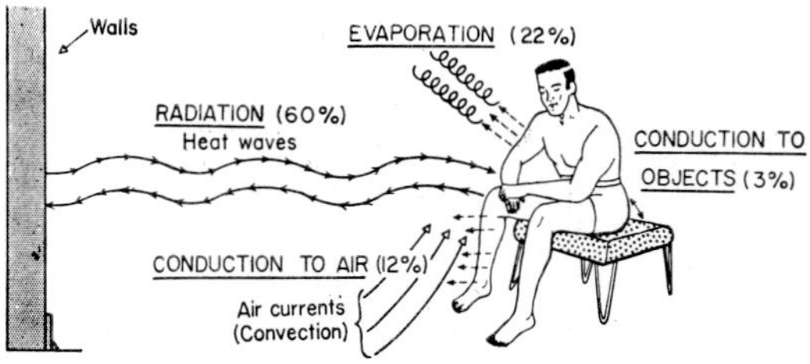

FIGURE 74. The mechanisms of heat loss from the body include radiation, conduction, convection, and evaporation. The very fine balance of body heat maintained by the integrating mechanisms to sustain a constant core temperature is remarkable in the face of environmental demands. (From Guyton, A.C.: *Textbook of Medical Physiology,* 3rd ed. W.B. Saunders Co., Philadelphia, 1966.)

increased body temperature because of the increase in energy production, the episode leaves the individual exhausted. Conserving energy that is needed for use is one thing, but physical exhaustion is another; such an expense of energy must be guarded against. The increased temperature and the more rapid metabolic rate are useful to the individual when they supply the additional energy without the sequelae of excessive muscular work or the danger of a body temperature that threatens the tissues and their biochemical activity. Thus, every effort is made to regulate the febrile level within the limits of effective physiological work. The first step is always knowledge of the temperature level, and this requires frequent measurement of the body temperature. Whenever a patient is running a temperature above the normal mean, tradition indicates that it be checked and recorded every four hours. However, when temperature control is being used by the nurse as a criterion for nursing intervention, the traditional pattern may not provide enough information to offer care successfully. Taking the individual's temperature and *merely* recording it, even with prompt reporting of unusual readings, is not utilizing this measurement sufficiently to plan care. The nurse must know the *pattern* of temperature change in that specific patient, and with that knowledge anticipate his care. The periodic change in the body temperature is a normal dimension of physiological action, but the period changes with a febrile condition and must be identified anew in the individual himself. With this kind of information, the nurse is able to make the decisions that will determine the care required by the patient. If, for example, a patient running a febrile course has repeatedly demonstrated a persistent high temperature during the night hours when the temperature ordinarily falls, then the intervention necessary to regulate the temperature can be anticipated, and the individual can be spared the threat of excess fatigue or tissue damage that accompanies a very high temperature reading. It is essential that the individual's temperature be measured immediately *following* an episode of chilling. It will reach its highest point at this time, and the prompt institution of measures to limit it may be undertaken on the basis of this information. Control of the external environmental exchange during a chilling episode may pose some difficult nursing problems. The patient feels very cold and is therefore very uncomfortable. He will want external heat applied to minimize and eliminate the discomfort of his sensations of cold. However, this must be done judiciously. The provision of hot water bottles and many extra blankets to warm him may or may not be advantageous. If the individual's basal temperature at the onset of the chill is already quite elevated, the fever may become very high afterwards. When external heat is applied, the loss of heat from the body surface is restricted. The chill itself is self-limiting and will cease when the blood temperature reaches the hypothalamic setting. But if the external covers continue to prevent the free movement of heat from the body surface, the body temperature may be raised past the self-limiting level. The gradual return of comfort accompanies the reduction of muscular activity (shivering) that is characteristic of a chill. Such a patient should be constantly attended, and external applications of heat should be gradually removed as his comfort level increases with the termination of the chill.

The regulation of the body temperature depends to a large degree on the evaporation of fluid from the body surface. There is often a marked decrease in perspiration during the chill itself, but as the body temperature regulates at its higher setting the increase in perspiration is an indicator of the regulatory effect that serves to stabilize the body temperature. Fol-

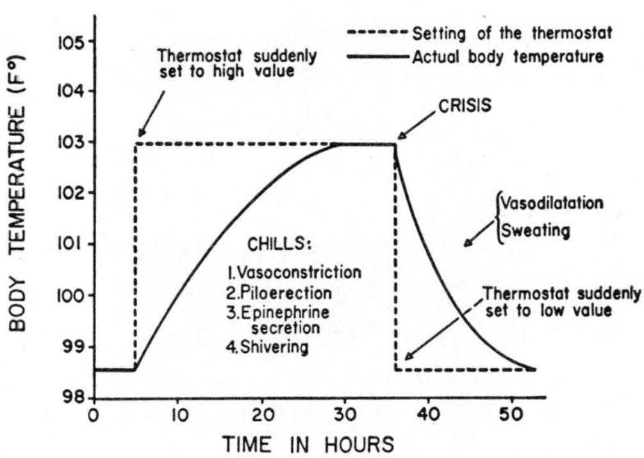

FIGURE 75. The setting of the "hypothalamic thermostat" is accompanied by physiological response of the entire body, so that the core temperature is altered by a change in the thermostat setting. (From Guyton, A.C.: *Textbook of Medical Physiology,* 3rd ed. W.B. Saunders Co., Philadelphia, 1966.)

lowing a chill, the increase in perspiration may become progressively more noticeable; when the external applications of heat are not removed, the amount of fluid loss is remarkably increased. An exaggerated loss of body fluid by extreme perspiration is called diaphoresis (carry through). The human organism loses isotonic body fluids during perspiration; thus, such an excessive fluid loss involves not only water but essential electrolytes as well. As the thermostatic setting of the hypothalamus is lowered, either by natural physiological change or by the mediation of drugs, the excess heat energy produced during the chilling is lost by a tremendous increase in perspiration. The cooling effect of the liquid removes heat from the body by evaporation. Excessive perspiration is effective only when evaporation takes place, however, and during diaphoresis the flood of fluid results in retention of observable fluid on the body surface. If the external covers are not adjusted at this time, the free exchange of heat with the environment is restrained. The excessive loss of fluid is such that the bedclothes often become soaked. In such a situation, provision of a dry bed is necessary, but it is also very important that the nurse make an estimate of fluid loss so that the fluids and electrolytes can be replaced. Such an estimate based on the size of the area moistened by the fluid is, at best, only a guess. However, even a guess is better than no indication at all of how profusely the body has eliminated essential fluids. Left in the wet bedclothes, the individual will soon be chilled again because of the rapid interchange of heat with the environment. Obviously, such a situation defeats the purpose of therapy and control. It may be necessary to replace the bedclothes several times before the body temperature has stabilized and the excess perspiration has ceased. Every episode of diaphoresis requires active energy utilization by the patient's body too, and such experiences are often followed by physical exhaustion.

When there is a pattern of chilling in the febrile patient, the effort to prevent these episodes is worthwhile and represents an essential goal in energy conservation. This is accomplished by regulating the body's temperature thermostat with drugs. The best drug for the purpose is also the most common—aspirin, or acetylsalicylic acid. When such drugs (antipyretic analgesics) are used in a febrile patient, the effect of the drug itself promotes a cooling diaphoresis which, nevertheless, must be dealt with exactly as described above. The drug remains effective for two or three hours after administration; then, unless the fever is subsiding with the disease process, the body temperature will begin to rise again as the effects wear off. If one is regulating the energy expense as manifested in the body temperature, recording the temperature so that the individual's condition is accurately assessed demands that the temperature be taken with the effect of the antipyretic drug clearly in mind. The successful effect is often observable in the patient within thirty minutes to an hour after administration. He may begin to perspire and, because of the analgesic effect of the drug, will feel more comfortable. If there is such obvious evidence of relief, taking the temperature at this time may not be necessary. However, if the behavior of the fever is to be properly understood, the temperature should be repeated immediately *before* the drug is administered. It is thus possible to determine the effect of the medication over a period of time and also the patient's response to the disease itself.

The increase in metabolic rate reflected in the elevated temperature is also measurable in the pulse and respiratory rates. These are measured each time the temperature is taken; in fact, the pulse rate alone may give a rough estimate of the degree of activity being required of the individual's resource. When the tachycardia is clearly related to the febrile condition and not a result of other concurrent disease, as the temperature returns towards normal levels, the pulse rate also tends to slow down. This may be a quick, though approximate, method of assessing the patient's condition when, for example, he is resting, and the nurse chooses not to disturb him at that moment to take a temperature reading. Cardiac activity, as reflected in the pulse, is a valid parameter of energy utilization, and changes in the pulse rate which attend activity on the part of the individual are indices that permit regulation of allowable activity.

The loss of fluids through the body's efforts to lower its temperature is only one of the reasons for assuring that the individual receives an adequate fluid intake. The increased metabolic rate in itself requires increased fluid intake, and, unless some other aspect of the patient's condition prevents it, the individual with an acute inflammatory disease is often ordered to force fluids. Any fluid will do, although replacement of electrolytes suggests that fruit juices and milk should be part of the additional fluid intake. When fluids are taken orally, the prescription for forcing intake means that the individual always has an available source of fluids at his bedside and that he is encouraged to consume them. Forcing fluids is always attended by a diuresis; when the individual is in bed and must use a urinal or must frequently go to the bathroom, he may be reluctant to drink fluids in the volume that requires this extra activity. Actually, forcing fluids is aimed at adequate hydration, and diuresis is an indication that hydration is satisfactory. His intake should therefore be adjusted so that he does not have to spend too much energy in micturition. It is usually easier to encourage the individual to take fluids than to succeed in getting him to eat, because anorexia is a frequent component of the systemic response to infection. There may be additional difficulty inasmuch as the folklore relating to food intake during a fever is extensive. The nutrients are very important, because there is an additional demand for protein and the vitamins associated with healing during an infection. If the diet does not supply them, the body substance itself must do so. If the individual refuses food, the diet should be planned so that he may have small meals at intervals during the day. The food should be relatively bland but with a protein content providing sufficient nutrients for the inflammatory process and the healing that must follow. When the exudate has formed and drainage begins, there is a loss of protein by this means. If the drainage is limited in both quantity and duration, the loss may be compensated in the diet without unusual attention. When there is profuse drainage, however, or the wound persists in draining over a long period of time, the protein loss may be considerable. An estimate of the volume of fluid and protein loss is incomplete unless some effort is made to describe the amount of drainage produced by the inflammatory site. An excess of protein loss by this means requires a high protein intake. The preparation of eggnogs and other high-protein supplement drinks may permit an increased intake of protein when it is required.

The cardinal signs of redness and local heat indicate a focus of energy utilization at the inflammatory site. The goal of localization that is pursued by the body's own defense mechanism is also the goal of therapy. Localization, release of the exudate, and the beginning of the healing process are encouraged by the increase in the local blood supply. Thus, the application of heat to the local area involved may assist the organism in the task of localization and even speed the process somewhat. If the dressing is to be effective, however, the heat must be maintained, either by frequent changing or by the use of a radiant source of heat to keep it at the proper temperature. When the area is an open wound, the dressing is applied with strict surgical asepsis, including a moisture-proof and sterile outer covering to prevent ready access of microorganisms into, or out of, the dressing itself. Ideally, the dressing should be very light in weight to avoid additional pressure on an already painful area and to preclude maceration of the surrounding skin by a heavy wet weight. It should be replaced as often as the drainage demands and as often as necessary to maintain a constant, gentle warmth on the affected area. The temperature of the dressing must never exceed a safe limit because of the danger of burning the tissues and adding to the inflammatory area. As the wound is localized and drainage begins, the relief of the interstitial pressure frequently results in a marked decrease in pain.

The use of antibiotic drugs to speed the body's assault against the organism also aids in terminating the inflammatory process, thus limiting the energy expense demanded. Professional practitioners now know well that the "miracle drugs" perform their miracles only when they are used judiciously. Not all organisms are susceptible to antibiotics, and the increasing number of resistant organisms indicates that, as their environment altered, they survived selectively through mutations which rendered the antibiotic useless against them. The shotgun use of antibiotics is rare; when the infection warrants antibiotic therapy, the physician will often culture the organism causing the infection and request sensitivity tests on it in the laboratory to find the antibiotic which will destroy it. Certain antibiotic drugs are described as "broad-spectrum" because they are effective against many different pathogens. Most viruses are not susceptible to antibiotics at all. The use of these drugs by the physician requires individual consideration of both the patient and his microscopic assailant. Many antibiotics cause sensitivity reactions in the individual, and a history of allergic manifestations in the past suggests caution in prescribing antibiotic drugs. The intensity of some of these reactions is in itself life-threatening, and when the patient is receiving antibiotics the nurse has a responsibility to promptly identify the earliest signs of an untoward effect. Skin manifestations, such as a rash, itching, or hives, should be immediately reported to the physician. If the reaction is mild and can itself be controlled by the administration of other drugs, the antibiotic may be continued or another substituted for it. These are decisions to be made by the physician, but he depends upon the nurse's assessment of the patient's response to insure the patient's safety.

Those individuals who are unable to muster an adequate resource to fight an infection require special consideration in the conservation of their energy needs. The increase in the metabolic rate that accompanies a febrile condition may, for example, make demands on the cardiovascular system which the individual simply cannot afford. In such patients, reduction of the increased body temperature is necessary, and efforts are made to keep the temperature at a lower level than the inflammatory process itself might demand. If antipyretic drugs do not succeed in regulating the fever, more heroic measures must be undertaken. These measures involve manipulating the energy exchange with the external environment by cooling sponge baths, alcohol sponges, tepid tub baths, or in some instances, cold enemas. Such measures are always taxing and difficult for the patient, and their performance must take into consideration all of the needs of the individual. He must be cooled, but not chilled. His temperature must be reduced but not too fast or too suddenly. During the procedure, only repeated measurements of the temperature indicate whether or not the therapy is working. The use of such methods is frequent when the temperature tends to go as high as 104°F in any patient, but it may be ordered for a weakened individual with a temperature somewhat less than that. Reduction of body temperature by surface cooling is often necessary in young children. Their thermostatic control of body temperature tends to be quite labile, and youngsters often develop very high temperatures very quickly. Such high temperatures in children may cause convulsions, an indication of interference with nervous system function related to the high metabolic rate and interference with enzyme systems. The convulsions usually leave no permanent sequelae, but they must be terminated and cooling the entire body is the most effective means to accomplish this quickly.

The Conservation of Structural Integrity

There is no demonstration of the importance of structural integrity that is more compelling than the process of normal healing. The ability of the body to seal its injuries and to do so promptly creates even in the very young child the confidence that permits indifference to the wound once its initial presence has been acknowledged and, if necessary, treated. The minor wounds and injuries that are part of the accepted hazard of the environment *are* minor only because of the immediate response of the body to seal and heal them. The ordinary expectations that the integrity will be restored are poor preparation for those clinical events where the orderly replacement of wounded tissue does not occur. Moreover, the tacit assumption that healing will take its natural course does not acknowledge the complex and astonishing pattern that assures it. Within moments of the injury, the orderly replacement of the lost tissue begins. The most obvious indication of tissue injury is a prompt display of blood. The bleeding begins profusely but, unless a fairly large vessel has been entered upon, slackens quickly and stops altogether within five minutes. Although there is much variation depending on individual bleeding tendencies, the site of the wound, and the blood supply to the part, as well as the extent of the injury, the "minor" wound which bleeds can, with confidence, be expected to stop bleeding quite promptly. The ability of the blood to clot, that is, to quickly turn from a liquid to a solid, represents the first step in the normal healing process. The matrix of fibrin strands that is an essential part of the blood clot establishes in the injured tissue the framework upon which reconstruction will take place. But the clot itself seals the small wound. The sealing, which involves a network of fibrin, in effect results in a reapproximation of surfaces. When the wound is made by a very sharp instrument with minimal trauma to the tissues, such a seal very effectively brings the severed surfaces back together again. It is characteristic of healing that approximating surfaces heal more quickly and more satisfactorily than does a gaping type of injury where the wound edges remain far apart. The surgical technique recognizes the advantage in close wound edges, and suturing tissues together is the surgeon's method of enhancing the body's own inclination.

The progress of healing is an orderly and systematic formation of new tissue to replace that which was lost in the injury. Within an hour, the blood supply and thus an increased number of leukocytes have been brought to the injured area. There is a migration of epithelial cells from the wound edges across the injured region, and this is apparent within twenty-four hours of the injury. By the third day, a very active proliferation of the epithelial cells is taking place, reaching its peak within seven days. By the eighth day, the wound is completely restored by epithelial tissue, although the underlying area that was injured may still be granulation tissue which has not yet been organized (or cicatrized) into a fibrous scar. The blood supply to the area is restored with the growth of new capillaries; when the nerve supply has been disrupted, it too will ultimately be restored to the injured part. The maturing of the scar into a tough fibrous tissue may take considerably longer, but the restoration of the lost tissue is an accomplished fact by the end of a single week. The healing of clean, restricted, and close-edged wounds is called "primary union," or, to use the medieval phrase, "healing by first intention."

A wound which involves larger areas of tissue and in which the wound edges cannot be approximated is quickly sealed too, but the defect caused by loss of tissue may not be entirely filled for some time. The seal is initiated by the clotted blood, but it consists of a layer of granulation tissue covering the defect from one edge to the other; ultimately, the laying down of fibrous tissue takes place, so that the defect itself is largely replaced by scar tissue. This is called "secondary union," or "healing by second intention." So long as the wound remains uninfected and clean, the process, though prolonged, is nevertheless organized and persistent. The pink granulation tissue, richly supplied with blood, is very friable, however, and the wound must be carefully protected from the encroachment of microorganisms. In both the time and the risk involved, it is vastly preferable to have a wound heal by primary union. Only this normal process really assures immediate restoration of structural integrity.

All of the skill and ingenuity of the modern operating room are devoted to establishing an environment where the individual whose defenses are being deliberately broached will, nevertheless, be able to have a wound that heals by primary union—quickly, neatly, and thoroughly. In a process as complex as that which leads to healing, however, a failure to insure optimal conditions invites a failure in wound healing. Many times, control of all of the essentials does not rest with the surgeon or the nursing staff. Some procedures inevitably must be performed where infection is already present, or where the possibility of introducing infection is great. Surgery, for an inflamed appendix, for example, may successfully remove the infected organ, but the conditions for infection are already established. The individual's state of nourishment influences his ability to heal, and though it is desirable to postpone surgery so that nutrition can be improved, this is not always possible. The presence of other disease entities interferes with healing too, although the physician naturally makes every effort to control these factors. There are also technical problems that may interfere with normal healing. The sutures which approximate the wound edges must be tight enough to hold them together, but not sufficiently tight to cause inflammation and edema in the wound. Occasionally a patient will develop an allergic reaction to suture material so that it does not hold. But none of these problems is as threatening to the normal healing of the wound as are the hazards in the environment established for the individual during his postoperative convalescence.

The control of the microbial population in the hospital ward is the fundamental problem which dictates administrative and nursing policies. The responsibility to provide a clean and pathogen-controlled environment for every patient admitted to the hospital is a heavy one; it can be honored by the institution only in direct proportion to the individual participation of every person who functions in that institution. It was not until antisepsis became an established fact that the hospital was a place where healing was possible. The pesthouses and poor farms, which were the hospitals before knowledge of microorganisms was available, were repositories of virulent infection, and the death toll in those institutions reflected the terrible price

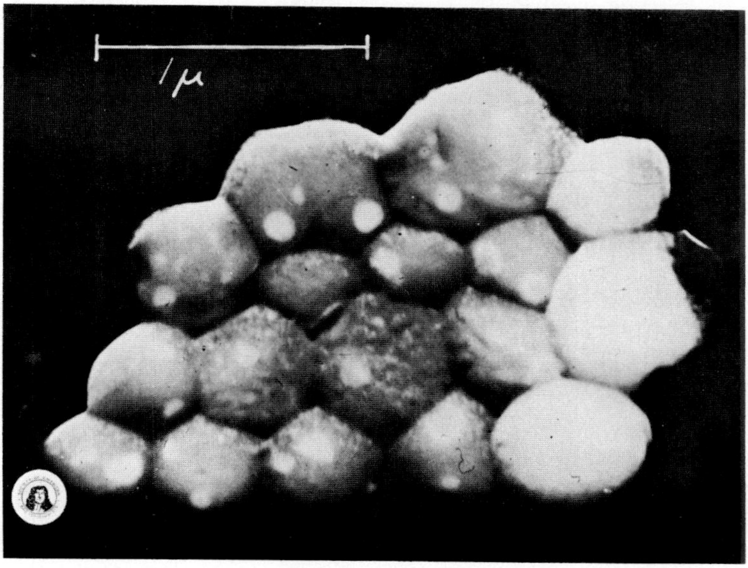

FIGURE 76. Electron micrograph of Staphylococcus aureus, the organism which has demanded a constant vigilance against cross-contamination in the hospital. (American Society of American Bacteriologists.)

of cross-contamination. All nursing care is designed to break the chain of such contamination. Every individual in the hospital—doctor, nurse, aide, or scrubwoman—is a link in the important and continuing task of protecting the patient from cross-contamination. Every professional person must develop an extremely active "aseptic conscience," arising not only from the manipulative skills that insure asepsis but equally from a deep commitment to the patient which is a moral necessity. The microorganism cannot be seen, and the prevention of spreading pathogens is therefore invested in a mastery of the ritualistic skills that alone insure the patient's safety. The most minor break in technique must arouse in the nurse (or doctor) an intolerable anxiety that forces the individual to begin again in order to establish an absolutely perfect pattern of aseptic technique. Asepsis and the skill that assures it must become an almost palpable recognition of safety. A tactile awareness based on sound knowledge and perfect technique is the only guarantee to the patient that he is adequately protected. The conscientious performance of aseptic skills is a highly personalized and highly individualized responsibility that will NOT permit the nurse (or doctor) to break technique, whether there are witnesses present or not.

The first step in protecting the patient from infection is the individual's awareness of his role in the prevention of contamination, and that begins with the personal hygiene of the nurse. Much of the militaristic tone in the "rules and regulations" governing hospital dress first arose from the urgency of microbial control. But there is a sound and sensible reason for clean uniforms, polished shoes with washed shoelaces, clean nails, and a hair style that will not allow contamination to be carried to the patient. This cleanliness initiates the certainty that the nurse will not bring contamination to the ward. The use of modern "wash and wear" uniforms that are not sterilized in the laundering process may be a source of contaminants and emphasizes the importance of the attention required in the personal hygiene of the nurse.

Aseptic preparation of the environment is often described as medical or surgical asepsis. Such a division reflects the intent in each instance. Medical asepsis is undertaken to eliminate the presence of pathogenic organisms in the environment. Surgical asepsis demands that all organisms, pathogenic or not, be excluded from the environment. Although these techniques represent a difference of degree, in some instances the guidelines are beginning to fade. The extreme demands of surgical asepsis are based on the certain knowledge that the patient's defense system has been challenged and that an open wound must be protected from encroachment by microorganisms. Medical asepsis has rested on the assurance that the individual's ordinary defenses are intact, including a potential ability to protect himself from the possibility of infection. Even though a clean and pathogen-free environment is required in the hospital ward, when an individual has an infection which may be transmitted to others, he may be placed in some degree of isolation. The isolation varies with the organism, its means of transmission, and its portal of entry into the body. The patient and the artifacts required for his care are physically and aseptically separated from other patients. With the use of drugs that deliberately suppress the body's defense mechanisms, it has become increasingly common to place a patient in "reverse isolation" where the purpose is to protect him scrupulously from the danger of infection carried from other sources in the hospital. The use of isolation procedures mirrors the change in the treatment of infections that accompanied the use of antibiotic drugs. Many diagnostic entities which were formerly immediate indications for isolation of the patient are now treated on the open ward. The most sinister danger to personnel and other patients, however, is the presence in an open ward of a patient with an undiagnosed infection. When the diagnosis is known, personnel can take the necessary precautions to protect both themselves and the patients, but the hidden case still poses grave danger to all who come in contact with such a patient.

In spite of the skilled technique and knowledge and the increasing use of presterilized and disposable hospital equipment, the hospital ward still remains a dangerously contaminated place. The miracle drugs have compounded the problem to some degree because of the incidence of pathogens which have become resistant to them. The problem of staphylococcic infection in the modern hospital continues to be very serious. The dimensions of the problem are, of course, founded in the certainty that the population in the hospital is one that is unusually susceptible to infection. The patients are there because they are sick enough to be hospitalized in the first place; they are vulnerable because their illnesses increase the likelihood of contracting an infection and the danger of being unable to withstand it.

One area of particular sensitivity lies in the incidence of postoperative wound infection. The surgical wound is prepared so that normal healing will take place promptly and without incident. The amount of tissue damage during a surgical procedure is minimized by the skill of the surgeon. However, if a wound becomes infected, the pattern of healing is radically changed. The inflammatory process extends the amount of tissue damage. The systemic effects of the infection add to the already considerable demands made on the patient who has had a recent operation. And instead of a tight, closed wound in eight days, the individual may be faced with a wide, draining, and destructive inflammatory process that may persist for many weeks. The relatively simple task of restoring structural integrity in the operative site becomes a complex one that threatens the integrity of the surgical wound and may threaten the integrity of the entire surgical procedure. The nurse should be thoroughly acquainted with the appearance of a healing wound in all of its stages. Observation of the surgical patient includes an examination of the wound, when possible, and a precise description of its appearance on the patient's chart. The surgical nurse must learn to recognize the allowable amount of redness and induration (hard swelling) which accompanies healing in the early stages and to determine, as soon as possible, changes that indicate the possibility of a developing infection.

When the wound, whether surgical or traumatic, is frankly infected, every precaution must be made to prevent the spread of the causative organism in the ward. Frequent observation of the wound, its appearance and changes in it from day to day, must be made to assess the effect of treatment. Control of the inflammatory process and a rapid debridement contribute to a limitation of the amount of tissue damage that will take place. The sooner healing begins, the less likely it is that a structural insult will leave the patient with extensive scarring. The presence of a scar on the body always represents a structural change; though many are merely cosmetic and do not alter function, some may be extensive enough to create problems of function restoration. Since the therapeutic goal in the care of all infection is to terminate the inflammatory process as soon as possible, the active intervention of the nurse is an essential factor in limiting and restricting the amount of tissue damage accompanying an infection. In this sense, nursing care directly influences the conservation of structural integrity, and all nursing measures employed in the care of the patient with an acute infectious process are essential components of the therapeutic plan.

Protection from infection and the subsequent threat of structural damage is fundamental in the personal hygiene offered to all patients. It is this compelling threat that dictates the need for cleanliness, position change and mobilization, adequate nutrition, and aseptic precautions in the use and preparation of materials required in daily patient care. Protection from minor injury in the environment also rests on this concept as a break in the skin barrier will predispose an individual to a struggle to heal. And, of course, the introduction of disease by a nurse who has an upper respiratory infection, a hand or finger infection, or a gastrointestinal upset that may be infectious must always be zealously prevented. The potential for injury which attends carrying an infection to the ward should always be weighed carefully by the individual whose conscientious desire to go on duty tempts her to ignore her own illness.

The Conservation of Personal Integrity

In the jargon of the hospital, the infected patient is a "dirty case." The degree to which this description influences the nurse's view of the patient varies with the individual nurse. But there is inherent in such a description an element of disapproval and disdain that may, in silent ways, influence the care received by the patient. The offending organism can always hide from the observer, but the ugly effects of the infection are easily seen. The purulent exudate is a repulsive liquid and often evil-smelling as well. The tissue destruction creates a lesion where necrosis, sloughing, and inflammation combine to repel the observer. The patient is well aware of these factors too, and his ability to confront them may be even less than that of the nurse. It is always surprising when healing does not occur, because all of life's experiences encourage the expectation that it will. The postoperative patient who has successfully survived the operation only to face a long bout with a wound infection must be, at the very least, a disappointed man.

The systemic effects of an acute infectious process are almost always accompanied by a lethargy and withdrawal determined by the altered physiological function of the body. Malaise is not an uncommon experience, since it accompanies acute respiratory disease; most people have personally contended with the feelings of illness, weakness, discomfort, and discouragement that are characteristic of this response. It is difficult to muster confidence and enthusiasm when all of the biochemistry of the body is conspiring against it. For this reason, the acute phases of an infection leave a patient with an emotional tone over which he has very little control. It is certainly true that every human being responds to this experience in his own way, generally in a pattern of behavior predicated on his usual reaction to stressful situations. Some people want to withdraw completely and constantly beg to be "left alone." Others become extremely demanding and express their discomfort and disaffection as a kind of projection into every activity in which they are involved. In the first instance, the misery seeks annihilation in withdrawal; in the second, it seeks company, but in either case the defense of personal integrity has become an active process.

The individual with an infection soon identifies nursing activities that isolate him to some degree. Even if he remains on an open ward, the caution (wisely) stimulated by the infection takes the form of aseptic ritual; and though such is not intended this can easily be interpreted as rejection. If his infection requires actual isolation, the problems are exaggerated. Physical isolation of the individual removes him from the freedom to interact in his environment that provides the distraction and involvement so essential to the human organism. It also sets him apart and emphasizes that, for the time being, he represents a threat to other human beings. Isolation procedures involve time for the nurse and other personnel, and the widespread tendency is to limit contact with the isolated patient on the rationalization that time must be saved for other tasks. He is witness to the very special treatment accorded to the ordinary implements around him. Either his dishes are disinfected before they are removed, or else he is served a meal on disposable dishes that can be easily destroyed. No one enters his room who is not gowned and often masked as well. There is much to-do about "clean areas" and "dirty areas," and he is expected to understand these too. His own family members are as disguised behind the isolation costumes as are hospital personnel. He may or may not be allowed a radio or a television set. It is obvious that, in addition to the sickness which takes its physiological toll on him, the idea that he is being punished or unloved is easily fostered. The limitation of contact, even with the nurse and the physician, is an invitation to increased anxiety and dread. And if there is a genuine withholding of time and attention on the part of personnel, his suspicion that he is being shunted aside may have a firm footing in reality. The striking of a balance between recognizing the wisdom of isolation to restrain the infection, on the one hand, and a therapeutic approach to the individual's personal integrity, on the other, is obviously a considerable problem. The solution rests on the human interaction created in the nurse-patient contact. To the degree that the nurse can communicate continuing concern and interest in him, even in relatively limited time periods, the patient can recognize that the isolation is in his interest and somehow tolerate it better. Nurses frequently must participate with patients in treatment that is disagreeable or even painful. In such instances, it is never wise to ignore the reality or pretend that it is not there, and most individuals respond positively when their plight is recognized, even though it cannot be eliminated.

The prevention of infection is another definitive contribution to the conservation of personal integrity. For the hospitalized patient the assurance of safety from infection, while he struggles with the disease that brought him to bed, is a contribution to the personal goals of convalescense. The additional burden of infection means a prolonged hospitalization, with all of the social, economic, physiological, and physical dislocations that are involved. If recovery from surgery allows the individual to resume his normal life after ten days, the cost of an additional week is more than he should be required to pay. And if the additional disease threatens his life, as, indeed, it may, then the personal cost cannot be measured.

Conservation of Social Integrity

Isolation means separation from other human beings, and the implications of such an experience are best understood in the social context. The anxiety and feelings of rejection experienced by the patient are very easily communicated to the human beings with whom he normally has a social exchange. The wisdom of restricting the possibility of spreading his pathogen can hardly mean the same thing to the patient or to his family that it means to the professional practitioner. And in those instances when the infection arose directly from the fact of hospitalization itself, the devices that isolate the patient from his family are readily interpreted in hostile ways. The isolation may be a physical reality, requiring separate placement and treatment in the ward. But it may also be the continued isolation of hospitalization itself, arising from the necessity to remain in the hospital, because of an infection, well past the expectation that the patient and his family may have entertained before he entered. The additional burden on the family resource, both in actual cost and in continued removal from the family group, is an expense that nurses must understand. The further threat of an exaggeration of the illness and the implications for the patient's future constitutes another dimension of reaction in the family group.

The same naïveté that encourages the lay public to ascribe illness to "germs" characterizes their expectations that a miracle drug will wipe such an illness away. The concept of mutative strains of organisms that are not susceptible to antibiotic treatment is rather sophisticated, and the problem is compounded by the free publication of the results of incomplete research with its promise of magical cures. The increase of hospital-induced infection has not escaped the attention of the public media either, and indeed it should not. But all of these common attitudes come with the patient and his family to the hospital, and hospital personnel cannot ignore their influence in the treatment of the patient.

The highly specialized knowledge, which directs the activities of the nurse in the care of the patient with an inflammatory condition, places a special burden on nurses to assume a responsible role in the dissemination of essential information to the public. It is unthinkable that any child be denied the protection of a thorough immunization program. Where ignorance fosters this denial, knowledge must be spread; where immunization is a question of dollars and cents, the economy must be educated to support it. The central issues of health have moved away from the problem of infection towards the research effort directed at noninfectious disease entities. But the importance of knowledge concerning ways to control pathogenic spread of disease continues just the same, and in some social situations the threat persists in spite of the excellence of modern therapeutic intervention.

There is perhaps no area of infectious disease more threatening than the dissemination of venereal infections. The incidence of venereal disease showed a marked decline when the therapeutic methods became effective following the Second World War. But in recent years, the increase in these diseases, especially in adolescents and young adults, has created a justifiable alarm. Extensive public health efforts to spread information about the dangers of venereal infection deserve the support and active assistance of nurses. In this single disease there is evidence that relaxation and loss of interest in control of infection constitute an invitation to serious renewal of social and medical problems.

The social integrity of all patients is intimately associated with the larger integrity of the social group. Just as the individual nurse cannot abandon her aseptic skill for even a moment during the care of patients, the professional practitioners, as members of society, cannot abandon their continued interest and concern in the control of infectious disease. The ubiquitous microorganism has not surrendered to modern science, and only constant vigilance will insure the relative freedom presently enjoyed by twentieth century populations.

In a real sense, the aseptic conscience of the practitioner arises from his dedication to the social integrity of the patient. In the social system that characterizes human interaction in the hospital, the burden of knowledge must ultimately be translated into a recognition of social responsibility. Control of infection in the hospital ward stems, in the first place, from the social structure that identifies any group of human beings functioning collectively in the pursuit of mutually valuable goals. The patient comes to the hospital with the desire to be healed, and the practitioner is there because he has chosen the science of healing as a means of finding his own integrity as a human being. All asepsis is a product of the social integrity which is a goal of healing and in its broadest sense demands the personal commitment that alone insures the group welfare.

Model IX: Establishing an Aseptic Environment

OBJECTIVES

1. To understand and utilize the microbiological principles that determine the characteristics of the aseptic environment.
2. To understand and practice the principles guiding the role of the individual nurse in the establishment and maintenance of an aseptic environment.
3. To understand the threat to asepsis created by the nature and function of the hospital unit.
4. To understand the physiological functions which provide the body's defense against insult, injury, or infection.
5. To understand the specific behaviors of common pathogens so as to adapt the environment for the individual patient and thus limit the microbial population.
6. To recognize the legal and moral implications involved in bacteriological control in the hospital with particular emphasis on the development of an "aseptic conscience" by the individual nurse.
7. To understand the necessity for teaching individual patients the fundamental principles of asepsis as a means of limiting cross-contamination and insuring the safety of the individual in the hospital environment.

ESSENTIAL SCIENCE CONCEPTS

1. Microorganisms are ubiquitous in every environment.
   - 1.1 Normal body defenses protect the individual so that life processes are not threatened under ordinary conditions of health.
   - 1.2 Some microorganisms live in symbiosis with other living things.
   - 1.3 The ability of microorganisms to cause disease depends on many variables.
     - 1.31 Specificity of the host.
     - 1.32 Availability of susceptible hosts.
       - 1.321 Establishment of required modes of transmission.
       - 1.322 Individual ability of the host to defend himself.
         - 1.3221 An intact defense barrier against invasion from the external environment.
         - 1.3222 Age of the host.
         - 1.3223 Nutritional status.
         - 1.3224 Genetic capability.
         - 1.3225 Previous exposure to immunity-conferring infection.
         - 1.3226 Absence of concurrent disease.
       - 1.323 Environmental factors.

1.3231 Number of patients in a given area.
1.3232 Selection of diagnostic entities in the geographic placement of patients.
1.3233 Utilization and means for disinfection of equipment and personal possessions.
1.3234 Administrative policy and supervision to insure safe aseptic practice of all personnel concerned with the care of the patient.
1.3235 Accurate diagnosis and provision for isolation of infected individuals.
1.3236 Skill and conscience of practitioners.

1.33 Pathogenicity of microorganisms present in the environment.
1.331 Ability to cause disease in the human host is influenced by the virulence of the microbial strain.
1.3311 Virulence is increased by rapid transmission through a biological population.
1.3312 Virulence is decreased by rapid transmission through an artificial medium in the laboratory.
1.332 Ability to cause disease may result from an environmental factor which changes symbiosis to pathogenicity.

1.34 Infection with pathogens may be asymptomatic or symptomatic.
1.341 "Carrier" transmission of pathogens.
1.342 Prodromal infection without awareness of impending illness.
1.343 Portal of entry.
1.3431 Inhalation.
1.3432 Gastrointestinal tract.
1.3433 Break in skin or mucosa.
1.34331 Hematogenous spread.
1.34332 Ascending infection to vital organs.
1.34333 Localized infection.

2. Control of microorganisms in the environment depends on the knowledge and skill of the practitioner.

2.1 The ritual of asepsis is based on knowledge of the behavior of microorganisms.
2.11 Mechanical removal of microorganisms.
2.111 Handwashing techniques (including use of soaps and detergents to lower surface tension and increase solubility of contaminants).
2.112 Cleansing of implements used in patient care.
2.1121 Accessibility for thorough mechanical scrubbing (as in tubing, needles, etc).
2.1122 Cleansing technique designed for materials being used.
2.12 Maintenance of an absolutely dry field since fluids provide organisms with a transport system.

2.13 Control of air currents to prevent transmission of airborne contaminants as far as possible.

2.14 Identification of clean and contaminated working areas in the administrative structure of the ward to control populations of bacteria as far as possible.

2.15 Disinfection of surface areas and equipment.

2.151 Chemical disinfection depends on denaturation of proteins and permeability of bacterial cell membrane.

2.152 Sterilization by physical means results from denaturation of proteins of the bacteria by heat.

2.1521 Steam can be superheated only by an increase in the atmospheric pressure (autoclave).

2.1522 Boiling effectively kills some organisms.

2.15221 Length of time of exposure to temperature of boiling water.

2.15222 Tolerance to boiling of material being sterilized.

2.2 Establishment of an aseptic environment is a function of the purposes for which it is being done.

2.21 Medical asepsis is established whenever it is necessary to exclude pathogenic organisms from a prescribed area.

2.211 Evidence of infectious disease in a patient where transmission to others must be prevented.

2.2111 Factors in establishing limits of contamination vary with the nature of the pathogen.

2.2112 The administrative structure of the ward influences the method and techniques of isolation.

2.212 Failure of body defense that makes it necessary to protect the patient from microorganisms in the environment.

2.22 Surgical asepsis is established whenever it is necessary to exclude all microorganisms from a prescribed area.

2.221 Deliberate surgical interference with the natural barriers.

2.222 Protection from secondary infection during the healing period following surgical procedures or traumatic injury.

NURSING PROCESS

1. The nurse's individual role is crucial to the establishment of an aseptic environment.

1.1 The aseptic conscience.

1.11 The only test for adequacy of technique is by bacteriological sample—a procedure requiring a minimum of 24 hours.

1.12 The skilled performance of recognized technique offers indirect assurance of successful asepsis.

1.13 Awareness of possible contaminating factors is the scrupulous responsibility of the individual practitioner.

1.14 Legal and moral responsibility for the safety of the patient provides the practitioner with compelling need to observe aseptic excellence, whether it involves the nurse alone or the behavior of another practitioner.

1.2 Attention to personal hygiene of the nurse is a contribution to safeguarding the patient from infection.

1.21 Clean uniform, shoes, laces, and cap.

1.22 Proper nail care.

1.23 Frequent shampoos and hair style that precludes possibility of contamination from this source.

1.24 Persistent handwashing habits, on the ward and off.

1.25 Absenting the nurse from duty when she has an infection or infectious disease, including upper respiratory disease.

1.26 Current immunizations.

1.3 Knowledge of the characteristics of a variety of microorganisms so that decisions concerning patient care can be made sensibly and safely.

2. The technical skills insure safe practice of aseptic techniques.

2.1 Clear establishment and understanding of the designated clean and contaminated areas in any aseptic process.

2.2 Proper sterilization of supplies, with regular bacteriological testing procedures being used.

2.3 Planning the activities required in the successful performance of an aseptic technique in safe sequence, anticipating, by organization of materials, the steps to be followed in the procedure.

2.4 Zealous protection of the sterile field by movement around it.

2.41 The operator always faces the sterile field.

2.42 Never reach over a sterile field.

2.43 Use of masks to prevent airborne contamination.

2.44 Strict limitation of traffic and/or observers in the immediate vicinity (for example, close off a treatment room).

2.45 Conversation during the procedure is kept to absolute essential minimum.

2.5 All materials expected to remain sterile MUST be kept absolutely dry.

2.6 The line of division between sterile and contaminated areas must be scrupulously respected.

2.61 Instruments in disinfectant solutions are always held point down to prevent transmission of contaminants by fluid flow from sterile to contaminated end, and then back to the sterile area.

2.62 Even if the pouring lip of a container is known to be sterile, the surfaces of containers never touch each other during transfer of materials from one container to another.

2.63 The outer edge of a sterile field is defined as contaminated within a range of 2 to 6 inches, depending on the procedure being done.

2.64 Materials taken from the sterile area which have been used and contaminated are NEVER put back into the sterile field.

2.641 Bloody soilage on dressings or instruments represents a potentially excellent medium, so that such items are immediately removed from the sterile area.

2.642 Contaminated articles are promptly disposed of.

2.6421 Reusable instruments and implements are placed in a container away from the sterile field.

2.6422 Dressings and soiled disposable materials are immediately placed in a liquid-proof paper bag, the outer surface of which is kept clean to allow for ultimate closure.

2.6423 Proper cleansing procedures, dependent upon materials involved, precede the resterilization of articles used.

2.7 The cautious establishment of the sterile field is fundamental to a safe procedure.

2.71 The area chosen must itself be clean.

2.72 Draping of the area sets the limit of recognized sterility.

2.721 Draping materials must be nonporous.

2.722 Damaged materials of all kinds must be rejected.

2.723 Edges used to handle drapes are clearly contaminated.

2.724 Placement of the drape is always towards the operator when working over the contaminated area.

3. Isolation of individual patients to restrict transmission of known pathogens is accomplished by clear definition of clean and contaminated areas.

3.1 Definition of contamination includes the gowning of the nurse.

3.2 Decontamination of materials used is dependent upon the organism for which the isolation procedure is established.

3.21 Degree of isolation is determined by the portal of entry of the organism.

3.22 Body wastes and disposable materials may require preliminary decontamination before being discarded in a central sewage system.

3.23 Cleansing of nondisposable items requires sterilization procedures suitable to adequate removal of the organism.

3.231 Linen may be placed in specially marked bags before sending to the laundry.

3.232 Food service implements must be cleaned before removal to the usual washing site.

3.233 Reusable implements, such as bedpan, should be retained in the unit until isolation is discontinued, with cleansing and proper disposal of wastes after each use.

3.3 Entering the isolation unit is forbidden without proper gowning, handwashing, and observation of correct procedure.

3.4 Observation of clean and contaminated areas within the unit must always be precise.

3.41 Touching any area, such as doorknobs, should be performed with protective material such as paper towels or squares, to prevent contamination of defined clean areas.

3.42 An area of cleanliness must be provided for and protected within the isolation area.

3.5 Patient should be taught how to respect the isolation procedure within the limits of his ability to understand and perform.

4. Isolation of individual patients to protect them from microorganisms when their own defenses are impaired.

4.1 Aseptic techniques approach the rigidity of surgical asepsis for protective or "reverse" isolation.

4.2 Minimize traffic into the area to lessen the opportunity for cross-contamination.

5. Isolation for microbiological control results in social isolation for the patient.

5.1 Patient should understand the reasons for his isolation, if possible.

5.2 Diversional activity allowable in terms of the patient's condition and the restrictions of isolation should be provided.

5.3 Adjustments which jeopardize the isolation limits cannot be allowed (as removal of screens), but patient should be instructed in the importance of such restrictions.

5.4 Bedside contact can be emotionally supportive if the time is used wisely–true interaction is a function of quality, not quantity.

5.5 Visitor restrictions must be explained to patient and family members.

5.51 Family members should be assisted in gowning and disposal of gown following visit.

5.52 Family members should be supervised in handwashing after visit is terminated.

5.6 Intellectual understanding of the restrictions of isolation may not exclude emotional response of patient and family members.

5.61 Recognition of expressions of anxiety and fear in patient and family allows consideration of needs arising from isolation.

5.62 Explanation of restrictions in language that can be understood, offered sympathetically and reiterated as needed.

Vocabulary

antibiotic
aseptic conscience
attenuated vaccine
avascular
bacteremia
carrier
cellulitis
chemotaxis
cicatrization
debridement
diapedesis
disease reservoir
endemic
epidemic
fibrous tissue substitution
friable
healing
host
hyperemia
immunity
infection
inflammation
isolation
leukotaxine
localization
malaria
margination
medical asepsis
pathogens
prodromal
protective isolation
resistance
resolution
reverse isolation
scar
septicemia
specificity
surgical asepsis
susceptible
virulence

General Bibliography

MOORE, FRANCIS D.: Give and Take. Doubleday & Co., Inc., Garden City, N.Y., 1965.

NETER, ERWIN: Medical Microbiology, ed. 5. F. A. Davis Co., Philadelphia, 1966.

Articles

AGER, ERNEST A.: Current concepts in immunization. Amer. J. Nurs. 66:2004-2011, Sept. 1966.

BILLINGHAM, R. E.: Tissue transplantation: Scope and prospect. Science 153:266-270, July 1966.

BRAND, LUCY, AND KOMORITA, NORI: Adapting to long-term dialysis. Amer. J. Nurs. 66:1778-1781, Aug. 1966.

BRAUDE, A. I.: Bacterial endotoxins. Sci. Amer. 210:34-45, March 1964.

BUCHANAN-DAVIDSON, DOROTHY J.: A drop of blood. Amer. J. Nurs. 65:103-107, July 1965.

BURNET, SIR MACFARLANE: Concepts of autoimmune disease and their implications for therapy. Perspect. Biol. Med. 10:141-151, Winter 1967.

FREIMER, EARL H., AND MCCARTHY, MACLYN: Rheumatic fever. Sci. Amer. 213:66-74, Dec. 1965.

GORINI, LUIGI: Antibiotics and the genetic code. Sci. Amer. 214:102-109, April 1966.

GREENBERG, BERNARD: Flies and disease. Sci. Amer. 213:92-99, July 1965.
HARDER, HELEN I., AND CHRIST, NANCY: The peril of glove powder. Amer. J. Nurs. 66:761-764, April 1966.
KLINE, PATRICIA A.: Isolating patients with staphylococcal infection. Amer. J. Nurs. 65:102-104, Jan. 1965.
KRETZER, MARION L.: Another look at Typhoid Mary. Nurs. Sci. II:487-491, Dec. 1964.
LANGER, WILLIAM L.: The black death. Sci. Amer. 210:114-121, March 1964.
NOSSAL, G. J. V.: How cells make antibodies. Sci. Amer. 211:106-115, Dec. 1964.
SEIDLER, FLORENCE M.: Adapting nursing procedures for reverse isolation. Amer. J. Nurs. 65:108-111, June 1965.
SHEBELSKI, DOROTHY I.: Nursing patients who have renal homotransplants. Amer. J. Nurs. 66:2425-2428, Nov. 1966.
SPEIRS, ROBERT S.: How cells attack antigens. Sci. Amer. 210:58-64, March 1964.
TREXLER, P. C.: Germ-free isolators. Sci. Amer. 211:78-88, July 1964.

10 The Dimensions of the Organismic Response

The Individual Actively Participates in His Environment

Activity and living are almost synonymous terms. The staggering display of activity represented by the incessant chemical exchange within cells is only a little less breathtaking than the amazing ability of the separate systems to function together so that life is supported and the individual is recognizable as an integrated organism. It is, moreover, upon these two limits of life activity that the scientific community focuses concern. The molecular biologist, armed with knowledge of the intricate chemical structure of subcellular components of living systems, contributes the detailed and enlightening behavior of essential substances, and this same information explains and expands understanding of the functional organism. There are some scientists who believe that the unanswered questions of health and disease will eventually be expressed in chemical formulae and others who must view the interaction of many organized systems as the basis for understanding the issues of well-being. Both viewpoints are, of course, necessary. The pathophysiology becomes understandable both within the context of cellular change and within that of the effects of such alterations on the life-processes of the entire organism. Science education must turn increasingly towards the knowledge explored by the molecular biologist. The influence of this knowledge on diagnosis, therapy, and the prevention of disease makes it important to the modern nurse. But nursing, by its very nature, has always had to focus concern on the behavior of the individual, and the interaction which characterizes the nursing situation, by its very nature, demands understanding at the organism level as well. It is significant that the era of molecular biology has paralleled the era of environmental biology. The range of research that extends from the structural model of a chemical in the nuclei of individual cells to the study of the relationships of living organisms within their environmental milieu promises the nurse an equally broad range of professional practice.

Conceptually, the study of molecular exchanges and the study of environmental interactions are very similar. The chemical reaction is founded on energy exchanges and displacements. The orderly transaction that characterizes the chemical change is created out of the relationships existing between the parties to that change. When the participants are known and their behavior is, therefore, predictable, the result of their interaction also becomes predictable. The ability to predict often also means an ability to measure, and, of course, the measurement of observed phenomena is the foundation of all scientific inquiry. Arthur Compton, the Nobel prize-winning physicist, said, "Science is founded upon a belief that the world is reliable in its operations." To the scientist, reliability means a system of measurement which any observer can duplicate. Obviously, it is easier to apply such rigorous tests to inanimate systems and to have the confidence, necessary as a consequence of measurement, that duplication will constantly reflect the same results. Even very complex chemical reactions, such as those involving living tissues, are more susceptible to scientific certainty than are the complex environmental interactions which arise, at least in part, from the wilful choice of the organism. And yet, the environmental biologist can confidently describe the effects of individual interaction with environmental conditions and be reasonably certain that his generalization will be sound. Some of the certainty depends on the chemical and, therefore, energy exchange. Some reflects the reiteration of response that has previously been described under very similar environmental circumstances. In fact, the practice of the healing arts is clearly founded on learning to predict a response to a given set of circumstances, in the precipitating of a disease process or in prescribing treatment.

Just as the molecular biologist has provided new insight into the cellular interaction, the environmental biologist provides essential information that illuminates the organismic interaction. The individual is always within an environmental milieu, and the consequences of his awareness of his environment persistently influence his behavior at any given moment. There is nothing new in this idea. Everyday experience with temperature change, for example, soon teaches the individual how to seek comfort within a thermal continuum. If he is chilled, he learns to wear appropriate clothing; if he is overly warmed, he plans a day at the beach. The choices available to him are also products of his environmental milieu. How he defends the homeostasis of his internal temperature depends on where he lives. An individual who spends his life in a tropical climate adapts to the climatic demand and is aided in his adaptation by the availability of materials in his environment. Such a lifetime of adaptation may actually create alterations in the basic pattern of energy production and utilization in his body. In one study, for example, which contrasted the adaptations to temperature variation as evidenced by body structure and life-style in two very different ethnic groups living in Africa, the environmental challenge was faced in very different ways. A group of Caucasians living in a large and cosmopolitan city enjoyed environmental choice of solidly built homes, a wide choice of external clothing, and even air conditioning to temper the extremes of climate. A desert nomad tribe depended, instead, on the adaptations in their living pattern to sucessfully withstand the extremes of temperature in their environment. The surface area of the body compared to the total body weight provides a ratio (or relationship) that indicates the ability of the individual to conserve body heat or to transfer it freely. A low ratio of body surface to weight improves the individual's ability to conserve body heat and is directly related to the layer of fat that insulates the internal body structure. The layer of fat, in turn, depends on the diet. And the selection of foods in the diet is strictly limited by their availability in any given region. The city dwellers had a low ratio of body surface to weight. The members of the nomadic tribe, on the other hand, had a high ratio, indicating that they could freely lose body heat. In the seasonal change, however, the nomadic people did not have the choice of air conditioning or stoves to stabilize their thermal environment. During the hot summer, they wore only loincloths and always rested for long intervals during the middle part of the day. During the colder winters, they slept around a central fire, their bodies entirely covered with skin cloaks, huddling together to share their body warmth. Their alternative to turning on the stove, moreover, was more than enough to provide a "microclimate" immediately around their bodies to maintain their internal temperature as well as to provide adequate comfort. The thermostat of the nomadic tribesman is his feet, which he points towards the fire; as the fire dies during the night, the decreasing temperature of his feet awakens him, so that he can stoke his fire and thus insure the comfort of his family. Although many variables were measured in this study, the remarkable consistency in the ability of individuals to tolerate extremes of heat and cold with equal facility, in spite of their widely different life patterns, testifies to the plasticity of adaptation available to human beings. But it also does something more. It emphasizes that the final measure has a validity transcending the variables and permits the environmental researcher to make generalizations from his observations of widely divergent behaviors. The highly individualized solutions available to each of these groups of people are significant because of the uniqueness of their behavior. In addition, the choice or selection of the methods of temperature control was dependent entirely upon the environment in which they lived.

It is now apparent that a selection of artifacts in the environment and the use of the materials found there are possible only through an *assessment* and an *awareness* of the environment itself. The poetic aspects of mankind's capability to adapt and use the environment to his own purpose are exciting. Robinson Crusoe continues to fascinate the young reader because of his imaginative use of the resources available to him. But, satisfying as such solutions to unusual situations may be, the daily—even momentary—interchange between the environment and the individual, even in the most ordinary events, is far more amazing. The human organism is a sentient being, and the ability to interact with the environment seems ineluctably tied to his sensory organs. In the language of the modern automated machine, the scientist talks about "sensory input." The description of a passive receptor, receiving stimuli via the sense organs, and the wondrous computer in the brain, interpreting and collating the information so that behavioral decisions can be made, fails entirely to encompass the remarkable interaction that really takes place. The reception of sensory stimuli by the sensory organs is never—or very rarely—a discrete, simple, unified response. The organism is never—or very rarely—a passive recipient of environmental information. The knowledge that comes to the individual every moment from his environment is a summation of many simultaneous sensory responses, *many of which he actively seeks.* And furthermore, his presence in the environment also influences it and thereby the kind of information available from it. Tradition describes five senses: sight, hearing, smell, taste, and touch. The sense of balance is often added to this list. All that the individual knows of his environment and, in fact, all conscious awareness must come to him through his sensory apparatus. The evidence of the senses is all an individual has with which to identify himself in his environment. Whitehead said, ". . . our only exact data as to the physical world are our sensible perceptions. . . ."[3] The word "perception" (from the Latin *perceptio,* "gathering in") has come to mean awareness or consciousness. It is often used in a broader, social sense to imply the ability of the individual to make fine judgements; such individuals are described as "perceptive." In its stricter sense, however, perception is the reception of environmental stimuli via the sensory organs. Thus, perception is comprehension of the "physical world."

Experience alone must create some doubt as to the inviolability of sensible perception. Every child has been fascinated by optical illusions, and it is a matter of common knowledge that three witnesses to the same event will each reveal a very different account of what happened. The sensory organs play "tricks." If an individual listens to a watch tick and looks at a bright light at the same time, the tick of the watch is noticeably louder. The distinctive physiological characteristics of perception in the behavior of sensory organs have been studied, and many details of the physiological changes are well known. The visual perception of distances in space, for example, is related to the individual's determination of the size of objects within his visual field; experience soon teaches him that as the distance becomes greater the image becomes smaller. Many factors that influence the information provided by visual stimuli are understood. The study of specific organs, however, and a description of their specific function, does not provide enough information about the individual's perception of his environment. Such localization of attention denies the interaction between the kinds of sensory information actually sought by the individual and those aspects of the environment that influence his behavior by producing stimulation to several sensory organs at the same time.

The human organism is a terrestrial animal, adapted to breathe air within a specific pressure gradient. If a human being seeks to alter that fundamental relationship by flying into the sea of air or diving into the watery ocean, he can do so only if he brings his own environment with him. The escape from both the atmosphere and the gravitational effect has been achieved through space flight, but the most important information provided by these projects is related to the physiological response to these radically altered conditions. The firm earth is man's habitat. His body is adapted to the rigidity of solid ground underfoot. Upon the surface of the earth he stands and walks, and with every step he tests the solidity and rigidity of the support it offers him. He balances his body against the effects of gravity through a structural design that is mediated by his nervous system and accomplished by a skeletal-muscle system which can withstand the stress of moving against the gravitational force. The ability to move depends upon his ability to be aware of where he is, and he decides where he is going on the strength of what he *perceives*. This is not a simple matter of "seeing where he is going." The direction he chooses comes from the information brought to him by a talented and capable capacity to orient himself in his environment. In the larger task of orientation, the sensorium comprises, in Gibson's words, "energy receptors," which respond to the "modes of attention": listening, touching, smelling, tasting, and looking.

Gibson proposes that the behavior of the organism in its environment must be understood as mediated by "perceptual systems." Such systems indicate that the external senses are ". . . active, rather than passive," and that they ". . . function to pick up information, not simply to arouse sensations. . . ." The effect of all stimuli on the sensory organ itself represents an energy exchange; thus, the environmental effect on the organism represents, from an external source, a modification of the organism's very sub-

Table 13: The Perceptual Systems

NAME	MODE OF ATTENTION	RECEPTIVE UNITS	ANATOMY OF THE ORGAN	ACTIVITY OF THE ORGAN	STIMULI AVAILABLE	EXTERNAL INFORMATION OBTAINED
The basic orienting system	General orientation	Mechano-receptors	Vestibular organs	Body equilibrium	Forces of gravity and acceleration	Direction of gravity, being pushed
The auditory system	Listening	Mechano-receptors	Cochlear organs with middle ear and auricle	Orienting to sounds	Vibration in the air	Nature and location of vibratory events
The haptic system	Touching	Mechano-receptors and possibly Thermo-receptors	Skin (including attachments and openings) Joints (including ligaments) Muscles (including tendons)	Exploration of many kinds	Deformations of tissues Configuration of joints Stretching of muscle fibers	Contact with the earth Mechanical encounters Object shapes Material states Solidity or viscosity
The taste-smell system	Smelling	Chemo-receptors	Nasal cavity (nose)	Sniffing	Composition of the medium	Nature of volatile sources
	Tasting	Chemo- and Mechano-receptors	Oral cavity (mouth)	Savoring	Composition of ingested objects	Nutritive and biochemical values
The visual system	Looking	Photo-receptors	Ocular mechanism (eyes, with intrinsic and extrinsic eye muscles, as related to the vestibular organs, the head, and the whole body)	Accommodation Pupillary adjustment Fixation convergence Exploration	The variables of structure in ambient light	Everything that can be specified by the variables of optical structure (information about objects, animals, motions, events, and places)

(From Gibson: *The Senses Considered As Perceptual Systems*, Houghton Mifflin Co., New York, 1966.)

stance as definitive as the energy exchanges which characterize its "internal" life. The information brought to the individual by his senses is essential to his defense of his integrity as an individual. While mere sensation presupposes activity in the sensory organ, the structuring of a cogent message, of information, demands that the initiating change create a sequence of change that ultimately involves the entire organism. The eye is the sensory organ which responds to the energy of light because it possesses retinal cells that are photosensitive. But vision is considerably more than the effect of light energy on the retinal cells. The eye itself is structured to bend the light waves and direct them to the retinal receptors. It is a movable organ, even in its relatively fixed position in the bony cages of the skull, and thus has muscles which allow it to sweep back and forth across the "field" of the immediate environment. It can adjust its ability to bend the light waves to objects close at hand as well as to objects far away; in addition, it can detect the movement of objects in the environment, even if the head is held absolutely still. The range of motion of the head also increases the range of the visual field available to the receptor organ itself. Gibson indicates that the stabilizing of the eyes in the head depends, in turn, upon the sensory organ of stabilization in the inner ear. The individual eye can scan its own field, but two eyes not only scan a much wider area, but add stereoscopic information as well. He writes, ". . . the two-eyes-with-head-and-body system, in cooperation with postural equilibrium and locomotion, can get around in the world and look at everything." There is, thus, a very real distinction to be made between the simple reception of visual stimuli and the organism's ability to use the visual system to experience its environment.

The visual system is certainly an important one, and it often provides information which substantiates that available from the other perceptual systems. The auditory system responds to vibratory energy, according to Gibson, but the ears do not only detect sound. They also can detect the direction from which a sound is coming. The haptic system provides information that arises out of the pressure of touching. In this sense, while there is no specific organ that responds to touch, the entire body is a perceptual organ. The hands explore and thus provide information usually confirmed by the visual system. The taste-smell system responds to chemical stimuli and is essential to the nutrition of the organism. But mere odor and taste are not the only determinants in the selection and ingestion of food. Food brought into the mouth is also felt, and before it is swallowed, its characteristics are explored by a combination of haptic (touching) information as well as chemical (taste-smell) information. Gibson also describes the basic orienting system, in which the sensory organ is the balancing portion of the inner ear. This organ responds to position change in relation to gravity, as well as to changes in the acceleration, or movement, of the organism, including the beginning and the cessation of motion in any plane. The basic orienting system is essential to the proper function of all other perceptual systems, and it is described by Gibson as providing "a frame of reference for them."

The perceptual systems provide information to the individual; usually this is knowledge sought by the individual. The hungry organism searches for food. While this is relatively simple to understand in a predator stalking his prey, it is equally important to the human being when his body tells him it needs to be replenished with nutrients. He does not go out seeking his meal as the lion does by stalking, pursuing, and perhaps overpowering another animal. The smell of food cooking in the kitchen arouses his attention and begins to prepare him for the act of ingesting the food. If his physiological signal has been sent, and there is no smell or sound of preparation, he may make a trip to the refrigerator, survey its contents, make his decision, and select the food he hungers for. Even when the specific object of exploration of the environment is not as definite as the satisfaction of hunger, the individual is constantly and actively seeking information which indicates where he is, what he is doing, and, often, whether he is safe. The process of gaining information from the environment is continuous, perhaps operative to some degree even during sleep. Certainly some of the information that incessantly enters upon his conscious awareness is reiterative, and therefore reassuring, and serves to establish the dimensions of the reality as he perceives it. Familiarity decreases the need for some kinds of information or simply renders them into a background of reference which previous experience has taught the individual poses no threat to him.

This view of the individual in persistent exchange with the environment is an important consideration in the care of the hospitalized patient. First, of course, there are the obvious situations in which the disease process obstructs the function of a perceptual system and thus limits the reception of information by the patient. Specific disease may afflict a sense organ so that the reception of the initiating energy required to establish the perceptual information is blocked at the source. Diseases of the eye or ear which either temporarily or permanently prevent the reception of information about the environment immediately alter the perceptual capabilities of the individual. In fact, much of the emphasis in the nursing care of such patients must be concerned with the environmental adaptations required by this altered perception of the environment. The importance of the visual system in gaining information about the environment is very apparent in the helplessness felt by newly blinded individuals.

Cerebral disease is another frequent cause of interference with perceptual systems. Quite beyond the effects of damage to brain tissues that are essential to interpretation of information from the environment, the frequent paralysis of parts of the muscular-skeletal system also causes interference with perceptual systems. The hemiplegia which is so often a part of the clinical picture in cerebral vascular accidents immediately destroys the basic orienting system and often the haptic system too. The problem of maintaining the balance of the body for skeletal-muscular movement, when half of it is paralyzed, is further complicated by the loss of the sensations of touch and of body position in space. The contribution of the basic orienting system and the haptic system to other essential perceptual systems, such as the visual, also serves to markedly alter the way in which such patients perceive their environment.

Any restriction of free movement through the environment accomplishes, in effect, the same shrinkage in the amount of information received by perceptual systems. Lying flat in bed, or on a wheeled stretcher, the individual is not able to use his visual system to freely perceive all of the immediate environment. In addition, the angle of vision that is permitted when the patient is in a supine position does not provide much information to the earth-bound organism. Orienting himself accurately requires the establishment of his position relative to others in the same plane. If, in addition, the individual is lying on a wheeled stretcher en route to the operating room or even to another area where therapy will be carried out, the passage through the environment into unfamiliar areas, without the opportunity to gain information about it, stirs an anxious reaction. Perhaps the initial placement of a patient in the strangeness of the hospital ward without the freedom to explore and thereby define the environment is equally anxiety-provoking. The variety of sensory stimuli that characterize the sights, sounds, odors, and feelings (he is, after all, in a strange bed) which he is unable to adequately perceive because of limitation on his activity is another source of basic anxiety to the newly hospitalized individual. Even after he has learned, through experience, how to interpret the information conveyed to him by the sights and sounds of the hospital, some guarding of his safety in this threatening environment must persist. The individual protects and defends himself within his environment by gaining all the information he can about it. When illness alters the function of his perceptual systems or when the necessary treatment interferes with the adequacy of the information he receives, the reassurance that he is safe has to come from other sources. This is why explanation is so essential to the successful completion of a nursing task, even when the procedure is familiar and often repeated. The verbalized information that the patient is about to be turned, for example, increases his own feelings of safety, even though his perceptual systems are not recording enough information to give him the necessary confidence.

The nursing measures that conserve his muscle tone and the range of motion in his joints are dedicated to the assumption that renewed activity will restore well-being, and at least a part of the well-being represents the independence of the individual in the information-gathering of perception. But perhaps one of the most interesting problems associated with perception is the diminution of the ability to use perceptual systems when the sensory organs are not adequately stimulated. The immobilization of the body which leads to atrophy of muscle and alteration of the normal physiological patterns is analogous to the severe restriction of sensory experience which results in a kind of atrophy of perception and awareness. It must be emphasized that restriction of sensory experience does NOT mean that the sensory organs are incapable of receiving stimuli. There is no interference with the ability of the senses to function. The individual is not blind or deaf. However, if he is long deprived of the interaction that brings environmental information to him, the human organism characteristically loses some of his ability to perceive and may withdraw so that there is every evidence that he is no longer oriented to reality. This atrophy of response is often called "sensory deprivation." It may be more accurate to call it "social deprivation." The factors involved in such deprivation are undoubtedly complex and involve the dynamics of the personality, but the research in sensory deprivation clearly demonstrates that essentially healthy individuals must have a constant exchange of information with their environment or they lose some of their ability to engage in such an exchange. In research situations in which individuals were placed in an entirely darkened and silent environment, after only a day or two they began to experience hallucinations—visual, auditory, and even of taste and smell. Because such information was unreal, their perceptions of the dark silence represent the threat which a cessation of perceptual information creates in the individual. Some degree of this manufacturing of environmental experience is seen in patients who are not able to participate in the reality of their environment. Long hospitalization with limitation of human interaction, often coupled with the restriction of bedrest, may be as depriving as the dark, silent room in the laboratory. Just as muscle tone is maintained only by muscle use, perceptual tone is maintained by the use of perceptual systems. Deprivation shrinks the muscle, but it also shrinks the spirit of a man. This is a particular danger in older patients, and the predisposing deprivation that may characterize their lonely existence outside of the hospital creates a disorientation and inability to assess reality, which considerably complicates their nursing care.

The interlocking perceptual systems in the individual combine to safeguard him in his environment. The nurse's concern for manipulation of the environment in order to make it one in which healing can take place cannot succeed without recognition of the perceptual systems and the ways in which the patient's illness has altered them or without a responsible effort to bring information to the patient to compensate for that which he is unable to seek for himself.

The Individual's Territorial Claim Defines Him in the Social Group

"Individuals," wrote Thoreau, "like nations, must have suitable and broad boundaries, even a considerable neutral ground between them." Not every person can retreat, as Thoreau did to Walden Pond, to establish a "considerable neutral ground" and to surround himself, thereby, with inviolate space. Yet every individual requires space, and both the establishment of his personal boundaries and their defense are essential components of his behavior.

There are many boundaries that are marked only by the intense feeling which erected them in the first place. Certainly this is true of nations; even when there is no threat to the boundary line that separates two nations, the intensity of affect is apparent when the line is crossed. The borders that create the United States are quiet borders, but nevertheless constructed of patriotic fervor. Nations with threatened borders live in an atmosphere of political uncertainty. The peace that reigns inside the American boundary lines ill equips a citizen of this country to understand the anguish that is a daily experience for an Israeli who lives in a kibbutz on the Syrian border. In every political arena where border dispute is a persistent fact, the dislocation of the group is reflected in the individuals who compose it. There are boundaries, too, of cultural allegiance that influence the political and social goals of the entire populace. Until very recently, the immigration laws of the United States reflected cultural boundaries that excluded Central Europeans and Orientals from joining the "melting pot" of American life. And social boundaries may be the most subtle, but the most powerful, of all. The civil rights movement is directed at social boundaries, and these walls which cannot be seen have proven to be the most difficult to tumble. Social boundaries are woven of the cloth of shared value systems, and irrational and ignorant as such restrictive devices may be, such borders are defended with a ferocity which even exceeds that of the patriot. The old saying that "a man's home is his castle" is incorporated into the American Constitution, in which the right to search and seizure without due process of law is expressly forbidden.

Thus, the defense of territory is not an uncommon aspect of group life. It is far less common to recognize the establishment and defense of territory in individuals, and yet it is a fact of everyday life. When students are not assigned a seat in the classroom, they nevertheless quickly stake

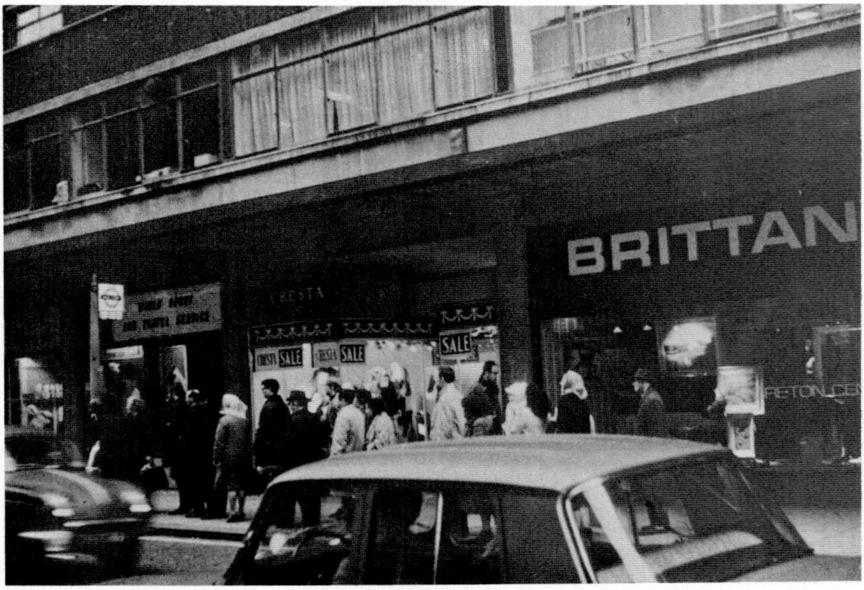

FIGURE 77. The London bus commuters space themselves politely along the curb, forming a line that is often a block long, while awaiting the bus. However, all the restraint and order apparent on the curb disappear in the scramble to get a seat inside the bus. (Photo by Assoc. Prof. Rachel Bliss, University of Illinois College of Nursing, Chicago.)

out their individual territories, and return class after class to the same seat they occupied the first time. In fact, the rare maverick who upsets the order by sitting in the "wrong" place is very likely to be notified that he is usurping someone else's territory.

The way in which London commuters queue up for their bus is almost legendary. They establish themselves along the curb, perfectly spaced one from the other, and it would be unthinkable for anyone to impose himself into the line. But once the bus arrives, the same considerate spacing and separation is lost in an aggressive struggle for a seat which is so fierce as to have no counterpart in the civilized world—even in the New York subway. This apparent difference in behavior is testimony to the single motivating force that is responsible for both the polite queue and the aggressive struggle. In each instance, the individual's territory is at stake. Out on the curb, the territory is readily identified. Inside the bus, the defensible territory is a seat. The losers must stand in close contact with each other. Now, actually, even in a crowded bus, the individual continues to defend his territory. The contact with other persons creates a kind of muscle tension that is almost like an effort to pull one's skin inside. In addition, the eyes are focused on infinity. They never engage the gaze of the individual standing a hairsbreadth away, and thus staring into the distance the personal involvement in the crowded crush of other bodies is effectively limited.

The commuter queued along the curb behaves much like the birds that line the lamp post. Such behavior reflects the territorial claim of the individual, but only within the context of the group. Each bird assumes his own space, but he does so as a member of a social organization. The territory of the individual arises out of the necessary discipline that defines his place in a social structure. The space he claims for himself both separates him from, and integrates him into, the social organization.

The behavior of individuals as members of a group is easiest to study in nonhuman populations, and much of the interest in territory has centered on animal populations. However much dog lovers insist that their pets possess human attributes, the variety of perceptual experience that distinguishes various kinds of animals indicates that the environment is

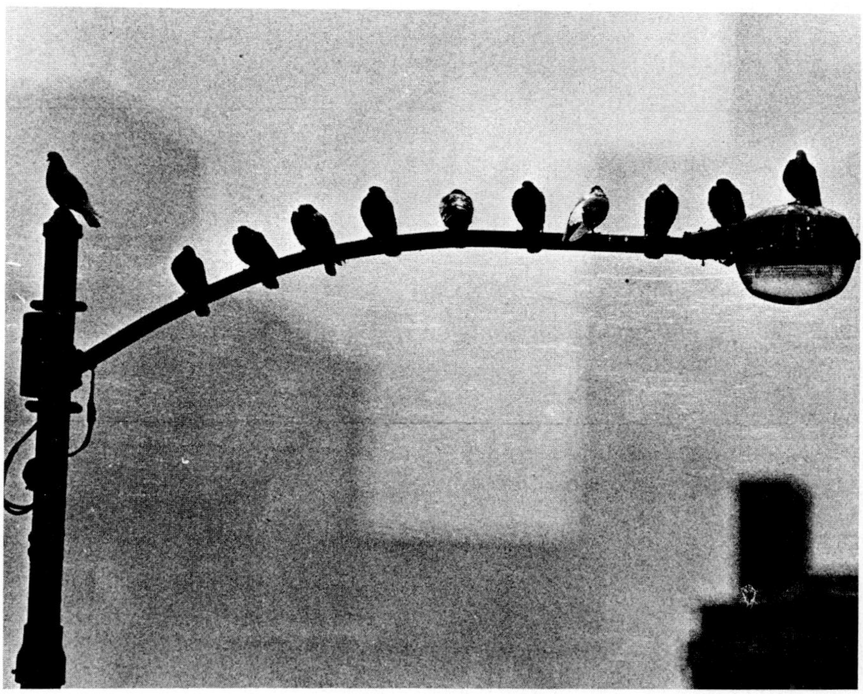

FIGURE 78. On a cold and foggy day ,the birds roost on a lamp post, meticulously spaced although a sharing of body warmth might have brought them comfort. (Chicago Sun-Times photo by Bob Langer.)

interpreted very differently by nonhuman organisms. And because the spacing that is so wilful a behavior in animal groups must depend upon their perception of their environment, including its living inhabitants, it is not possible to assume that human territorial needs arise from the same motivations. The ascription of human behavior and intent to animals is called anthropomorphism (the shape of man). Mickey Mouse and his entourage are delightful and funny because their antics stir the observer to recognition, but their human traits would be less lovable in human form. Thus, even though most of the research in territory has described animal behaviors, it cannot be adapted, *ipso facto,* to human populations.

Students of human groups have, however, begun to explore the territorial needs of individuals. In 1959, Sommer studied personal space in a group of hospitalized mental patients in Saskatchewan. The sociologist Goffman has hinted at the use of space by individuals in several studies of social interaction. The major contributor to this research, thus far, is the anthropologist, Edward Hall, who defined territorial needs for human populations based on the perceptual information which determines spacing behavior and emphasized that cultural determinants markedly influenced the territorial definitions used by individuals. It is Hall's description of territorial behaviors that is offered here.

The establishment of a defined boundary must involve a distance, that is, a measurable space. The use of specific distances to describe territorial spacing was introduced by Hediger, a zoologist and animal ethologist. Hediger distinguished between the spacing taking place between individuals of the same species and that used by individuals of different species. Those distances involving different species were described by Hediger in specific measurements, and the consistency in the measurements for a variety of organisms was remarkable. But human contacts with non-domesticated species are limited in the civilized world to zoological parks; perhaps the most common exchange is the stereotyped (but convincing) behavior of the female in the presence of a mouse. All in all, the distances that influence the behavior of members of the same species are the important ones in human interaction.

The birds on the lamp post and the Londoners in their bus line demonstrate the behavior of noncontact species (a terminology introduced by Hediger). Some species require physical contact. The seals that cluster together illustrate a "contact" species. The adult human being is a noncontact organism, but there is compelling evidence that the newborn infant requires contact. The influence of cultural determinants is apparent even in this kind of behavior; the conservation of heat by contact, as practiced by the African desert nomads, is an illustration of a cultural variant in which contact is practiced by adults.

Hall has coined a word to describe human territorial behavior. He calls this study "proxemics," and defines it as ". . . the interrelated observations and theories of man's use of space as a specialized elaboration of culture." Hall divides the functional use of space into four "distance zones," and subdivides each zone into a close and a far phase. The distinguishing characteristics of each distance are established by the perceptual information available within the measured distance. The *interpretation* of the perceptual information by the individuals results in behaviors which are culturally prescribed.

In the *intimate zone,* the close approximation of the bodies of the two individuals insures the perception of body heat, odor, and movement. At this close range, the visual system provides little useful information; in fact, visual perceptions are distorted by the nearness of the other individual. The breath sounds and odor, as well as the movement of the breath, are also clearly perceptible. Hall describes the close phase of the intimate zone as the distance of "love-making and wrestling." The use of the voice at this range is unnecessary, and even whispering has the effect of increasing the distance. The far phase is measured as a distance of 6 to 18 inches. The bodies are not in contact at this distance, but the individuals can easily hold hands. If the voice is used, it is very quiet. Visual perceptions are distorted, so that the head seems "larger than life-size," and at this close range, the nose appears quite big. There is still a transmission of heat and odor from the body, as well as from the breath. Very fine details of the skin are easily seen. The intimate zone is not a distance that is acceptable in public places, with the possible exception of the beach. Thus, the crowded subway or bus, in forcing contact of this kind, creates tension and defense in the individual trapped in it. Hall also indicates that Americans feel very threatened when individuals of other cultures infringe on their intimate zones. In some countries, the tendency for the American to back away from this kind of contact creates a failure of communication that leaves both of the parties dissatisfied with their encounter.

The second zone described by Hall is that of *personal distance,* that is, the distance defended by the noncontact behavior of the individual. The close phase is from 1½ to 2½ feet, and the far phase extends the distance to 4 feet. The establishment of this zone of space around the individual was described by Hall as the placing of a "bubble" of space which really represents an extension of the body surface of the individual. He calls the personal distance "an internalized version of territory," and it represents, in a real way, an extension of the individual's definition of "self." The close phase defines relationships, so that, as Hall indicates, a wife may enter the personal distance of her husband, but such behavior is not socially permitted to another woman. Perceptual information becomes chiefly visual at this distance, the distortion is gone, and the head size and details of the face are life-size and quite clear. The odor of the body is not apparent unless the individual has used "colognes to create an olfactory bubble." This practice, incidentally, is not approved of in the deodorized American society; its widespread use in other cultures is often offensive to Americans. The voice level is moderate.

The third zone is that of *social distance,* with a close phase of 4 to 7 feet and a far phase of 7 to 12 feet. Perceptual information becomes much less detailed; the importance of visual perception is increased, since the individual can now see more of his partner than just the head and face. The gaze, in fact, must shift, and this behavior is another culturally determined one. Americans tend to shift their gaze from the eye to the mouth, and if the gaze wanders, it is interpreted as a lack of attention. The social distance is the one usually selected for impersonal business transactions. The voice level in Americans is such that conversations can be heard up to 20 feet away. It is interesting that alterations in the voice level often create boundaries of emotional response that do not parallel the actual distance involved. Raising the voice level in the social distance has the effect of shrinking it to personal distance. This manipulation of relationships is not unfamiliar; aggressive, autocratic individuals often use the voice level to establish their dominance.

The final zone is that of *public distance,* in which the close phase ranges from 12 to 25 feet, and the far phase extends beyond that. In this distance, individuals are involved with each other only in the most impersonal way. The perceptions of the other individual result in a figure that appears less than life-size. The voice must be raised or projected, subtleties of facial expression are lost, and much communication in this zone is nonverbal.

The consideration of space needs of the individual as a determinant of nursing intervention is an expression of the influence of other living beings in the environment as part of the perceptual information received by the individual. There is little doubt that space requirements are influential in human behavior and that such interpretations are culturally induced and socially prescribed. When an individual comes into the hospital, he discovers that an entirely new set of space definitions are an established fact of the cultural determinants in the hospital itself. His personal territorial claim is immediately restricted to the boundaries of his "unit." If he must remain in bed, his territory has shrunk to the limits of the bed itself. "His" bedside table and chair and perhaps "his" half of the closet or dresser space establish the limits that are now his boundaries. He must learn rather promptly that encroachment on the space in the hospital is especially dangerous because the aseptic ritual establishes safe and unsafe zones, and the walls that separate them are invisible. The concern for asepsis is real, but the frequency with which he may be enjoined to respect the territorial limits of aseptic safety may be threatening in itself. If, for example, he has been "taught" not to touch a sterile dressing on his own body, the inroad on his territorial prerogative may be considerable. The unusual intensity with which many patients defend the artifacts in their immediate environment may well be related to their need to establish a bubble of "self" that supports their sense of integrity, both personal and social. Nurses are often impatient with individuals who refuse to allow a wheelchair out of their sight, even when they have no plan to use it for a length of time. But when the bedridden patient is finally given permission to expand his territory and the success of such a move depends on the ready access of a wheelchair, his defense is more than a selfish focus on his own needs.

It is hardly possible to provide nursing care without entering the personal zone of the individual. And there is never an assurance that the interpretation of such an infringement will mean the same things to all patients. They will bring their own cultural values to the hospital with them, and even though they must adopt those of the hospital during their stay, the emotional impact of this demand may be a telling one. The use of space is, of course, equally a factor in the nurse's behavior, and thus the interaction between patient and nurse may involve their mutual concerns about spacing. From Hall's analysis of the zones of interaction, the nurse can use territory as a positive contribution to the patient's comfort and well-being. One obvious source of control is the voice level. Some of the subjects of conversation between nurse and patient require the emotional level of the personal or even the far phase of the intimate zone. Raising the voice level in the personal or intimate zone has the effect of widening the distance, whereas the same behavior in the social zone decreases the distance. The essential communication involving the personal factors in the patient's care may be projected into a personal zone by the use of the voice, even if the distance maintained is a social one and thereby more comfortable for the patient. The direction of the gaze is another means of controlling the distance; during those aspects of care that require encroachment on the personal zone of the patient, the nurse can reduce the anxiety by directing her eyes away from the patient's face. In fact, this is precisely the outlet used by many patients during the bathing procedure. They rarely engage the gaze of the nurse, and by looking at a far point, reduce the distance to a tolerable level.

The culturally determined territorial rules of the hospital are temporary as far as the patient is concerned, even though the nursing personnel subscribes to them without analysis or understanding. There are instances

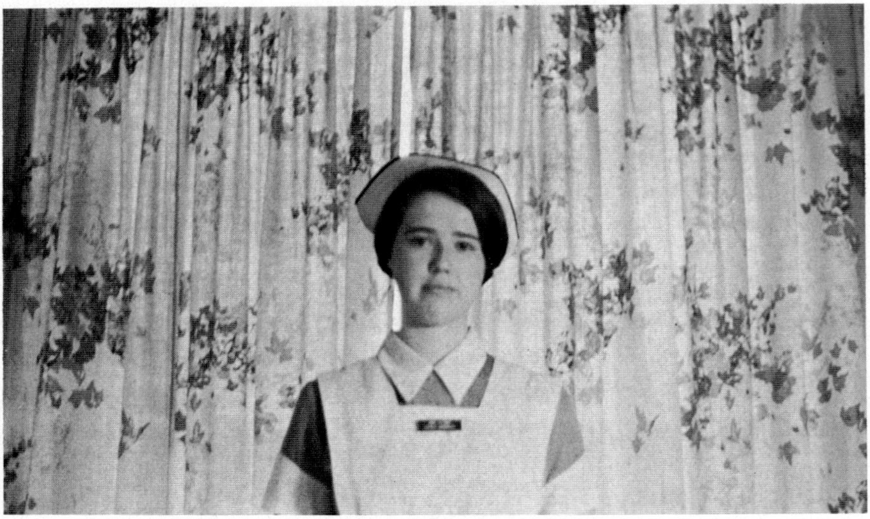

FIGURE 79. The nurse from a patient's pillow-based view. Standing within his social zone at the foot of the bed (six feet away), the top half of the nurse's figure is visible, as well as the background of the surrounding environment. Here communication is relatively impersonal, and the gaze would wander from eye to mouth as patient and nurse converse. (Photo by David Mandrgoc.)

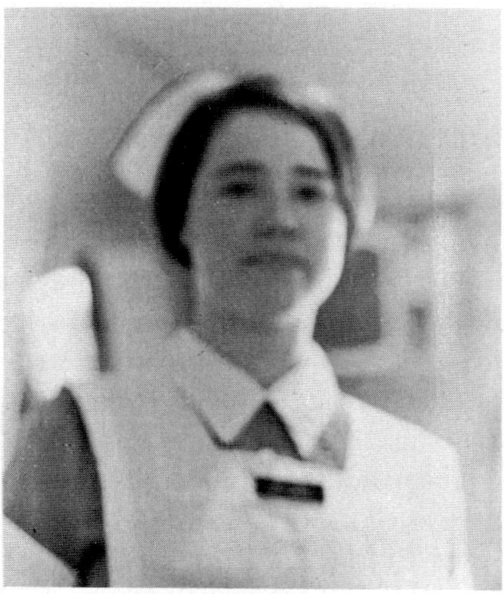

FIGURE 80. As the nurse enters the personal zone of the patient, approaching him from the side of his bed (three feet away), less of the detail of her figure is visualized, and her facial features are larger than life-size. Many transactions take place within this zone, and many kinds of procedures are performed within this range. (Photo by David Mandrgoc.)

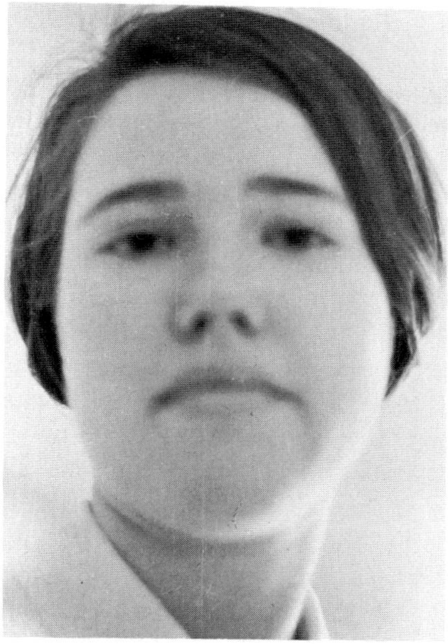

FIGURE 81. From a distance of eighteen inches, and within the far intimate zone of the patient, only the nurse's facial features are visible to him. Some distortion is apparent, similar to the childhood game of viewing another person's face from an upside down position. At this distance, the nurse and the patient tend to defend themselves from encroachment by refusing to lock gaze, but nursing activities are carried on at this distance. (Photo by David Mandrgoc.)

when nurses recognize the behavior that tells them the patient is uncomfortable, but this is rarely attributed to territorial demand. Some conversations with patients, involving doctors or nurses, would produce very different results if the distance zones were understood. For example, inquiries about personal problems and needs of the patient directed from the foot of the bed may be responded to in one way, whereas the same conversation at the patient's head level will be quite different. This, too, must vary with the cultural antecedents which influence the patient's behavior. The defense of territory is an essential aspect of personal and social integrity. When the bubble of territory is challenged and disrupted as often it must be during hospitalization, the individual must mount his defense in another way or sacrifice a portion of his feelings about himself. If, in addition, his defense is not understood or tolerated, then the effect on the therapeutic process may become measurable. The patient who demands that his chair be left in sight is defending his integrity. The nurse who stubbornly ignores his request may well be defending hers.

The Individual's Biological Rhythms Mirror the Rhythms of His Environment

The most striking characteristic of the environment is the periodic cycling that is at once a frame of reference and an inexorable reminder of change. Day passes into night, and there is confidence in a new dawn. Winter becomes spring; the days grow longer and summer comes. Summer slips into autumn, and winter returns. The rhythm of change in the world, as experienced by man, establishes the rhythm of life.

There is a cosmic rhythm as the earth, tilted on its axis, revolves around the sun every 365 days, 5 hours, and 48 minutes. There is a solar day as the earth rotates on its axis relative to the sun every 24 hours. There is a lunar day as the earth rotates on its axis relative to the moon every 24 hours and 50 minutes. There is a synodical month as the moon returns to its same position relative to the earth and sun every 29.5 days. The annual cycle establishes the seasons. The daily cycle creates darkness and light. The monthly cycle is measured by the rising and falling of the tide on the ocean shores. Inevitably, the cyclic changes that dominate the lives of all creatures have left their imprint on every living thing. Throughout the evolutionary history of self-replicating substances, the environmental influence of periodic change in temperature (heat energy) and light (radiant energy) has dictated the structure and function of the organism. Just as the blood that courses through the human body bears the remembrance of the sea, the entire body depends upon the ebb and flow of periodic change in the environment as it is written in the very essence of the life-force itself. The dependable periodicity of the external environment is inscribed in a dependable periodicity in the internal environment. Men have made clocks that measure the cyclic variation in their environment, but the biological clocks which pace the activities of life are timepieces more exquisitely tuned than the finest watch.

There is, of course, an awareness of the periodic variations in each day's activities. Every person has a period of wakefulness and a period of sleep. The recurrent need for food is also common experience. And the vague, but nevertheless essential, recognition that every individual has "good" times and "poor" times during a day may influence the choice of a job, or even the more fundamental selection of a career. The monthly cycle of the menses (often colloquially called the "period") represents another periodicity in body function that is familiar and expected.

The periodic fluctuation in the body temperature has also been an aspect of familiar acquaintance with cyclic change affecting body physiology. On the strength of long experience, in fact, it is widely known that the body temperature peaks in the late afternoon and reaches its lowest level during the small hours of night. When, in a hospital, the patient's temperature is recorded only once a day, the time selected is always close to that of the expected peak reading. It is, of course, essential that the body temperature of homeothermic organisms be maintained within the homeostatic range, but the recognized variation in the body temperature (and the research scientist always means the *core* temperature) is not related to alterations in environmental temperatures themselves. In other words, such a range occurs, regardless of the external temperatures to which the individual is exposed. Thus, the cyclic variation in the body temperature is not a function of external temperature, but an internal alteration related, instead, to physiological function.

The 24-hour clock which is the common instrument for the measurement of time as experienced by human beings is a conventional agreement allowing a synchronization of social behavior. The exact time period of 24 hours does not, of course, quite agree with the earth's rotation on its axis, but it serves quite well to organize human activity. The daily clock of internal origin is not quite 24 hours long either. It is slightly less, averaging out to about 23.6 or 23.8 hours per day. On the basis of this slight variation, Franz Halberg named the "physiological day" circadian (almost a day). The circadian rhythm is only one of the periodic cycles which characterize physiological function, but it is an important one. Not only do many of the cyclic changes in the body follow a circadian cycle, but the laboratory investigation of periodicity is enhanced when the alteration is circadian. Much of the investigation of cyclic change in the organism has, for this reason, focused on the circadian span. There are other cycles, of course, of which the menses are only one example.

The most obvious cycle in a day's turning includes the definitive periods of light and dark. Therefore, it was entirely logical that the study of circadian cycles would explore the effects of alternate light and dark on the function of the individual organism. The influence of these alternative periods was quickly apparent. If the periods of light and dark are switched so that the laboratory animals (usually mice) experience day when it is night and night when it is day, the periodic cycle of their body temperature gradually switches too, and within twelve days is completely reversed. The influence of these environmental factors must be one of synchronization. That is, the external stimuli hold the periodic variation in its usual sequential pattern. If a cycle is visualized as a line graph with peaks and valleys, the phase is equal when the distance between peaks (or between valleys) is equal. A perfectly equal graph may be said to be "in phase" and, therefore, synchronized. When inequalities exist in the distance between peaks, the graph is "out of phase," or desynchronized. Since the circadian cycle is only about 24 hours, the removal of the usual external synchronizer alters the graphic representation of the variation in body temperature, leaving it "out of phase" or desynchronized. The continued exposure to the same environmental influence (such as the reversal of light and dark) will finally resolve into a synchronized rhythm once again, even though it is now completely reversed from the original pattern. The peaks have become valleys, and the valleys have become peaks—but the phase remains in tune.

If the body temperature were the only physiological parameter that demonstrated a circadian cycle, the concern which arises when it is out of phase, or desynchronized, might be quite casual. Actually, however, many of the biochemical functions of the body are also subject to circadian cycling. While the specific cycle of each measured function may have its own quite distinctive pattern of synchronization, the "melodic" unity of all of the circadian patterns together represents an interaction that supports optimal physiological performance. If only one such pattern is out of phase —like the violinist who is off-key—the total interaction is somewhat disturbed and, instead of harmonic sound, there is a clearly identifiable "noise."

Not all of the circadian rhythms in man have been identified, but there is, nevertheless, a noble list deserving attention. The body temperature of man is a reflection of energy production and is therefore an indicator of the rate of metabolic activity. It is not surprising that the maximum physical activity, and with it the feeling of well-being, occurs when the core temperature is at its highest level, whereas the opposite behavior is both manifested and recognized by the individual when the reading is at its low point. Not all individuals peak in the afternoon. Many a perfectly healthy human being describes himself as a "morning type," and his body temperature substantiates his own feeling of maximum energy. The "night owls" probably peak much later in the day than do most people; the selection of employment involving night activity is influenced by this fact. Some individuals rouse easily and quickly from a night's rest, whereas others are unbearable until well past lunch. These consistent behaviors reflect circadian cycling which is individualized in the human organism. The number of granulocytes circulating in the blood is at a peak at midnight and again during the afternoon. The hemoglobin, hematocrit, and total plasma protein are lowest after 10 P.M. but bear no relation to bedrest. The urinary excretion of water, chlorides, urea, and potassium ion peaks in the early afternoon. The minute volume of the heart (that is, cardiac output per minue) is highest from 6 P.M. to midnight and lowest from 4 to 6 A.M. The blood pressure is also highest in the evening and lowest in the morning. The vital capacity of the lungs is greatest in the afternoon and lowest around 2 A.M. And the mitosis of normal skin cells is highest from noon to midnight but virtually quiescent in the morning—when most skin biopsies are done. This listing is far from exhaustive. There is a cycling of hormonal substances, too, and undoubtedly many other essential physiological functions. The liver, responsible for at least 70 vital regulatory functions in the body's metabolism, also operates on a circadian cycling. However, even with the limited number of cyclic events described here, it is apparent that desynchronization produces a disturbance of the rhythm which will be recognized by the individual in his sense of well-being.

The most common source of desynchronization of the circadian rhythms, aside from disease and the effects of hospitalization which will be discussed later, is the rapid movement by jet airplane across many time zones. Even a 4-hour trip across the United States moves the external time one-fourth of a cycle of the clock, and a trip across the ocean is even more disrupting. If the tourist is possessed of knowledge concerning circadian cycles, he may muster the wisdom to restrict his activity until his body has resynchronized to the time zone in which he is a visitor. During the time that he is out of phase, he feels tired and irritable and is unable to enjoy himself. Business men who are often involved in international meetings have learned to allow for time to resynchronize and arrive soon enough to insure that they will not be out of phase when they must be alert to events around them. But the difficulties that confront the pilot and crew of the jet airliner have been of sufficient concern to stimulate a government-supported investigation of the effects of rapid travel across several time zones and its influence on the performance of these people. The same problems confront individuals who must alter their work pattern so that they are sometimes working on night shifts. No group faces this change more often than nurses; although doctors often work on night shifts, they usually have the alternative of resting or sleeping during the intervals when they are not needed. The doctors have a very special problem related to total loss of sleep in a 24-hour period, but the nurse assigned to the night shift must suddenly adapt to the alteration in her pattern and yet remain alert and functional throughout the 8-hour period. The shift to nights always means a shift in the synchronizing of the circadian cycles and an inevitable period when the individual is out of phase. When the night work is limited to one or two weeks, by the time resynchronization has taken place, the change back to a day shift upsets the pattern again, producing another period out of phase which must drain the resources of the nurse considerably. It seems likely, on the basis of this knowledge, that nurses who are natural "night owls" should select and remain on a night shift. Placing a nurse on this shift for a limited period of time should either allow her at least a month or should not be required for more than two or three nights at a time, with sufficient time between such scheduling to allow complete resynchronization. The same reasoning is valid, of course, for all essential night workers.

Policemen are often assigned to night hours for limited periods of time, and the wisdom of such personnel policies needs to be examined in the light of information now available about circadian cycling.

The unusual demands made on individuals who must work during the night expose them not only to an alteration in the environmental synchronizer of light-darkness but also to some very persistent synchronizers that are essentially social in nature. The social synchronizers represent the group expression of individual recognition of periodic cycling. The social tradition of three meals a day arises out of the need to replenish the body with nutrients, but the decided characteristics of the meals are purely culturally induced. At least part of the dislocation felt by sometime night nurses is their inability to know how to choose a meal. Long-standing habit suggests specific foods for the morning meal, but after a night's work, the possibility of enjoying a dinner meal at 8 A.M. is not remote. Nurses who always work at night solve this problem after a time, but the most frequent complaint, related to the lack of well-being in general, of nurses who occasionally work the night shift is the anorexia and disruption of dietary selection that make this stint a little more miserable. The additional social influences which dictate important relationships create further disaffection. The young nurse on a date, like Cinderella, must rush home before midnight. Even an attentive young man may object to that.

The lackluster and apathetic feeling of individuals who are out of phase does not, in itself, constitute a dramatic threat. However, certain research efforts have indicated that the circadian rhythm may, indeed, have serious implications for the individual. The ability of some laboratory animals to survive toxic dosages of drugs, or noxious dosages of pathogens, has shown a decided relationship to a circadian pattern. Halberg has called these vulnerable times the "hours of diminished resistance." A group of mice injected with a highly noxious pathogen at noon survived the insult, whereas their brothers who received the dosage at midnight promptly succumbed to it. The circadian cycle that regulates adrenal secretion may also influence the individual's ability to respond to stress. Since adrenal hormone levels are very decidedly related to the stress response, as elicited by Selye, the low ebb period of adrenal activity should contraindicate a surgical procedure during that period of time. Much elective surgery is scheduled for the morning hours, but some individuals do not peak their adrenal output at that time. There is a consistent statistical pattern in the hours of birth and death as well; such a repeated finding certainly suggests that the influence of circadian rhythms is much more important than the interference with well-being alone would suggest. Drug administration may also be susceptible to investigation of the physiological response to medications during various periods of the circadian cycle.

Both the environmental and the social synchronizers are quickly upset when the individual becomes ill and are further compromised when he enters the hospital. Illness in itself alters the physiological function sufficiently to force some of the circadian rhythms out of phase. The problem of an elevated temperature, in fact, poses an interesting adjunct to the circadian influence. Many individuals are able to depend upon their internal clock. They arouse themselves moments before the alarm rings. Or, having decided to awaken early the next morning, for some important reason, they achieve this with little difficulty. The passage of time, as measured in clock-hours, is more than an external fact of life. Some "time" passes swiftly, whereas some seems to go on and on. Awareness of the passage of time is thus a highly variable, subjective experience. Precisely what the clock mechanism is within the human body is not known, but it is apparent that the measure of passing time is somehow achieved by the brain. Some investigators have suggested that the rate of oxidation in the brain tissue determines the sensation of passing time. If this is true, then an increased rate of oxidation, such as occurs in a febrile condition, would result in a more rapid passage of physiological time compared to clock time. Such an individual would perceive that, as far as his clock was concerned, time was dragging. A lowered body temperature and a lowered metabolic rate should produce just the opposite effect. Clock time would appear to pass quickly compared to physiological time. Thus, an individual with a fever would come early to an appointment, whereas a person with a lowered temperature would come late. One investigator, in fact, asked febrile subjects to count off 60 seconds, and these individuals consistently counted faster than clock time. Obviously a great deal remains to be learned in this area, but the possibility that time (on the clock) is painfully slow for the sick individual may provide insight useful to nurses.

The drawing of various laboratory specimens, usually during the day shift when technicians are available, may also influence the conclusions drawn from the results. Repeated laboratory analysis of many specimens over a period of time would certainly be more meaningful than analysis of single specimen. The question persists of the accuracy of certain laboratory analyses using specimens drawn during periods in the circadian cycle when the level was either up or down, depending on the precise time of the drawing. If the laboratory analysis is a very important one, it appears inviting to establish the individual's circadian pattern as part of the evaluation of the results.

There is no resemblance between the hospital routine and that ordinarily followed by an individual at home. The desynchronization that invariably results during the first few days of a hospitalization may contribute in a substantial way to the patient's response to treatment. Hospital routine is established for the convenience of the people who work in hospitals, never for those who have the misfortune to require hospitalization. Many nurses have objected to the barbarity of the early rousing of patients so that the night nurses might check their temperatures (elevated or not) and provide wash water and oral hygiene before the breakfast trays appear. The fact that these trays often come at precisely the time the report is being given to the on-coming shift simply makes the early performance of the morning ablutions more certain. The hours at which meals are served are dictated by the diet kitchen staff on the rigid pattern that the last meal must be early enough to allow the dishwashers to go off duty on time for *their* supper. A breakfast tray between 7 and 8 A.M. is often followed by a lunch tray before noon. Or, if the lunch tray arrives closer to 1 P.M., then the supper hour often begins as early as 4:30 P.M. Unless the patient is fortunate enough to have an evening snack ordered for him as part of his diet, the long period between supper and breakfast is considerably more than most individuals would choose for themselves. The timing of treatments, dressing change, medications, and temperature or blood pressure taking is scheduled with the nurse in view, and the effect of such activity on the patient is rarely a consideration. It is hospital routine that insists that the bath is a morning procedure, although many, many people are habituated to bathing in the evening hours. Whatever the social synchronizers in the individual's "other" life, they are certain to be challenged when he is hospitalized. Nursing needs research in the area of circadian desynchronization arising from traditional hospital routines.

The one periodic rhythm which is recognized and treasured by most individuals is the opportunity to sleep sometime during every 24-hour day. The total number of hours spent in sleep varies considerably from one individual to another, but generally the human organism spends one-third of his life in slumber. The intense physiological need to sleep is not a demand that can be ignored, and the effort to remain awake requires a powerful exercise on the part of the individual. Everyone sleeps. Patients sleep. However, the information available on the physiology of sleep, some of it available for at least thirty years, has never been important to the nurse. Although nurses have long been concerned with the need to provide rest for patients, the sleep research suggests that traditional nursing techniques have hindered far more than they have helped, in insuring the patient the benefits of sleep. The poet has not ignored the wondrous promise of sleep, but the poetic interpretations have reinforced a widespread folk idea that sleeping and dying are similar states of being. Over 2000 years ago, Catullus wrote:

> Suns may set and rise again,
> But when our short day takes flight
> Sleep we must one endless night.

Sleep, on the other hand, far from resembling the stillness and peace of death, is a time of intense activity. Its place in the overall well-being of the individual is essential, not merely because it is a time of physical recuperation, but also because it provides a continuity of emotional life which is absolutely necessary for the health and welfare of the individual.

Most of the research on sleep has been done in the laboratory, where volunteers, wired to monitors that record many parameters, sleep for the sake of science. Numerous studies, involving many volunteers as well as many observers, have established some of the facts about sleep which can no longer be denied. The basic mechanism of sleep, however, is still a matter of theoretical conjecture. No one is certain why the body and spirit weary enough by the end of a day to require a third of a day for renewal. The reason for sleep, or for wakefulness for that matter, is still a secret somewhere in the central nervous system; eventually brain research will disclose it. But the descriptive characteristics of sleep, the physiological patterns of sleep, and many of the environmental influences on habits of sleep are clearly identified.

The success of monitoring devices, dependent upon electronic circuitry, rests with the fact that many body functions are attended by the development of extremely small electrical currents. The electronics explosion which has altered the technology of all science, incuding nursing, is based on the fact that these tiny electrical currents can be picked up, amplified, and thereby recorded or measured. The electrocardiogram does this for the activity of heart muscle. A pattern of consistency, making it possible to identify a specific physiological state by registering the typical electrical current, has vastly increased the knowledge of how many body processes are carried on. The search for unusual configurations has, of course, a valuable diagnostic purpose. The activity of brain cells can also be correlated with the distinctive electrical patterns that characterize aspects of cerebral function. Such a recording of the "brain waves" is called an electroencephalogram (EEG). Rather precise patterns are created by cerebral activity of various kinds. During wakefulness, the patterns show vigorous activity, and alterations in the patterns caused by disease can be identified. Since sleep is obviously an activity involving the central nervous system, the electroencephalographic patterns of sleep were soon identified.

On the basis of EEG tracings, it became apparent that there are at least four distinct stages of sleep. As sleepiness begins to overtake the individual, the waves of wakefulness (alpha waves) begin to disappear. At Stage 1 sleep begins, the brain pattern shows irregular, low-voltage waves, with occasional alpha waves intervening. After two or three minutes, the EEG pattern shows the development of bursts of rapid waves, called spindles; thus, Stage 2 is sometimes called spindle sleep. About a half-hour later, the spindle sleep waves begin to disappear, and the pattern

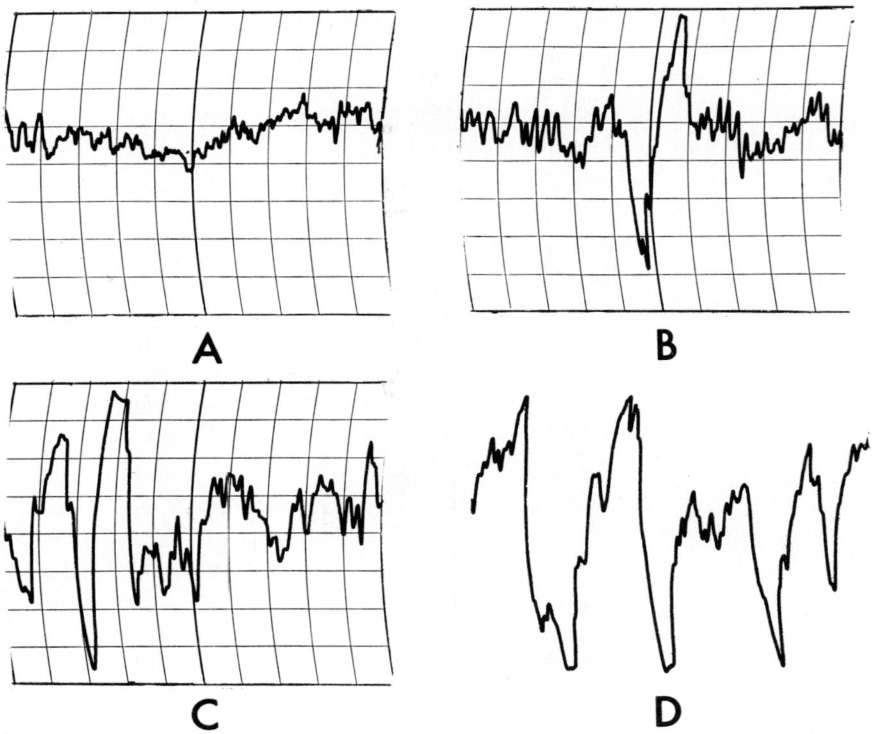

FIGURE 82. Electroencephalographic record of the stages of sleep. (A) descending stage one; (B) stage two, or spindle sleep. This tracing also demonstrates a K-complex, a tracing seen only in the sleeping individual, in response to some stimulus in the environment. (C) stage three and (D) stage four, the "deepest" stage of non-REM sleep. (Courtesy of Dr. Rosalind Cartwright, Director of the Sleep Laboratory, University of Illinois College of Medicine.)

traces large, slow waves (Stage 3). As the waves settle into a synchronous pattern, the sleeper has entered the depth of sleep, Stage 4. But it is not only the EEG patterns that are changing as sleep progresses through the four stages. Heart and respiratory rates are also modified. The brain temperature changes, as does the rate of gastric secretion. The body temperature falls and the muscle potential is altered. Contrary to every expectation, however, the descent into Stage 4, accompanied by a slowing and pacing of body activities, is not the final pattern of sleep. The passage into oblivion starts as the night's rest begins, but there is every evidence that the sleeper soon substitutes intense activity for the utter peace of Stage 4.

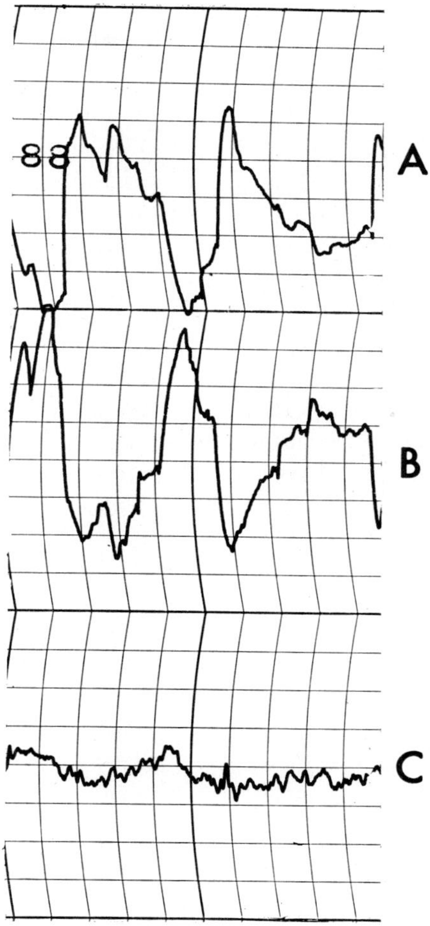

FIGURE 83. During the REM period, the eyes of the subject move behind their closed lids from side to side. (A) records the movement of the right eye; (B) records the movement of the left eye. In (C) the EEG tracing, simultaneously recorded, indicates that the REM sleeper is in stage one of the cycle. Most subjects awakened during this period indicate that they have been dreaming. (Courtesy of Dr. Rosalind Cartwright, Director of the Sleep Laboratory, University of Illinois College of Medicine.)

Kleitman is the dean of those physiologists who have studied sleep. In his laboratory at the University of Chicago, his associate, Aserinsky, made an observation on a sleeping subject that has opened wide the door of sleep research and its promised insights. He noticed that the soundly sleeping subject was rapidly moving his eyes from one side to the other behind their closed lids as if he were watching a swiftly unfolding movie. The possibility that these rapid eye movements accompanied a dream immediately occurred to the researcher. Thousands of observations later, it is an established fact that periods of rapid-eye-movement sleep (called REM sleep) occur regularly throughout the sleeping period in a recurrent pattern. It was soon established that REM sleep did coincide with dreaming, and that *everybody* dreams. Whereas all the other physiological measurements tend to decrease as the further stages of sleep are reached, the heart and respiratory rates not only increase during REM sleep, but also become variable. Muscle potential, especially of the muscles of the head and neck, disappears in REM sleep. The loss of muscle potential is recognized as the head drops when the individual is falling asleep. Electronic monitors record electrical potentials during the rapid eye movements; the incidence of REM sleep can thus be plotted, along with the EEG and other measurements which have established that the Stage 4 sleeper, after about 60 to 90 minutes, returns through the pattern of the stages of sleep all the way to Stage 1. Then he begins to dream.

From four to six times a night, the sleeper passes up and down through the stages of sleep and enjoys a REM period. The Stage 4 sleep tends to dominate the early part of the night, whereas REM sleep is most apparent in the latter half of the night. No two individuals have the same cycle of REM-nonREM sleep. Every individual has a pattern of REM periods as distinctive and unique to him as his fingerprints. The observer, having identified the sleep pattern in his subject, can predict almost to the minute when the next REM period will occur. Every adult spends an average of 24% of his sleep time in REM even those who are positive they never dream. Jouvet has called REM sleep "paradoxical sleep." All of the physiological measurements seem to indicate that the individual is close to wakefulness, but it is much easier to awaken an individual from nonREM than from REM sleep. In fact, several investigators have indicated that, when the individual is awakened during a nonREM period and asked what he is doing, the response invariably is: "I was awake." When the same question is asked of an individual aroused during a REM period, most subjects are able to recount certain details of their dream. The dream process does not consist of four to six isolated and separated dreams. The first dreams of the sleep period tend to reflect the reality of events which the individual had experienced, or was thinking about, before he fell asleep, or about which he was concerned. As the REM periods proceed through the night, the dreams become more and more bizarre. They are hallucinatory, cannot be tested against reality, and the individual is quite apt to respond to them with a visible display of emotion. But when all of the dreams of a night's sleep are recounted to the investigator, it is clear that there is a persistent thread of unity appearing in all of the REM periods. Some pattern, or unifying content, characterizes the total REM experience in a night of sleep. The increasing intensity and unreality of the progressing dream process suggest that the REM experience possesses a unique psychological state or tone. It is also a necessary aspect of sleep and contributes to the health and well-being of the individual.

The extreme importance of REM sleep has been demonstrated in individuals who have been deprived of REM periods. Such an interference with the normal sleep cycles is called dream deprivation, and the implications of the research are very important to nurses. In the laboratory, dream deprivation was first achieved by conscientiously awakening the individual each time he began to enter a REM period. When he was allowed to go back to sleep, the interval preceding the next REM period was noticeably shortened. The time between REM cycles was compressed; the individual appeared to be more and more insistent on entering the REM phase and more and more resistant to being aroused from it. Such a resistance to arousal as well as a compression of REM periods can occur in only one night of interference with REM sleep. When, finally, the individual is allowed to sleep without being aroused, the total percentage of sleep time spent in REM sleep is markedly increased. The REM phase of sleep *must* be compensated for sooner or later. After dream deprivation, the time spent in REM sleep remains increased over a period of time until it has been made up, and then the normal cycling is resumed. There is, thus, some truth to the folk idea that lost sleep must be made up—although it is the lost dreams that demand their moment. Evidence is increasing that intereference with REM sleep finally results in behavioral changes during the waking hours. The changes in behavior, in fact, may be very bizarre and suggestive of utter disorientation from reality.

The importance of REM sleep for general well-being has been demonstrated in individuals who have remained awake for prolonged periods of time. The longest recorded period without sleep is about eleven days; in two individuals closely observed during the sleepless time, profound behavioral changes were apparent. In one instance, these changes persisted well past the time that the individual had made up his REM loss. The profound personality changes that accompany lack of sleep testify to the integration of the organism in definitive ways. When the sleep pattern must be altered, the nearer it comes to the normal cycle for the individual, the better the possibility that his sleep will be profitable. This problem was specifically illustrated in the space program, when the flight plan called for four hours of sleep and four hours of duty, thus providing that there would always be one astronaut awake. In spite of the rigorous training they had undergone, the astronauts found that they were unable to rest under that regime and decided themselves to revert to the sleep cycle to which they were habituated. Although this meant both men were asleep at the same time, they recognized that the usual routine afforded them the safety of rest and that the other plan was interfering with their level of operation.

By far the most serious source of REM deprivation, however, is the effect, now widely documented, that sedative drugs have on REM sleep. Alcohol depresses REM sleep; in fact, just two cocktails can curtail REM periods by 15%. The possibility that delirium tremens represents a REM attack, or a flooding of hallucinatory material in an individual long deprived of dream periods, is being studied. Every sedative drug in common use in the hospital, moreover, has been shown to decrease REM time. Since sleeping medications are designed to promote sleep, this effect on REM time poses a serious clinical question. Many drugs have been tried to increase REM sleep, but none of them, including the psychedelics, have yet proved effective. Individuals who use sleeping medication over long periods of time continue to lose REM sleep, and a long recovery period is necessary to make it up.

Beyond expending every skill and effort to promote the patient's comfort so that he will be able to sleep, the nurse has very little control over the use of sedative drugs. Assessing the relative difficulties arising from their use is the doctor's responsibility; as sleep research continues, the modification in usage will doubtless follow. But the research in sleep does indicate a number of areas that directly affect nursing decisions and over which the nurse exercises considerable control.

It is apparent that when it is absolutely necessary to rouse a patient in order to perform a treatment or give a drug (not a sedative!), the individual's interest is best served if he is not awakened at the beginning of a REM period. Although this may be difficult to determine, the rapid eye movements *are* observable. That is how they were first discovered. A moment's careful observation may well provide the information that indicates whether or not a REM period is in progress. There may be a variation in pulse rate at the onset of a REM period too, although obviously the nurse would need to know the base rate in order to judge whether it has increased. The time may come when observation of the sleeping patient will require the noting of REM periods of sleep. The usual nursing position in reference to the sleeping patient, however, often excludes really careful observation altogether. The night nurse is much more interested in, and involved with, those patients who are obviously not sleeping; thus, she is much more apt to make accurate observations on the sleepless than on the sleeping. The frequency with which patients report to the physician that they did not sleep, although the night nurse as adamantly insists that they did, because she saw them asleep, may also have its explanation in the research findings. One is relatively easily aroused from nonREM sleep, and such patients insist that they were awake all the time. If some kind of signal, such as a sudden or unusual noise or the turning on of a light in the vicinity, should disturb an individual so that he is awakened from nonREM sleep, his testimony to the physician is not untrue. It is simply the often repeated claim of most individuals who are awakened in nonREM sleep. The observations must be more than merely perfunctory, however, if the nurse is really concerned about the patient's sleep pattern. While the individual may seek a favorite position in order to induce sleep, most individuals move about during a night's rest; it is, in fact, unusual if the position is not changed several times during the night. This can certainly be easily determined by the nurse. In addition, talking during sleep, while vigorously denied by most people, has been recorded so often in sleep research that it seems quite certain that everybody does it at one time or another. It does not, however, occur in REM sleep but often immediately before the REM period begins. This may also assist the nurse in deciding whether or not a patient should be aroused. The agitation apparent in the tone of the individual who is talking in his sleep sometimes provokes a nurse to awaken the individual on the grounds that he is having a "bad dream." The nurse may be reassured of the universal occurrence of sleep-talking and comforted, too, by the knowledge that the individual is about to enter a REM period. Sleepwalking, incidentally, never starts in REM sleep. The treatment for this occurrence is complex; its significance to nursing care is only that, when a patient is a sleepwalker, this information should be communicated to the nursing staff so that the patient can be protected from injury.

Quite apart from the nurse's interest in helping the patient to have a good night's sleep, the incidence of pathophysiological changes that are often initiated during sleep suggests that closer observation of the sleeping patient is well worthwhile. In normal individuals, for example, the secretion of gastric juice stops during REM sleep. However, in individuals with diagnosed peptic ulcers, the gastric secretions increase from four to ten times during REM sleep. There is a consistent finding of disturbances in cardiac rhythm at that time, and the uncomfortably high incidence of coronary artery disease during the early hours of morning suggests that understanding the sleep cycles will ultimately contribute important information on the etiology of these events. The incidence of convulsive seizures in epilepsy has also been documented in the small hours of the night, a fact that should encourage cautious observation of such individuals by the nurse. Some symptoms are so definitively associated with sleep that they are described as nocturnal. Paroxysmal dyspnea in individuals with congestive failure often occurs shortly after the patient has fallen asleep and has frequently been associated with alterations in cardiac output and vital capacity. There may be many manifestations of disease that are not sufficiently noted, because sleeping patients are seldom carefully observed.

The relationship of sleep patterns to disease processes is so persistent that one of the questions always asked when the doctor interviews a patient for his past history concerns his sleeping patterns and any alterations that have occurred in them. Sleeplessness or insomnia is not an uncommon complaint, and it is probably even a fairly normal response in times of great tension or excitement. But persistent failure to sleep accompanies many disease entities, and is, in fact, a common symptom in emotional disorders. The nurse should make observations of the patient's sleeping pattern so that his behavior in this important third of his day is as familiar to the staff as his waking behavior. While many events conspire against a decent night's sleep in the hospital, an individual who is insomniac deserves more than a hasty phone call to the physician for a sedative order.

With all of nursing's historic concern for providing an environment in which a patient can sleep, the provision for sleep is sometimes inadequate because of nursing activity. Many a patient has left a modern hospital bemoaning the impossibility of really resting during a hospitalization. The convalescent patient may have the strength to struggle for his night's sleep. But the very sick patient, who needs it the most, is the least likely to receive it. He is both the beneficiary and the victim of modern science. The placing of very sick medical and surgical patients into intensive care units provides them with all of the skill and technology that can be centered there. But such a patient has a very hard time getting any sleep. He is constantly aroused because various nursing measures and treatments must be performed. If he succeeds in dozing off, his chance of remaining asleep for longer than an hour is remote. And the constant activity required in such a ward conspires against relaxation. In open-heart cardiac surgery, the intensive care and attention received by the patient is important to his recovery. The monitor that beeps with every heartbeat is soon barely heard. But the care is required throughout the 24 hours of the day, and there is never a time for a long sleep. In one study, the postoperative patients who developed severe mental symptoms, including disorientation and hallucination, were found to have been nursed with such incessant fervor that they never really slept. Adjustment of the necessary procedures to allow for uninterrupted sleep periods is essential to the individual's recovery, and failing to provide for them may compromise all of the efforts devoted to his care.

From childhood on, everyone practices a ritual that serves to induce the onset of sleep. How people prepare themselves for a night's rest is a highly individualized matter, but if they are not allowed the ritual in the hospital, they will have difficulty in falling asleep. The individual ritual is not always possible, of course. But certainly those activities that *are* possible should be allowed and even encouraged. The blanket rule that lights go out at a certain hour may leave a person tossing half the night when 30 minutes more of reading would have lulled him to sleep. For an individual whose usual bedtime is close to midnight, insisting that he go to sleep at 9:30 P.M. will rarely work. If he *does* fall asleep, he may awaken, fully refreshed, hours before dawn. The usual sleep habits of the individual are important information for his nursing care, and the closer his usual pattern is approximated, the less likely that he will have a sleep disturbance while he is hospitalized.

Sleep research emphasizes that, throughout his life, the individual is constantly reacting to, and interacting with, his environment. During spindle sleep, a brain wave called the k-complex (because it resembles the shape of the letter on the graph) is observed in response to stimuli in both the internal and external environments. The k-complex has never been seen in the waking state; thus, it is entirely a response of the sleeping organism. While a full bladder, or pressure on an arm of the sleeping individual, may stimulate a k-complex, in one sleep laboratory it was elicited by a strictly external stimulus. As dawn approached, the birds outside the laboratory, stirred from their own sleep, began to signal the approaching day. And every chirp of the bird was registered in a k-complex on the moving EEG graph of the sleeping subjects. In that quick movement of the pen on the paper, the integration of all living things was recorded.

Vocabulary

assessment
awareness
biological clock
circadian
deprivation
desynchronized
dream deprivation
dreams
electroencephalography
haptic
hypnotic
information
intimate distance
monitors
paradoxical sleep
perception
perceptual system
periodicity
personal distance
proxemics
public distance
REM sleep
sedative
senses
sensory deprivation
sleep
social distance
synchronization
territoriality

General Bibliography

BAKER, PAUL, AND WEINER, J. S.: The Biology of Human Adaptability. Clarendon Press (Oxford University Press, Inc.), Fair Lawn, N.J., 1966.

DUBOS, RENE: Mirage of Health. Doubleday & Co., Inc., Garden City, N.Y., 1959.

DUBOS, RENE: Man Adapting. Yale University Press, New Haven, 1965.

FIENNES, RICHARD: Man, Nature and Disease. New American Library, Signet Science Series, New York, 1965.

GIBSON, JAMES J.: The Senses Considered as Perceptual Systems. Houghton-Mifflin Co., Boston, 1966.

GOFFMAN, ERVING: The Presentation of Self in Every Day Life. Doubleday & Co., Inc., Garden City, N.Y., 1959.

HALL, EDWARD T.: The Hidden Dimension. Doubleday & Co., Inc., Garden City, N.Y., 1966.

KLEITMAN, NATHANIEL: Sleep and Wakefulness, ed. 2. University of Chicago Press, Chicago, 1963.

LORENZ, KONRAD: On Aggression. Harcourt-Brace & World, Inc., New York, 1966.

LUCE, GAY GAER, AND SEGAL, JULIUS: Sleep. Lancer, New York, 1967.

Recent Research in Sleep. Publication No. 1389, U.S. Public Health Service, Washington, D.C., 1966.

SELYE, HANS: The Stress of Life. McGraw-Hill Book Co., Inc., New York, 1956.

Articles

AMVORE, JOHN E.: The stereochemical theory of odor. Sci. Amer. 210:42-49, Feb. 1964.

ANDREW, RICHARD J.: The origin of facial expressions. Sci. Amer. 213:88-94, Oct. 1965.

ASCHOFF, JÜRGEN: Circadian rhythms in man. Science 148:1427-1432, June 1965.

BENDER, RUTH E.: Communicating with deaf adults. Amer. J. Nurs. 66:757-760, April 1966.

BERLYNE, D. E.: Curiosity and exploration. Science 153:25-33, July 1966.

BROWN, FRANK, JR.: Living clocks. Science 130:1535-1544, Dec. 1959.

COHEN, JOHN: Psychological Time. Sci. Amer. 211:116-124, Nov. 1964.

CROMBIE, A. C.: Early concepts of the senses and the mind. Sci. Amer. 210: 106-116, May 1964.

HALBERG, FRANZ: The 24 hour scale: A time dimension of adaptive functional organization. Perspect. Biol. Med. III:491-527, Summer 1960.

HALL, EDWARD T.: The anthropology of manners. Sci. Amer. 192:84-90, April 1955.

HELD, RICHARD: Plasticity in sensory-motor systems. Sci. Amer. 213:84-94, Nov. 1965.

HESS, ECKHARD H.: Attitude and pupil size. Sci. Amer. 212:46-54, April 1965.

IRVING, LAURENCE: Adaptation to cold. Sci. Amer. 214:94-101, Jan. 1966.

JOUVET, MICHEL: The states of sleep. Sci. Amer. 216:62-72, Feb. 1967.

KLEITMAN, NATHANIEL: Biological rhythms and cycles. Physiol. Rev. 29:1-30, Jan. 1949.

PALMER, JOHN D.: How a bird tells the time of day. Natural History LXXV:48-53, March 1966.

ROCK, IRVIN, AND HARRIS, CHARLES S.: Vision and touch. Sci. Amer. 216:96-104, May 1967.

SOMMER, ROBERT: Studies in personal space. Sociometry 22:247-260, 1949.

SORENSON, KAREN M., AND AMIS, DOROTHY V.: Understanding the world of the chronically ill. Amer. J. Nurs. 67:811-817, April 1967.

STEPHENS, GWEN J.: The time factor – Should it control the patient's care? Amer. J. Nurs. 65:77-82, May 1965.

WYNNE-EDWARDS, V. C.: Population control in animals. Sci. Amer. 211:68-74, Aug. 1964.

Index